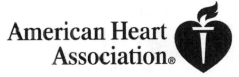

American Heart
Association®

Fighting Heart Disease and Stroke

Monograph Series

CEREBROVASCULAR DISEASE:
Momentum at the
End of the Second Millennium

Library of Congress Cataloging-in-Publication Data

Cerebrovascular disease: momentum at the end of the second millennium / edited by Dennis W. Choi .. [et al.]
    p.   cm.
    21st Princeton Conference on Cerebrovascular Disease, held at Union Station in St. Louis on May 7–10, 1998.
    Includes bibliographical references and index.
    ISBN 0-87993-484-0 (hardcover : alk. paper)
        1. Cerebrovascular disease—Pathophysiology—Congresses. 2. Cerebrovascular disease—Treatment—Congresses. I. Choi, D. W. (Dennis W.) II. Princeton Conference on Cerebrovascular Disease (21st : 1998: St. Luois, Mo.)
        [DNLM: 1. Cerebrovascular Accident —diagnosis—Congresses. 2. Cerebrovascular Accident—therapy—Congresses. WL 355 C413424 2001]
    RC388.5 .C423 2001
    616.8'1—dc21

                            2001040702

Copyright © 2001
Futura Publishing Company, Inc.
135 Bedford Road
Armonk, New York 10504
www.futuraco.com

ISBN #:0-87993-494-8

Every effort has been made to ensure that the information in this book is as up to date and accurate as possible at the time of publication. However, due to the constant developments in medicine, neither the author, nor the editor, nor the publisher can accept any legal or other responsibility for any errors or omissions that may occur.

Printed in the United States of America on acid-free paper.

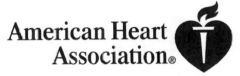

American Heart Association®

Fighting Heart Disease and Stroke

Monograph Series

CEREBROVASCULAR DISEASE:
Momentum at the
End of the Second Millennium

Edited by

Dennis W. Choi, MD, PhD
Department of Neurology
Washington University School of Medicine
St Louis, MO

Ralph G. Dacey, Jr., MD
Department of Neurological Surgery
Washington University School of Medicine
St. Louis, MO

Chung Y. Hsu, MD, PhD
Department of Neurology
Washington University School of Medicine
St. Louis, MO

William J. Powers, MD
Departments of Neurology and Radiology
Washington University School of Medicine
St. Louis, MO

**Futura Publishing
Company, Inc.**
Armonk, NY

Acknowledgements

The Local Organizing Committee of the 21st Princeton Conference consisted of Dennis W. Choi, Ralph G. Dacey Jr., Michael N. Diringer, Alexander W. Dromerick, Mark P. Goldberg, Chung Y. Hsu, Daniel K. Kido, Edward M. Manno, and William J. Powers. The Organizing Committee was wisely guided by a Scientific Advisory Board consisting of Pak H. Chan, Michael Chopp, Myron D. Ginsberg, Fletcher H. Mc-Dowell, Michael A. Moskowitz, Fred Plum, James T. Robertson, Bo K. Siesjö, Gary K. Steinberg, Justin A. Zivin, and R. Suzanne Zukin.

Primary conference funding was generously provided by the National Institute of Neurological Disease and Stroke. Other Major Supporters were Boehringer Ingelheim Pharmaceuticals, Hoffmann-La Roche, Janssen Pharmaceutics, and McDonnell Center for Cellular and Molecular Neurobiology at Washington University. Other Conference Supporters were the American Heart Association, Bristol-Myers Squibb, Genentech, Interneuron Pharmaceuticals, Park-Davis, Quintiles CVA, and Wyeth-Ayerst. Conference Grants were kindly provided by Alkermes, Cephalon, La Jolla Pharmaceutical Company, Pfizer, SmithKline Beecham, and Zeneca.

Outstanding staff support was provided by Micki Wilderspin and Patti Nacci from the Department of Neurology at Washington University School of Medicine. Assistance with travel arrangements by Alysa Kowalsky at The Travel Experts was most appreciated.

Preface

The 21st Princeton Conference on Cerebrovascular Disease was held at historic Union Station in St. Louis, on May 7–10, 1998. It was hosted by Washington University, and supported by grants from the National Institutes of Health, the American Heart Association, and many pharmaceutical and biotechnology companies active in the development of stroke therapies.

This Conference, the last in the millennium of a distinguished biennial series going back to the 1950s, provided an opportunity for an eclectic mix of junior and senior investigators to meet for a weekend, take stock of the stroke field at the millennial closure, and peer across Y2K into the future of stroke diagnosis and therapy. These invited investigators represented a broad array of clinical and basic disciplines, united by an interest in cerebrovascular disease. For some investigators, it was their nth Princeton Conference, and they knew what to expect; for many, it was their first. But all participated enthusiastically in the Conference's traditional emphases on pithy dialogue, lively argument, critical analysis, and brainstorming.

To catalyze discussions, a series of brief presentations were arranged around eight selected themes, each followed by extensive group discussions. Understanding that comprehensive coverage of topics could not be achieved in a 2-day meeting, the Organizing Committee selected these eight themes for their currency and impact. The meeting began with inspiring perspectives from the long-standing chief of the stroke and trauma program at NINDS, Michael Walker, and the then new NINDS Director, Gerald Fischbach. Both NIH officials emphasized the central importance of stroke research to the mission of NINDS, and the opportunity for major advances now unfolding.

The first theme of the Conference was an old issue revisited: extra-cranial-intracranial bypass surgery. Drs. Ralph Dacey and William Powers led the exploration, which beyond its intrinsic specific clinical importance, provided general insight into how a valid management conclusions based on earlier clinical study may be altered by technological advances (in this case, in diagnostic procedures). The second theme was pharmacological mediator and modulators of ischemic injury. Drs.

Richard Traystman and Peter Lipton led discussion of the pipeline between advances in understanding pathogenic mechanisms of neurodegeneration, and the identification of novel neuroprotective therapies – or *vice versa*. The third theme was white matter injury. Drs. Mark Goldberg and Vladimir Hachinski led discussion of an important and relatively under-investigated component of ischemic brain damage, likely influenced by different genes and different degenerative mechanisms than those predominant in grey matter injury. The fourth theme was inflammation. Drs. John Hallenbeck and Michael Chopp led discussion of how inflammatory reactions, triggered by infection or ischemic injury itself, likely contribute to the pathogenesis of further brain injury, as well as to stabilization and repair. The fifth theme was brain imaging. Drs. Marc Fisher and Justin Zivin led discussion of frontiers in positron emission tomography (PET) and magnetic resonance approaches of evolving brain ischemia, techniques that promise to offer powerful insights into pathogenesis as well as the means to identify tissue at risk for infarction while intervention is still possible. The sixth theme was programmed cell death. Drs. Matthew Linnik and Michael Moskowitz led discussion of rapidly growing evidence that apoptosis contributes to brain cell loss after ischemic insults, with attendant therapeutic implications, and Dr. Stan Korsmeyer provided a powerful summary of emerging new information regarding modulation of apoptosis by a growing family of bc1-2- related molecules. The seventh theme was delayed neuronal death, another old topic, recognized for 15 years but taking on new twists in the era of molecular biology. Drs. William Pulsinelli and Myron Ginsberg led discussion of how changes in glutamate receptor subtype expression may alter neuronal vulnerability to delayed death after ischemia, most obviously as a mechanism to increase this vulnerability but perhaps acting paradoxically to reduce apoptosis. The eighth theme was cortical reorganization and post-acute stroke treatment. Drs. Larry Goldstein and Alexander Dromerick led discussion of brain adaptation and recovery after ischemic injury, a topic of enormous importance, in its infancy now but certain to be a dominant research focus in years to come.

There were two superb and timely plenary lectures. The first, "Free Radicals and Ischemic Brain Injury" by Dr. Bo Siesjö; the second, "'CNS Stem Cells: Biology and Potential Utility for Promoting Recovery" by Dr. Fred Gage. The conference also benefited from a masterful update on recent clinical trials of drug treatments for stroke, from Dr. Greg Albers, and two no-holds-barred dinner debates on two controversial clinical issues. One debate, "'Heparin should be used to treat patients presenting with acute stroke or stroke-in-evolution'" was tackled by Dr. Louis Caplan (affirmative) and Dr. Roger Simon (negative); the other, "'MRI is a good endpoint for determining the efficacy of stroke treatment trials" by Dr. Steven Warach (affirmative) and Dr. Joseph Broderick (negative). It is fair to say that other conference participants also did not hold back their views on these topics.

The conference concluded with all participants discussing directions for the future. Dr. Murry Goldstein, initiated discussion by offering some ideas based on his many years as past Director of NINDS. He was assisted in the essential role of provocateur by an expert panel, consisting of Drs. Nicolas Bazan, Pak Chan, Fletcher McDowell, J.P. Mohr, Gary Steinberg, Michael Walker, and Justin Zivin.

The present volume captures some of the information presented during the conference. It cannot capture the dynamic interchanges occurring throughout the weekend in formal and informal settings, but in a series of brief chapters does provide a strong summary of the formal presentations. Although some time has elapsed between the conference, and the availability of this volume, the forward-looking template that guided the conference ensures that virtually all of the ideas and discussions contained in the volume are still in the foreground today. Bill Power's proposal for a major multicenter re-study of the utility of extracranial-intracranial bypass surgery in light of additional diagnostic information available through PET scanning has just received favorable review by Study Section and NINDS Council and will hopefully begin soon. Work is also now proceeding in many laboratories to advance understanding of how processes such as apoptosis, inflammation, free radicals, poly(ADP-ribose) polymerase activation, and alterations in glutamate receptor function contribute to the pathogenesis of ischemic brain injury, as well as how estrogens or cholesterol-lowering agents might be used therapeutically. The perspectives presented in this volume on topics such white matter injury, newer imaging approaches, delayed neuronal death, and recovery after stroke continue to guide current investigations, and continuing disagreements on the value of heparin or MRI endpoints in the management of stroke patients can still rouse a group of expert clinicians to vigorous debate. Furthermore, as a snapshot of topics considered important at the end of the second millennium, this volume will have lasting importance to medical historians and medical libraries.+   The editors note with sadness that one distinguished speaker and chapter author, Dr. Julio Garcia, passed away in the fall after the Conference; a eulogy by Dr. Marc Fisher follows.

Dennis W. Choi
Ralph G. Dacey
Chung Y. Hsu
William J. Powers

In Memory of Julio H. Garcia, MD

Comprehending the pathological substrate of ischemic injury is an important underpinning for determining the pathophysiology of ischemic stroke and for the development of acute stroke therapy. The career of Julio H. Garcia was dedicated to all these laudable endeavors. The review chapter in this volume by Pantoni and Garcia on the neuropathology of ischemic white matter lesions exemplifies the invaluable contributions provided by Dr. Garcia during his long and distinguished career. As a neuropathologist with a deep and abiding interest in focal brain ischemia, Dr. Garcia provided a unique and perhaps irreplaceable perspective to the stroke field.

A widely recognized and internationally acclaimed neuropathologist, he had obvious expertise concerning the pathological consequences of focal brain ischemia, publishing a multitude of important articles on this topic, in addition to widely-read neuropathology textbooks. Dr. Garcia also contributed to the experimental stroke literature. He maintained an experimental stroke laboratory for many years, exploring many important topics about stroke pathophysiology. In recent years, his efforts focused on the cellular, pathological evolution of ischemic brain injury, the role of inflammatory cells and their mediators and white matter ischemic injury. Although a neuropathologist, Dr. Garcia maintained a keen awareness of clinical neurology and the issues encountered by his clinical colleagues in neurology and neurosurgery. These insights were invaluable both for his work as a busy practicing neuropathologist and in his role as a stroke experimentalist. Dr. Garcia had a vast network of friends and collaborators around the world who turned to him for help with research projects and for valuable discussions about stroke pathology and pathophysiology. I consider myself lucky to have had access to Dr. Garcia's expertise in both of these areas, as well as enjoying his friendship, valuable insights and good humor on many occasions.

With the passing of Dr. Julio H. Garcia in the fall of 1998, ironically from the complications of a subarachnoid hemorrhage, his family, friends, colleagues and the stroke community at large have all suffered an irreplaceable and tragically premature loss. Dr. Garcia was the pre-eminent neuropathological contributor of his generation to the field of cerebrovascular disorders. We can only hope that his trainees such as Dr. Pantoni will now honor his legacy by building upon the foundations Dr. Garcia provided and maintain the important contributions of neuropathology to the understanding and treatment of ischemic stroke.

Mark Fisher

Contributors

Gregory W. Albers, MD   Director, Stanford Stroke Center
Stanford University Medical Center, Palo Alto, CA

Nabil J. Alkayed, MD, PhD   Dept of Anesthesiology & Critical Care
Medicine, Johns Hopkins University School of Medicine, Baltimore, MD

Jaroslaw Aronowski, PhD   Department of Neurology
University of Texas Health Sciences, Houston, TX

Stephen A. Back, MD, PhD   Assistant Professor of Pediatrics and
Neurology, Oregon Health Sciences Univ, Portland, OR

Henry J.M. Barnett, MD   Robarts Research Institute, London, Ontario

Frank C. Barone, PhD   Department of Cardiovascular Pharmacology, SmithKline Beecham Pharmaceuticals, Philadelphia, PA

Michael V.L. Bennett, PhD   Professor for Department of Neuroscience, Albert Einstein College of Medicine, Bronx, NY

Sondra Bland, BA   Dept of Psychology & Institute for Neuroscience
University of Texas at Austin, Austin, TX

Marie-Germaine Bousser, MD   Service de Neurologie
Hopital Lariboisiere 2, Paris, France

Joseph Broderick, MD   Stroke Research Center
University of Cincinnati College of Medicine, Cincinnati, OH

Agata Calderone, MD   Department of Neuroscience
Albert Einstein College of Medicine, Bronx, NY

Louis R. Caplan, MD   Beth Israel Deaconess Medical Center
Neurologist, Harvard University, Boston, MA

Hugues Chabriat, MD   Service de Neurologie
Hopital Lariboisiere 2, Paris, France

Pak H. Chan, PhD   Professor of Neurosurgery
Neurosurgical Labs, Stanford University, Palo Alto, CA

Dennis Choi, MD   Department of Neurology
Washington University School of Medicine, St. Louis, MO

John A. Connor, PhD   Department of Neuroscience
University of New Mexico, Albuquerque, NM

Barbara J. Crain, MD, PhD   Department of Neuropathology
Johns Hopkins University School of Medicine, Baltimore, MD

Ralph G. Dacey, Jr., MD   Department of Neurology
Washington University School of Medicine, St. Louis, MO

Ted M. Dawson, MD, PhD   Department of Neurology
Johns Hopkins University School of Medicine, Baltimore, MD

Valina L. Dawson, PhD   Associate Professor of Neurology
Johns Hopkins University School of Medicine, Baltimore, MD

Gregory J. del Zoppo, MD   Associate Professor, Department of
Molecular & Experimental Medicine, The Scripps Research Institute,
La Jolla, CA

Colin P. Derdeyn, MD   Division of Radiation Sciences
Washington University School of Medicine, St. Louis, MO

Alexander W. Dromerick, MD   Division of Neurology
Duke Center for Cerebrovascular Disease, Durham, NC

Julie A. Ellison, PhD   Department of Cardiovascular Pharmacology
SmithKline Beecham Pharmaceuticals, Philadelphia, PA

Matthias Endres, MD   Stroke & Neurovascular Regulation Laboratory, Harvard Medical School, Massachussetts General Hospital,
Charlestown, MA

Giora Z. Feuerstein, MD   Deptartment of Cardiovascular Pharmacology, SmithKline Beecham Pharmaceuticals, King of Prussia, PA

Seth P. Finklestein, MD   Department of Neurology
Massachussetts General Hospital, Harvard Medical School, Boston, MA

Mark Fisher, MD   Department of Neurology
University of Southern California School of Medicine, Los Angeles, CA

Joseph A. Frank, MD   Laboratory of Diagnostic Radiology Research
Clinical Center, National Institute of Health, Bethesda, MD

Kathleen M. Friel, MS   Department of Molecular and Integrative
Physiology, University of Kansas Medical Center, Kansas City, KS

Susanne Fritsch, RN   Department of Neurology & Neurological
Surgery, Washington University School of Medicine, St. Louis, MO

Julio H. Garcia, MD   Department of Pathology (Neuropathology)
Henry Ford Hospital, Detroit, MI

Myron D. Ginsberg, MD   Department of Neurology
University of Miami School of Medicine, Miami, FL

Larry B. Goldstein, MD   Division of Neurology
Duke Center for Cerebrovascular Disease, Durham, NC

Anders C. Greenwood, PhD   Department of Neurosciences
University of New Mexico, Albuquerque, NM

James Grotta, MA   Department of Neurology
University of Texas Health Sciences, Houston, TX

Robert L. Grubb, Jr., MD   Department of Neurology & Neurological Surgery, Washington University School of Medicine, St. Louis, MO

E. Mark Haacke, PhD   Department of Radiology
Washington University School of Medicine, St. Louis, MO

John M. Hallenbeck, MD   Chief, Stroke Branch, National Institute
of Neurological Disease and Stroke, National Institutes of Health,
Bethesda, MD

Chung Y. Hsu, MD   Department of Neurology
Washington University School of Medicine, St. Louis, MO

J.Leigh Humm, MA   Department of Psychology & Institute for Neuroscience, University of Texas at Austin, Austin, TX

Patricia D. Hurn, PhD   Deparments of Anesthesiology & Critical Care Medicine, Johns Hopkins Hospital, Baltimore, MD

Theresa Jones, PhD   Department of Psychology University of Washington, Seattle, WA

Anne Joutel, MD   INSERM, CHU, Paris, France

Daniel Kido, MD   Department of Radiology Washington University School of Medicine, St. Louis, MO

Jeffrey A. Kleim, PhD   Department of Molecular and Integrative Physiology, University of Kansas Medical Center, Kansas City, KS

Bryan Kolb, PhD   Department of Psychology University of Lethbridge, Lethbridge, Aleberta, Canada

Tibor Kristian, PhD   Senior Researcher, Center for Study of Neurological Diseases, The Neuroscience Institute, Queen's Medical Center, Honolulu, HI

Ulrich Laufs, MD   Cardiovascular Division, Brigham/Women's Hospital, Harvard Medical School, Boston, MA

Benjamin Lee, MD   Department of Radiology Washington University School of Medicine, St. Louis, MO

Ping-An Li, MD, PhD   Senior Researcher, Center for Study of Neurological Diseases, The Neuroscience Institute, Queen's Medical Center, Honolulu, HI

James K. Liao, MD   Cardiovascular Division, Brigham/Women's Hospital, Harvard Medical School, Boston, MA

Rick C.S. Lin, PhD   Department of Neurobiology and Anatomy Allegheny University, Philadelphia, PA

Weili Lin, MD   Department of Radiology Washington University School of Medicine, St. Louis, MO

Allen S. Mandir, MD, PhD   Department of Neurology
Johns Hopkins University School of Medicine, Baltimore, MD

John Markman, MD   Department of Neurology, Massachussetts
General Hospital, Harvard Medical School, Boston, MA

Venkata S. Mattay, MD   Clinical Brain Disorders Branch
National Institute of Mental Health, Bethesda, MD

Marc Mayberg, MD   Department of Neurosurgery
The Cleveland Clinic, Cleveland, OH

Alan C. McLaughlin, PhD   Clinical Brain Disorders Branch
National Institutes of Health, Bethesda, MD

Michael A. Moskowitz, MD   Stroke & Neurovascular Regulation
Laboratory, Massachusetts General Hospital, Charlestown, MA

Randolph J. Nudo, PhD   Asst. Professor, Department of Molecular & Integrative Physiology, University of Kansas Medical Center,
Kansas City, KS

Keiji Oguro, MD, PhD   Department of Neuroscience
Albert Einstein College of Medicine, Bronx, NY

Thoralf Opitz, PhD   Otto-von-Guericke University
Institute for Physiology, Magdeburg, Germany

Yi-Bing Ouyang, PhD   Senior Researcher, Center for Study of Neurological Diseases, The Neuroscience Institute, Queen's Medical Center, Honolulu, HI

Leonardo Pantoni, MD   Department of Neurological & Psychiatric
Sciences, University of Florence, Florence, Italy

Jeffrey J. Petrozzino, PhD   University of Medicine and Dentistry
of New Jersey, Robert Wood Johnson Medical School, Piscataway, NJ

Domenico E. Pellegrini-Giampietro, MD, PhD   Department of
Pharmacology, University of Florence, Florence, Italy

William J. Powers, MD   Department of Neurology and Radiology
Washington University School of Medicine, St. Louis, MO

Seddigheh Razani-Bourouterdi, PhD Department of Neurosciences, University of New Mexico, Albuquerque, NM

Jing Mei Ren, MD Department of Neurology Massachusetts General Hospital, Boston, MA

Renata Rusa, MD Department of Anesthesiology & Critical Care Medicine, Johns Hopkins University School of Medicine, Baltimore, MD

Kenji Sampei, MD Dept of Anesthesiology & Critical Care Medicine, Johns Hopkins University School of Medicine, Baltimore, MD

Masahiko Sawada, MD Department of Anesthesiology & Critical Care Medicine, Johns Hopkins University School of Medicine, Baltimore, MD

Timothy Schallert, PhD Department of Psychology University of Texas at Austin, Austin, TX

Bo K. Siesjö, MD, PhD Center for the Study of Neurological Diseases, The Neuroscience Institute, Queen's Medical Center, Honolulu, HI

Roger P. Simon, MD Department of Neurology University of Pittsburgh, Pittsburgh, PA

Peter K. Stys, MD, FRCP(C) Professor of Medicine (Neurology) University of Ottawa; Loeb Health Research Institute, Ottawa, Ontario,

Thomas JK. Toung, MD Department of Anesthesiology & Critical Care Medicine, Johns Hopkins University School of Medicine, Baltimore, MD

Elizabeth Tournier-Lasserve, MD INSERM, CHU, Paris, France

Richard J. Traystman, PhD Dept of Anesthesiology & Critical Care Medicine, Johns Hopkins University School of Medicine, Baltimore, MD

Steven Warach, MD, PhD Chief, Section on Stroke Diagnostics & Therapeutics, National Institute of Neurological Disorders & Stroke, Bethesda, MD

Daniel R. Weinberger, MD Clinical Brain Disorders Branch National Institute of Mental Health, Bethesda, MD

Frank Q. Ye, PhD   Clinical Brain Disorders Branch
National Institute of Mental Health, Bethesda, MD

Justin A. Zivin, MD, PhD   Department of Neurosciences
University of California, La Jolla, CA

R. Suzanne Zukin, PhD   Department of Neuroscience
Albert Einstein College of Medicine, Bronx, NY

Contents

SECTION III. White Matter Ischemia—Unique Mechanisms of Injury?

SECTION IV. Inflammation

SECTION V. Beyond Diffusion: Imaging Measurements of Cerebral Blood Flow and Metabolism

SECTION VI. Delayed Neuronal Death

SECTION VII. Cortical Reorganization and Post-Acute Stroke Treatment

SECTION VIII. Clinical Treatment Trials

Section I

Extracranial/Intracranial Bypass Surgery: Time for a New Clinical Trial?

Chapter 1

Overview

Ralph G. Dacey Jr., MD, and
Williams J Powers, MD

During the discussion period several important issues regarding extracranial/intracranial bypass surgery and the need for a new clinical trial were raised. The mechanism by which strokes occur in the patients with hemodynamic compromise has not been resolved by current studies. Although, it is tempting to conclude that improving hemodynamics may improve outcome, other factors may be involved. Drs. Yatsu and DeGraba pointed out that inflammatory responses may be important in the pathogenesis of stroke and may be different in the patients with hemodynamic compromise. The issue of postoperative morbidity in patients with hemodynamic compromise was raised. There are no published data regarding the postoperative morbidity in this group. Dr. Yonas suggested that in his experience, it was not prohibitively high. However, Dr. Baron commented that they had tried performing extracranial/intracranial bypass surgery on these patients in the early and mid eighties and the operative morbidity was extremely high such that they abandoned the surgery. Dr. Caplan suggested that it would be worthwhile to considering operating on patients in the very acute phase since there were a group of patients who presented with fluctuating neurological deficits who may benefit from acute surgery as opposed to the patients in the St. Louis Carotid Occlusion Study who are all at least several weeks away from any accute cerebral infarction. The necessity for state-of-the-art medical treatment in any subsequent surgical trial was pointed out. This should include careful attention to blood pressure control (with perhaps 24-hour monitoring), careful glycemic control and the use of lipid lowering drugs. Dr. Baum pointed out that

From: Choi D, Dacey RG, Hsu CY, Powers WJ. *Cerebrovascular Disease: Momentum at the End of the Second Millennium.* Armonk, NY: Futura Publishing Company, Inc., © 2002.

outcome endpoints should include assessments of disability and quality of life as opposed to simply recurrence of stroke. A question was raised as to whether there are data to demonstrate that extracranial/ intracranial bypass surgery will improve the hemodynamic deficit demonstrated by positron-emission tomography (PET). Studies from the early and mid-1980s from a variety of centers around the world have demonstrated that this is the case. Dr. Steinberg made a plea to determine if there was any method other than PET for establishing hemodynamic risk in patients with carotid occlusion. He pointed out that PET was not generally available and it would be advantageous to perform this measurement in another way.

In conclusion, there was general consensus among the attendees at the Princeton Conference that further investigation into the value of extracranial/intracranial bypass surgery to prevent subsequent stroke in patients with hemodynamic failure due to carotid occlusion was warranted.

Chapter 2

Cerebral Hemodynamics and Stroke Risk

Robert L. Grubb, Jr., MD, Colin P. Derdeyn, MD, Susanne Fritsch, RN, and William J. Powers, MD

The role of hemodynamic factors in the pathogenesis and treatment of ischemic cerebrovascular disease remains unclear.[1,2] In the typical patient with atherosclerosis of the carotid or vertebrobasilar systems producing focal ischemic symptoms, the relative impact of embolic and hemodynamic factors on the subsequent occurrence of stroke has been difficult to determine. Observations of platelet thrombi both in retinal vessels and in surgical specimens removed at carotid endarterectomy have given support to the idea that platelet emboli are of primary importance in patients with minimal or minor degrees of carotid stenosis. Recent observations of a high percentage of intracranial arterial occlusion in patients undergoing ultra-early carotid arteriography in patients with acute ischemic stroke further substantiates this view.[3-5] Results from the North American, VA, and European trials demonstrating marked superiority of carotid endarterectomy over medical therapy for symptomatic patients with 70%–99% carotid artery stenosis make the differentiation of hemodynamic from emboli causes a moot question for these patients.[6-8] The recently completed Asymptomatic Carotid Atherosclerosis Study demonstrated a small, but definite, reduced 5-year risk of ipsilateral stroke in patients with 60% or greater carotid artery stenosis who underwent prophylactic carotid endarterectomy.[9]

From: Choi D, Dacey RG, Hsu CY, Powers WJ. *Cerebrovascular Disease: Momentum at the End of the Second Millennium.* Armonk, NY: Futura Publishing Company, Inc., © 2002.

There remain, however, a large number of patients with complete carotid artery occlusion for whom there is no therapy proven effective for preventing subsequent stroke. These patients comprise approximately 15% of those with carotid territory transient ischemic attacks or infarction.[10-12] Twelve prospective follow-up studies of angiographically documented symptomatic carotid occlusion of 1,261 patients, followed for a mean of 45.5 months, found an overall risk of subsequent stroke of 7% per year and a risk of stroke ipsilateral to the occluded carotid artery of 5.9% per year.[13] Platelet inhibitory drugs and anticoagulants have not been evaluated specifically in this group. Superficial temporal artery-middle cerebral artery bypass (STA-MCA) surgery was not effective in a large randomized trial of surgery versus medical therapy.[14] The relative importance of hemodynamic and embolic factors in these patients remains unclear. These patients may suffer stroke from hemodynamic insufficiency distal to the carotid occlusion or from emboli arising from several sources including the stump of the occluded internal carotid artery in the neck, the tail of the stagnation thrombus that forms distal to the occlusion or the contralateral carotid artery. This distinction is of more than just academic interest since treatment with antithrombotic drugs such as aspirin or warfarin is unlikely to prevent hemodynamic stroke. Surgical revascularization procedures have the potential to improve regional cerebral perfusion pressure (rCPP) and regional cerebral blood flow (rCBF) and prevent hemodynamic infarction. Since these patients are at risk for both hemodynamic and embolic stroke, a better understanding of the relationship between cerebral hemodynamics and stroke risk is critical for the proper design of studies to evaluate both medical and surgical therapies to prevent stroke. Therapeutic trials are most effective when restricted to those patients who will benefit. This approach improves statistical power, decreases the likelihood that benefits in small subgroups will be overlooked, and permits more specific applications of the results to clinical practice. Trials of anticoagulant and platelet inhibitory drugs should ideally exclude patients with hemodynamically mediated cerebral ischemia.

Consideration of hemodynamic factors is, perhaps, even more important in the proper design of trials of surgical therapy for cerebrovascular disease. Superficial temporal artery-middle cerebral artery bypass surgery was developed to improve CBF in patients with complete carotid occlusion or intracranial carotid stenosis not amenable to conventional endarterectomy. Since this surgery is unlikely to provide protection from embolic stroke, its efficacy in preventing stroke should be greatest in those patients in whom hemodynamic factors are important in the pathogenesis of cerebral infarction. Although a large prospective randomized trial has demonstrated no value for this surgery in preventing subsequent stroke,[14] this trial has been criticized for failing to identify and separately analyze the subgroup of patients with reduction in perfusion pressure in whom surgery might be more beneficial.[15-17] In addition, STA-MCA bypass has been criticized for not providing adequate augmentation of flow to restore hemodynamics to normal. This has led to the development of other surgical revascularization strategies based on the premise that hemodynamic factors are important.[18] Thus, a better understanding of the importance of cerebral hemodynamics is also critical in determining future research directions into improved methods for stroke prevention.

Relationship of Cerebral Perfusion Pressure and Cerebral Hemodynamics

In order to determine what role hemodynamic factors play in the pathogenesis, prognosis, and choice of treatment of patients with carotid artery occlusion, a method for determining the hemodynamic status of the cerebral circulation, accurately and in awake subjects under normal conditions, must be available. It is obviously impractical to directly measure the perfusion pressure in the distal arterial bed of the cerebral circulation. It has been necessary, therefore, to rely on indirect assessments.

Measurements in the cervical carotid artery have demonstrated that reductions in flow distal to a stenosis occur only when the lumen diameter is reduced by more than 60%-65% producing a residual lumen of less than 1-2 mm in diameter.[19-21] The presence of such a hemodynamically significant carotid artery lesion is often used as an indication that the hemodynamic status of the cerebral circulation is impaired. Emphasis on the hemodynamic significance of a carotid artery lesions ignores the possible contribution of collateral circulatory pathways in maintaining cerebral perfusion.[22-26] The importance of collateral channels in maintaining CBF distal to an occluded or stenotic carotid artery is well recognized, but its relationship to the subsequent risk of stroke is less clear. Previous attempts to address this question based on analysis of the incidence and extent of cerebral infarction in patients with varying degrees of stenosis and different patterns of collateral flow have been inconclusive,[27-31] since collaterals were assessed some time after, not before the infarct occurred.

To gain a better idea of the effect of proximal atherosclerotic lesions and collateral circulation on cerebral hemodynamics, a variety of indirect methods for evaluating the status of the distal cerebral vasculature have been developed. The rationale for these methods is based upon the compensatory responses made by the brain to progressive reductions in CPP.

When CPP is normal, CBF is regulated by changes in arteriolar size. Under these conditions, CBF is also closely matched to the resting metabolic rate of the tissue. Gray matter areas with higher metabolic rates have higher CBF and white matter areas with lower metabolic rates have lower CBF. A fairly uniform value for the ratio between CBF and metabolism exists in all areas of the brain. As a consequence of this resting balance between flow and metabolism, the oxygen extraction fraction (OEF) from the blood shows little regional variation. The actual value for OEF will vary from person to person and from measurement to measurement within the same person, but it is approximately one-third for normal individuals.[25,26,32-35]

Changes in CPP over a wide range have little effect on CBF.[36,37] This phenomenon is known as autoregulation. Increases in mean arterial pressure produce vasoconstriction of pial arterioles and decreases produce vasodilation, thus altering resistance and maintaining a constant CBF. These changes are accompanied by corresponding changes in intravascular cerebral blood volume (CBV). Thus, there is an increase in CBV as CPP falls.[38,39]

When the capacity for compensatory vasodilation has been exceeded, autoregulation fails and CBF begins to decline. Measurements of arteriovenous oxygen differences in both animals and humans have demonstrated the brain's capacity to increase OEF when oxygen supply is diminished due to decreasing CBF.[40-43] A progressive increase in OEF now maintains cerebral oxygen metabolism ($CMRO_2$). Once this mechanism becomes maximal, further declines in blood flow cause disruption of normal cellular metabolism and infarction may result.

Determining the Hemodynamic Effects of Atherosclerotic Occlusive Carotid Artery Disease

The measurement of multiple physiologic variables is necessary to accurately assess cerebral hemodynamics. Measurements of CBF alone are inadequate for this purpose, since they cannot detect reductions in CPP when CBF is maintained by compensatory vasodilation. Furthermore, they cannot differentiate decreased CBF caused by reduced blood supply from that caused by reduced metabolic demands. While these latter two causes of reduced CBF may not be difficult to distinguish in areas of known infarction demonstrated by computed tomography (CT) or magnetic resonance (MR) scans, there can be real problems in the interpretation of CBF measurements when the reduction in metabolic demand occurs in structurally normal brain tissue.

Destruction of afferent or efferent fibers pathways by a cerebral lesion may cause reductions in both CBF and metabolism in regions which show no abnormality on CT or MR scans. Such areas of reduced blood flow are commonly seen overlying subcortical lesions as well as in more distant structures such as contralateral cerebellum.[25,33] Determination of the hemodynamic status of such areas of preserved brain when supplied by a stenotic or occluded vessel is not possible with simple measurements of CBF.

Two basic approaches have been created to assess regional cerebral perfusion pressure through utilization of knowledge of the normal compensatory responses of the brain. These approaches are accurate only with uninfarcted brain tissue studied at a time that is remote from a cerebral ischemic event. Cerebral blood flow, blood volume, oxygen metabolism, and cerebrovascular reactivity can be profoundly changed in a complex manner in recently ischemic or infarcted brain tissue. These changes may not be appropriate to determine that hemodynamic changes have occurred in the cerebral tissue due to reduced cerebral perfusion pressure caused by larger vessel atherosclerotic occlusive disease.[33,44-47] The first approach uses paired rCBF measurements with the initial measurement obtained at rest and the second measurement obtained following a cerebral vasodilatory stimulus. Hypercapnia, acetazolamide, and physiologic tasks such as hand movement have been used as vasodilatory stimuli. Evidence of a preexisting autoregulatory cerebral vasodilation due to reduced cerebral perfusion pressure is inferred if there is impairment of the normal cerebral blood flow increase caused by vasodilatory stimuli. A variety of methods to determine rCBF (including Xenon-133 inhalation, intravenous Xenon-133, stable Xenon CT, transcranial Doppler, SPECT, positron-emission tomography [PET], and MR) have been used to make the paired measurements of blood flow needed for this approach.[16,22,28,48-61] An advantage of this approach is that simpler, less expensive methodologies than PET can be used to acquire the needed data, since only measurements of rCBF are needed. However, some investigators have reported inconsistent results with the use of acetazolamide as a vasodilatory stimulus.[56,62-65] The response of the blood flow in the brain to acetazolamide is dependent on the dosage administered and the timing of the blood flow measurements.[65] Acetazolamide may dilate both the trunk of the middle cerebral artery in addition to dilating the small resistance cerebral arteries. Thus, a constant cross-sectional area of the middle cerebral artery trunk is not certain with acetazolamide testing, which may confound the interpretation of cerebral vasoreactivity testing utilizing acetazolamide and transcranial Doppler. Women have been found to have an increased vasodilatory response to acetazolamide compared to men.[56] A recent study found a poor correlation between ipsilateral CO_2 reactivity and acetazolamide reactivity in 24 symptomatic patients with unilateral occlusive lesions of a major cerebral artery.[62] This study indicated that these patients may show preserved CO_2 reactivity, but an absent or inverse response to acetazolamide.

A second approach combines measurements of rCBV and rCBF in the resting brain to determine the rCBV/rCBF ratio. Combining rOEF measurements with the rCBV and rCBF measurements increases the information available to accurately assess cerebral hemodynamics.[24,66-68] We have used PET measurements of rCBF, rCBV, and rOEF to classify changes in regional cerebral hemodynamics into three stages.[24] At normal levels of cerebral perfusion pressure, rCBF, rCBV, rCBV/rCBF ratio, and rOEF are all normal. We have labeled this stage as Stage 0. At milder levels of cerebral perfusion pressure reduction, the cerebral resistance vessels will dilate to maintain brain blood flow. rCBF is normal to mildly reduced (depending on metabolic demand), rCBV is elevated, and rOEF remains at normal levels. This stage is labeled as Stage 1. If cerebral perfusion pressure falls to lower levels, the capacity of the cerebral resistance vessels to dilate and maintain blood flow is exceeded and rCBF will begin to decline. The rCBV, the rCBV/rCBF ratio, and rOEF will all increase. The ability of the brain to increase the extraction of oxygen from the blood, reflected by the increased rOEF, enables the brain to maintain oxygen utilization at normal levels. We have called this stage, which reflects a more severe decrease in cerebral perfusion pressure, Stage 2. The ratio of rCBV/rCBF is felt to be a more sensitive index of reduced cerebral perfusion pressure than increased rCBV alone, as rCBV may remain in the upper range of normal, even though the rCBV/rCBF ratio is increased. However, the CBV/CBF ratio may increase without changes in CPP.[69] Assessment techniques such as SPECT or PET can be used to measure both rCBF and rCBV.[24,66,67,70,71] Although SPECT assessment of rCBV/rCBF is an attractive modality for determining cerebral hemodynamics because it can be performed with conventional nuclear medicine equipment and radionuclides, it suffers from some drawbacks. SPECT has poor quantitative accuracy (although this is improving) and there is currently a lack of validated tracer techniques that permit accurate, quantitative measurements of CBF in both physiologic and pathologic circumstances. PET provides more accurate quantitative regional measurements. In addition, measurements of rOEF and $rCMRO_2$ can be made only with PET. Thus, patients cannot be classified into less severe (Stage 1) and more severe (Stage 2) stages of cerebral hemodynamic compromise without PET at this time.

Studies comparing the two different approaches of assessing cerebral hemodynamics with PET in atherosclerotic carotid occlusive disease have found variable results. The correlation between the rCBV/

rCBF ratio and cerebral CO_2 reactivity was found to be significant by Herold and coworkers.[54] However, another study did not find as good correlation, as 3 of 10 patients with high rCBV/rCBF ratios had normal cerebral CO_2 reactivity.[72] Four studies found a linear relationship between cerebral CO_2 reactivity and rOEF, with the highest levels of rOEF occurring in areas of the brain that had lost their CO_2 reactivity.[52,54,72,73] However, two other studies did not find a good correlation between the degree of CO_2 reactivity and rOEF.[74,75]

Impaired cerebral vasoreactivity to vasodilatory stimuli such as hypercapnia and acetazolamide has been shown to spontaneously improve over time in some patients with carotid artery occlusion or stenosis, probably due to the development of collateral circulation through the circle of Willis and leptomeningeal anastomoses. In one study 28 of 55 patients with an internal carotid artery occlusion and impairment of cerebrovascular reactivity at the time of their initial study demonstrated spontaneous improvement in cerebrovascular reactivity during follow-up studies.[76] In patients with normal or moderately stenotic contralateral carotid arteries, the percentage of improved CO_2 reactivity was 64%, whereas CO_2 reactivity improved spontaneously in only 22% of patients with bilateral carotid artery occlusion. In this group of patients, the improvement in cerebral hemodynamics occurred mainly in the first few months following carotid artery occlusion. Similar spontaneous improvement in cerebrovascular reactivity has been reported in 5 of 7 patients with internal carotid artery occlusion[77] and 3 of 6 patients with cerebrovascular occlusive disease.[78] Another recent study found that 11 of 24 patients with impaired cerebrovascular reactivity due to a variety of atherosclerotic cerebrovascular lesions, had spontaneous improvement at an average of 2 years.[79] The development of intracranial collateral circulation with time after carotid artery occlusion has been shown experimentally. A spontaneous improvement in CO_2 reactivity 1 month after carotid artery ligation was demonstrated in a rat model.[80] A significant increase in the diameter of the anterior communicating artery was seen during the first 6 weeks after unilateral carotid artery ligation in rats.[81]

Cerebral Hemodynamics and the Prognosis of Atherosclerotic Occlusive Carotid Artery Disease

Several methods have been used (Table 1) to assess the impact of cerebral hemodynamics on the pathogenesis and treatment of stroke.[2] However, follow-up information about patients studied with these

Table 1

Cerebral Hemodynamics and Stroke Risk.

Author	Study Design	No. of Patients	Follow-up (months)	Technique	Cerebral Vasoreactivity (No. of Patients) (Ipsilateral Annual Stroke Risk)		
					Normal	Moderate Impairment	Severe Impairment
Kleiser-1992[59]	Prospective	*85	38	Transcranial Doppler CO_2 Reactivity	48 0	26 7%	11 24%
Widder-1994[76]	Prospective	*86(111)	a19 b31.7	Transcranial Doppler CO_2 Reactivity	b(48) 1%	b(37) 1%	a(26) 8%
Yonas-1993[16]	Retrospective	*41	24	Xenion-CT CBF acetazolamide	25 0	16 16%	
Webster-1995[82]	Retrospective	*64	19.6	Xenon-CT CBF acetazolamide	26 0	38 13%	
Yamauchi-1996[84]	Prospective	40	12	PET OEF	33 6%	- -	7 57%
Yokota-1998[79]	Prospective	105	32.5	SPECT CBF acetazolamide	50 4%	55 4%	- -
Grubb Powers-1998[85]	Prospective	*81	31.5	PET OEF	42 3%	- -	39 13%

*Only ICA occlusion patients ( ) No. of cerebral hemispheres

techniques has been limited and is insufficient to allow any definitive conclusions to be drawn from too many of these studies.

One small longitudinal study found a relationship between cerebral hemodynamics and the subsequent risk of stroke in patients with atherosclerotic occlusive carotid artery disease.[16] Cerebrovascular reserve was tested in these patients by paired CBF measurements obtained with the stable Xenon/CT scanning method, with the cerebral vasodilatory agent acetazolamide given intravenously 20 minutes prior to the second study. The patients were placed in one of two groups based on the vascular territory found to have the lowest cerebral vasoreactivity and a relatively low baseline CBF. This categorization was done retrospectively based on assessment of the characteristics of the patients who went on to develop a stroke. The first group (n = 27) had baseline blood flow values > 45 ml · 100 g^{-1} · min^{-1} or cerebrovascular reserves ≥ 5%. The second group (n = 41) had initial blood flow values < 45 ml · 100 g^{-1} · min^{-1} and cerebrovascular reserves < 5%. Sixty-eight patients with either carotid artery stenosis of ≥ 70% or carotid artery occlusion were followed for a mean of 24 months. There were two contralateral strokes in the first group and eight ipsilateral strokes in the second group (12.6 times greater chance of stroke). Forty-one of the 68 patients in the study had internal carotid artery occlusion. None of the 25 patients with internal carotid artery occlusion in the first group had an ipsilateral stroke, whereas 5 of 16 patients with internal carotid artery occlusions in the second group suffered a subsequent ipsilateral stroke (31% stroke risk). In a subsequent report by these authors, 27 additional patients were included in an analysis of 95 patients with either stenosis of ≤ 70% or carotid artery occlusion.[82] The patients were followed for a mean of 19.6 months. In the second group with the more severe impairment of cerebral vasoreactivity, 8 of 38 patients with occlusion of the internal carotid artery had a subsequent ipsilateral stroke (21% stroke risk). These patients were classified into two groups based only on a paradoxical response of CBF to the cerebral vasodilatory agent acetazolamide, different criteria than those used in the first study. The authors do not state whether these criteria were decided prospectively or retrospectively after reviewing the results. Three of the five new strokes that occurred did so in patients who would not have met criteria for the first study. Only two of these five new strokes were in the hemodynamically compromised territory of the occluded vessel. Thus, their previously retrospectively derived criteria for identifying patients at high risk failed when subjected to a prospective test on a new group of patients.

Another group investigating the response of the cerebral circulation to a vasodilatory stimulus, also found a relationship between cerebral hemodynamics and the subsequent risk of stroke in patients with carotid artery occlusion.[59] This longitudinal study tested the cerebrovascular reserve capacity in 85 patients with internal carotid artery occlusion using transcranial Doppler sonography. Middle cerebral artery (MCA) blood flow velocity and end-tidal PCO_2 were monitored during steady states of normocapnia, hypercapnia induced by breathing 5% CO_2 in 95% O_2, and hypocapnia produced by voluntary hyperventilation. The results of CO_2 reactivity studies were classified into three categories. Sufficient CO_2 reactivity was defined as an increase of MCA blood flow velocity of 10% during hypercapnia and a decrease of 10% during hypocapnia; diminished cerebrovascular reactivity was characterized by a marked decrease or lack of increase in flow velocity during hypercapnia with a normal response to hypocapnia; and exhausted CO_2 reactivity was defined by a marked decrease or lack of change in blood flow velocity during hypercapnia combined with a diminished response during hypocapnia. There were 81 angiographically proven unilateral and four bilateral internal carotid artery (ICA) occlusions in the study group. At the time of entry into the study, 46 patients were asymptomatic on the ipsilateral side of the ICA occlusion, 13 had presented with reversible symptoms, and 26 had had a minor stroke. Two patients had a transient ischemic attack (TIA) and eight had a stroke contralateral to the ICA occlusion. The patients were followed for a mean of 38 ($\pm$15 SD) months. A total of eight patients had an ipsilateral stroke and eight patients had an ipsilateral TIA or prolonged reversible ischemic neurologic deficit (PRIND) during the follow-up period. There were four contralateral strokes and one contralateral TIA, which occurred in conjunction with progression of an ICA stenosis on the same side in three cases. In the group with sufficient cerebrovascular reserve, four of 48 patients had an ipsilateral TIA or PRIND, but no patient had a stroke. Six of 26 patients with diminished CO_2 reactivity had an ipsilateral ischemic event (three strokes [12%], three TIAs), and three patients had a contralateral event (two strokes, one TIA). In the group with exhausted cerebrovascular reserve capacity, five of 11 patients (45%) had an ipsilateral stroke and one patient had an ipsilateral TIA. Two patients had a contralateral hemisphere stroke. During the follow-up period, 10 patients died of noncerebral causes. In this study a significant correlation was found between diminished CO_2 reactivity of the cerebral circulation and ischemic events ipsilateral to an internal carotid artery occlusion. There was no significant relationship between patients with and without a history of neurological symptoms at the time the ICA occlusion was discovered. This is puzzling since the prognosis of asymptomatic carotid occlusion is relatively benign.[83] The increased risk of contralateral stroke in the patients with a diminished or exhausted CO_2 reactivity suggests that the two groups were not matched with the normal CO_2 reactivity group for other stroke risk factors, and this may explain the differences observed. In a subsequent report by these authors, 86 patients with carotid artery occlusion were followed for variable periods of time.[76] A stroke ipsilateral to an occluded internal carotid artery occurred in 3 of 26 patients with an exhausted CO_2 reactivity, corresponding to an annual stroke rate of 8% (mean follow-up time of 19 months). The annual stroke rate in patients with exhausted CO_2 reactivity was much lower in this study, compared to the group of patients previously reported by these investigators. In 37 patients with diminished CO_2 reactivity and 48 patients with sufficient CO_2 reactivity, only one patient in each group developed an ipsilateral stroke (mean follow-up time of 31.7 months). There are a number of potential problems with the interpretation of the results of these two studies. In the first study, 46 of 85 patients were asymptomatic. In the second study, the number of asymptomatic patients is not given. The 86 patients in the second study were selected from 452 patients with ICA occlusion studied with transcranial Doppler cerebrovascular resistance studies. The criteria for selecting the patients in the second study was not given. The dates of data collection in the two studies overlap. How this impacted the results of the two studies was not given.

A recently reported small longitudinal study also found a relationship between cerebral hemodynamics and the subsequent risk of recurrent stroke.[84] PET measurements of rCBF, rCBV, rOEF, and $rCMRO_2$ were performed in 40 patients with symptomatic occlusion or intracranial stenosis of the internal carotid or middle cerebral arterial system treated medically. During the period in which these patients were studied, 12 other symptomatic patients with internal carotid artery or middle cerebral artery occlusive disease underwent PET studies, but were excluded from this study because they underwent vascular reconstructive surgery. Seven patients had an STA-MCA anastomosis and 5 patients had a carotid endarterectomy. Patients were divided into two categories based on the absolute mean hemispheric value of oxygen extraction in the symptomatic cerebral hemisphere: patients with normal OEF and those with increased OEF. Six patients had TIAs and 34 patients had minor infarctions. The intervals between the most recent cerebral ischemic event and the PET studies was 1 to 55 months, with 17 of the 40 patients studied 30 to 90 days following the most recent cerebrovascular event. All patients were treated with antiplatelet therapy. All patients were followed for at least 12 months. At one year following the PET studies, 5 of 7 patients with increased OEF had developed a stroke; 4 strokes were ipsilateral, and 1 was contralateral. Four of 33 patients with normal OEF had developed a stroke. Two strokes were ipsilateral and two were contralateral. In patients with increased OEF, 3 of 4 ipsilateral strokes were watershed infarctions corresponding to an area of increased rOEF. All the patients with a stroke in the follow-up period had had a minor stroke at entry into the study. After the first year of follow-up, one ipsilateral stroke and one contralateral stroke occurred, with both of these strokes occurring in patients with normal OEF.

A recent prospective study failed to demonstrate a relationship between cerebral hemodynamics and the risk of subsequent stroke.[79] One hundred and five patients with evidence of ischemic cerebrovascular events, minimal infarct on a CT scan, and unilateral occlusion or severe stenosis (> 75% in diameter) of the ICA or proximal MCA confirmed by cerebral angiography had a SPECT study of cerebral perfusion using I-123 IMP and measurement of cerebrovascular reactivity using acetazolamide. Based on the local cerebral perfusion reactivity to acetazolamide, the patients were divided into two groups, those with normal cerebrovascular reactivity and those with impaired cerebrovascular reactivity. Risk factors for stroke at entry were recorded and included in the final data analysis. The primary endpoint was stroke occurrence. The median follow-up period in the study was 32.5 months. Fifty-five patients had an abnormal cerebral vasoreactivity response to acetazolamide and 50 patients had a normal response. There was no significant difference in the stroke risk factors between the two groups, except the group with an abnormal response to acetazolamide had a higher systolic blood pressure at entry into the study. The sites of the vascular lesions were comparable between the two groups. During the follow-up period, 13 patients had a stroke, 11 died, 16 had surgical cerebral revascularization procedures (9 extracranial/intracranial [EC/IC] bypasses and 7 carotid endarterectomies), and 11 were lost to follow-up. Eight of the 13 patients with subsequent stroke had stenosis of the ICA or MCA at entry into the study. Follow-up SPECT studies with acetazolamide testing showed that cerebrovascular reactivity became normal at an average of 2 years in 11 of 24 patients with initially impaired response to acetazolamide. There was no significant difference in the rate of subsequent stroke in the two groups during the period of follow-up. When stroke recurrence and death were combined, the two groups again had no significant difference. There are a number of potential problems in this study. The SPECT cerebral perfusion measurements were qualitative, and there is a possibility that the measurements of cerebrovascular reactivity in this study failed to differentiate a group of patients with severe impairment of cerebral hemodynamics. The patients in the study had a variety of extracranial and intracranial cerebrovascular lesions and included only a small number of patients with ICA occlusion. A relatively large number of patients were censored from the study because of subsequent cerebrovascular surgery and a significant number of patients were lost to follow-up. Thus the validity of the negative results of this study is not certain.

We carried out a blinded, prospective study to test the hypothesis that Stage II hemodynamic failure (increased oxygen extraction) in the cerebral hemisphere distal to complete carotid artery occlusion is an independent predictor of the subsequent risk of stroke in symptomatic medically treated patients.[85] Inclusion criteria were occlusion of one or both common or internal carotid arteries demonstrated by contrast angiography or MR angiography in patients with transient ischemic neurological deficits (including transient monocular blindness) or mild to moderate neurological deficits (stroke) in the territory of the occluded carotid artery. Patients who had undergone ipsilateral external carotid endarterectomy (CEA) or contralateral CEA prior to PET were eligible whether or not they had had recurrent symptoms. Any subsequent cerebrovascular surgery after the initial PET caused the patient to be censored from the study at the time of surgery. All subjects were studied at the Washington University Medical Center. Just prior to PET, each underwent neurological evaluation including detailed questioning regarding any symptoms. Focal ischemic symptoms in the territory of the occluded carotid artery were categorized as cerebral TIA (< 24 hours duration), cerebral infarct (> 24 hours duration), or retinal event (any duration) and as single or recurrent episodes. Time from most recent symptom was recorded. Pertinent medical records, CT scans, and angiograms were reviewed. The following baseline risk factors were specifically determined: age, gender, hypertension, previous myocardial infarction, diabetes mellitus, smoking, alcohol consumption, and parental death from stroke. The degree of contralateral carotid stenosis and collateral arterial circulation to the ipsilateral middle cerebral artery (MCA) was determined from arteriograms if available.[24] Blood samples were collected for determination of hemoglobin, fasting lipid levels (triglyceride, HDL-cholesterol, LDL-cholesterol) and fibrinogen levels. A noncontrast CT scan of the brain was performed if a CT had not been done as part of usual clinical care sufficiently long after an ischemic event to permit accurate definition of infarct location. This CT was used only to determine the site of tissue infarction so as to exclude these regions from subsequent PET analysis (see below).

PET measurements of CBF, CBV, $CMRO_2$, and OEF were carried out. Regional OEF was measured by the method of Mintun et al. using $H_2^{15}O$, $C^{15}O$, and $O^{15}O$.[86,87] For each subject, 7 spherical regions of interest 19 mm in diameter were placed in the cortical territory of the middle cerebral artery in each hemisphere using stereotactic coordinates.[24,88] Any regions in well demarcated areas of reduced oxygen metabolism which corresponded to areas of infarction by CT or MR imaging and their homologous contralateral regions were excluded. The mean OEF for each MCA territory was calculated from the remaining regions and a left/right MCA OEF ratio was calculated. The maximum and minimum ratios from 18 normal control subjects were used to define the normal range. A separate range of normal for $H_2^{15}O/O^{15}O$ images was determined. Patients with left/right OEF ratios outside the normal range were categorized as having Stage II hemodynamic compromise in the hemisphere with higher OEF. These categorizations were made without knowledge of the side of the carotid occlusion or of the clinical course of the patients since the initial PET study. No information regarding the PET results was provided to the patients, treating physicians or the investigator responsible for determining endpoints.

Patients were followed for the duration of the study by the study coordinator via telephone contact every 6 months with the patient or next of kin. The interval occurrence of any symptoms of cerebrovascular disease, other medical problems, and functional status were determined. Interval medical treatment on a monthly basis was recorded as warfarin (with or without other medication), antiplatelet drugs (without warfarin), or no antithrombotic medication. The occurrence of any symptoms suggesting a stroke was thoroughly evaluated by a single designated, blinded investigator based on history from the patient or eyewitness and review of medical records ordered by the patient's physician. If necessary, follow-up examination and brain imaging were arranged. This investigator remained blinded to the PET data. All living patients were followed for the duration of the study.

The primary endpoint was subsequent ischemic stroke defined clinically as a neurological deficit of presumed ischemic cerebrovascular cause lasting greater than 24 hours in any cerebrovascular territory. Secondary endpoints were ipsilateral ischemic stroke and death. Subjects were divided into two groups: those with Stage II hemodynamic compromise and those with normal (symmetric) OEF. Comparison of 17 baseline risk factors and subsequent medical treatment between the two groups was performed with unpaired t-tests and Chi square analysis. Bonferroni adjusted p values of $0.05/18 = 0.003$ were used as the criterion of statistical significance. The primary analysis compared the two groups with respect to the length of time before reaching the primary endpoint by means of the Mantel-Cox log rank statistic and Kaplan-Meier survival curves. A value of $P < 0.05$ was used as the criterion of statistical significance. Secondary endpoints were analyzed in a similar manner. No interim analysis was planned or performed.

The Cox proportional hazards model was used to test nineteen candidate predictor variables in a univariate analysis. This included seventeen baseline variables, PET categorization of Stage II hemodynamic compromise, and subsequent medical treatment. All variables except medical treatment were treated as time-constant variables whereas medical treatment was treated as a time-dependent variable. All variables with $P < 0.05$ in the univariate analysis were included in a subsequent multivariate analysis. Both forward and backward stepwise selection based on maximum partial likelihood estimates were used. Those variables that remained significant at $P < 0.05$ in the multivariate analysis were included in the final model. Statistical analyses were performed with SPSS 7.0 for Windows and SAS.

Eighty-one patients successfully underwent initial data collection and PET measurements and were enrolled in the study. Thirty-nine patients had Stage II hemodynamic failure (increased OEF) in one hemisphere and 42 did not. In all 39 patients with Stage II hemodynamic failure, the hemisphere with increased OEF was ipsilateral to the occluded carotid. There were no subjects with bilateral carotid occlusion. There were no significant differences between the two groups in baseline risk factors or subsequent medical treatment. Arteriographic collateral circulation did not permit distinction between the two groups. Three subjects who underwent contralateral carotid endarterectomy prior to occurrence of ipsilateral ischemic stroke were censored after being followed for 13 months, 29 months, and 29 months, respectively. Two had not reached any endpoint and one had experienced a vertebrobasilar stroke. A fourth patient who had experienced an ipsilateral stroke underwent subsequent endarterectomy and was censored at 13 months.

Mean follow-up duration of the patients was 31.5 months. Fifteen total and 13 ipsilateral ischemic strokes occurred during the follow-up period. There were no hemorrhages. In the 39 stage II subjects, 12 total and 11 ipsilateral strokes occurred. In the 42 subjects with normal OEF, there were 3 total and 2 ipsilateral strokes. The Kaplan-Meier estimates for the risk of subsequent stroke at one and two years are given in Table 2. The risk of all stroke and ipsilateral ischemic stroke in symptomatic Stage II subjects was significantly higher than in those with normal OEF ($P = 0.005$ and $P = 0.004$ respectively). Twelve deaths occurred during the follow-up period. Ten deaths were due to non-stroke causes and two deaths resulted from large cerebral infarctions ipsilateral to a symptomatic occluded internal carotid artery. Both stroke-related deaths occurred in patients with increased OEF. There were six deaths in each group. No significant difference in the risk of death was demonstrated ($P = 0.942$). In the univariate analysis of the relationship to outcome of patient characteristics and subsequent medical treatment, only younger age and Stage II hemodynamic failure were significant predictors of both all stroke and ipsilateral ischemic stroke. Both variables remained significant in the multivariate analysis.

Table 2

Stroke Risk for Symptomatic Patients.[85]

	Total Patients (81)	Increased OEF (39)	Normal OEF (42)
All Stroke–1 year	7.7%	13.2%	2.4%
2 years	19.0%	29.2%	9.0%
Ipsilateral Stroke–1 year	6.4%	10.6%	2.4%
2 years	15.8%	26.5%	5.3%

Event rates were derived from Kaplan-Meier estimates of survival. The number of patients in each group is given in parenthesis. OEF = oxygen ejection fraction.

The age adjusted relative risk conferred by Stage II hemodynamic failure was 6.0 (95% CI 1.7 – 21.6) for all stroke and 7.3 (95% CI 1.6 – 33.4) for ipsilateral ischemic stroke.

We have demonstrated that Stage II hemodynamic failure (increased oxygen extraction) distal to a symptomatic occluded carotid artery is an independent predictor of subsequent ischemic stroke. This study was prospective, blinded and addressed the possible effect of treatment and other risk factors for stroke. As with any study which requires informed consent, these patients did not constitute a consecutive series and thus there remains the possibility of some bias in the selection which might limit the generalizability of the conclusions. However, the rates for stroke and ipsilateral ischemic stroke in the total group of 81 symptomatic patients are similar to those reported by others and the risk factor profile is typical for patients with carotid artery disease.[6,13,14]

The development of modern imaging techniques has made it possible to indirectly assess the hemodynamic status of the human cerebral circulation in vivo. Most of these methods rely on identification of preexisting autoregulatory vasodilation by the measurement of CBV or the CBF response to vasodilatory stimuli as a criterion for hemodynamic compromise.[2] Physiologically, this approach can be expected to detect less severely affected subjects than the measurement of OEF.[25] We therefore believe that it would be inappropriate to extrapolate our findings to other modalities.

The results of medical treatment of Stage II patients were poor and comparable to those reported for medically treated patients with symptomatic severe carotid stenosis.[6] Surgical approaches to improve cerebral hemodynamics, such as EC/IC arterial bypass surgery, are the logical treatment for these patients. However, in the absence of an empiric trial, it cannot be assumed that the stroke risk in operated patients would be equal to that in patients with normal OEF nor that the morbidity and mortality due to surgery would be outweighed by any subsequent reduction in stroke risk. A large, multicenter randomized trial conducted from 1977 to 1985 showed no benefit of EC/IC bypass surgery in preventing subsequent stroke.[14] At the time that this trial was conducted, there was no reliable and proven method for identifying a subgroup of patients in whom cerebral hemodynamic factors were of primary pathophysiologic importance. We have now established that such a subgroup can be identified and, furthermore, that they are at high risk for subsequent stroke when treated medically.

Cerebral Hemodynamics & Extracranial Intracranial Arterial Bypass Surgery

Several laboratories (including our own) have used PET to demonstrate postoperative improvement of cerebral hemodynamics by STA-MCA bypass surgery.[89-96] In patients with Stage II hemodynamic failure (increased oxygen extraction), EC/IC bypass surgery will return hemispheric OEF ratios to normal.[89-92] Several groups have reported improvement in impaired cerebral vasoreactivity to CO_2 or acetazolamide following EC/IC bypass for atherosclerotic occlusive cerebrovascular disease.[17,50,97-100] In most of these patients resting rCBF showed little change, although some patients with low resting rCBF demonstrated improvement in blood flow in the affected cerebral hemisphere following surgery. Some authors have recommended that EC/IC bypass be carried out in symptomatic patients with appropriate cerebrovascular lesions in whom impaired cerebral vasomotor reactivity to acetazolamide or CO_2 testing is demonstrated.[17,82,101] All of these studies were retrospective analyses of surgical patients. No prospective study of patients with occlusion of the internal carotid artery and impaired cerebral vasoreactivity to CO_2 or acetazolamide or increased oxygen extraction randomized to medical treatment or EC/IC bypass, with other risk factors for stroke controlled, has been carried out. The long-term benefit of using impaired cerebral hemodynamics in the selection of patients for EC/IC bypass to prevent stroke remains unproven at this time. It is appropriate at this time to consider performance of a new trial of EC/IC bypass surgery restricted to patients with Stage II symptomatic carotid occlusion.

References

1. Barnett HJM. Hemodynamic cerebral ischemia – An appeal for systematic data gathering prior to a new EC/IC trial. *Stroke* 1997;28:1857-1860.

2. Klijn CJM, Kappelle LJ, Tulleken CAF, et al. Symptomatic carotid artery occlusion: A reappraisal of hemodynamic factors. *Stroke* 1997;28:2084-2093.

3. Del Zoppo GJ, Poeck K, Pessin MS, et al. Recombinant tissue plasminogen activator in acute thrombotic and embolic stroke. *Ann Neurol* 1992;32:78-86.

4. Zanette EM, Fieschi C, Bozzao L, et al. Comparison of cerebral angiography and transcranial Doppler sonography in acute stroke. *Stroke* 1989;20:899-903.

5. Horowitz SH, Zito JL, Donnarumma R, et al. Computed tomographic – angiographic findings within the first five hours of cerebral infarction. *Stroke* 1991;22:1245-1253.

6. North American Symptomatic Carotid Endarterectomy Trial Collaborators: Beneficial effect of carotid endarterectomy in symptomatic patients with high-grade stenosis. *N Engl J Med* 1991;325:445-453.

7. Mayberg MR, Wilson SE, Yatsu F, et al. Carotid endarterectomy and prevention of cerebral ischemia in symptomatic carotid stenosis. *JAMA* 1991;266:3289-3294.

8. European Carotid Surgery Trialists' Collaborative Group: MRC European Carotid Surgery Trial. Interim results for symptomatic patients with severe (70-99%) or with mild (0-29%) carotid stenosis. *Lancet* 1991;337:1235-1243.

9. Executive Committee for the Asymptomatic Carotid Atherosclerosis Study: Endarterectomy for asymptomatic carotid artery stenosis. *JAMA* 1995;273:1421-1428.

10. Balow J, Alter M, Resch JA: Cerebral thromboembolism. A clinical appraisal of 100 cases. *Neurology* 1966;16:559-564.

11. Pessin MS, Duncan GW, Mohr JP, et al. Clinical and angiographic features of carotid transient ischemic attacks. *N Engl J Med* 1977;296:358-362.

12. Thiele BL, Young JV, Chikos PM, et al. Correlation of arteriographic findings and symptoms in cerebrovascular disease. *Neurology* 1980;30:1041-1046.

13. Hankey GJ, Warlow CP: Prognosis of symptomatic carotid artery occlusion. *Cerebrovasc Dis* 1991;1:245-256.

14. EC/IC Bypass Study Group: Failure of extracranial-intracranial arterial bypass to reduce the risk of ischemic stroke. Results of an international randomized trial. *N Engl J Med* 1985;313:1192-1200.

15. Day AL, Rhoton AL Jr, Little JR: The extracranial-intracranial bypass study. *Surg Neurol* 1986;26:222-226.

16. Yonas H, Smith HA, Durham SR, et al. Increased stroke risk predicted by compromised CBF reactivity. *J Neurosurg* 1993;79:483-489.

17. Schmiedek P, Piepgras A, Leinsinger G, et al. Improvement of cerebrovascular reserve capacity by EC-IC arterial bypass in patients with ICA occlusion and hemodynamic cerebral ischemia. *J Neurosurg* 1994;81:236-244.

18. Diaz FG, Ausman JI, Mehta B, et al. Acute cerebral revascularization. *J Neurosurg* 1985;63:200-209.

19. Archie JP Jr, Feldtman RW. Critical stenosis of the internal carotid artery. *Surgery* 1981;89:67-70.

20. Deweese JA, May AG, Lipchik EO, et al. Anatomic and hemodynamic correlations in carotid artery stenosis. *Stroke* 1970;1:149-157.

21. Brice JG, Dowsett DJ, Lowe RD. Haemodynamic effects of carotid artery stenosis. *Brit Med J* 1964;2:1363-1366.

22. Schroeder T. Cerebrovascular reactivity to acetazolamide in carotid artery disease. *Neurol Res* 1986;8:231-236.

23. Sillesen H, Schroeder T, Steenberg HJ, et al. Doppler examination of the periorbital arteries adds valuable hemodynamic information in carotid artery disease. *Ultrasound Med Biol* 1987;13:177-181.

24. Powers WJ, Press GA, Grubb RL Jr, et al. The effect of hemodynamically significant carotid artery disease on the hemodynamic status of the cerebral circulation. *Ann Intern Med* 1987;106:27-34.

25. Powers WJ. Cerebral hemodynamics in ischemic cerebrovascular disease. *Ann Neurol* 1991;29:231-240.

26. Grubb RL Jr, Powers WJ. Role of cerebral hemodynamics in ischemic atherosclerotic cerebrovascular disease. *Neurosurg Quart* 1993;3:83-102.

27. Pitts FW. Variations of collateral circulation in internal carotid occlusion. *Neurology* 1962;12:467-471.

28. Norrving B, Nilsson B, Risberg J: rCBF in patients with carotid occlusion. Resting and hypercapnic flow related to collateral pattern. *Stroke* 1982;13:155-162.

29. Alpers BJ, Berry RG: Circle of Willis in cerebral vascular disorders. *Arch Neurol* 1963;8:398-402.

30. Prosenz P, Heiss WD, Tschabitscher H, et al. The value of regional cerebral blood flow measurements compared to angiography in the assessment of obstructive neck vessel disease. *Stroke* 1974;5:19-31.

31. Schomer DF, Marks MP, Steinberg GK, et al. The anatomy of the posterior communicating artery as a risk factor for ischemic cerebral infarction. *N Engl J Med* 1994;330:1565-1570.

32. Frackowiak RSJ, Lenzi GL, Jones T, et al. Quantitative measurement of regional cerebral blood flow and oxygen metabolism in man using ^{15}O and positron emission tomography: Theory, procedure and normal values. *J Comput Assist Tomogr* 1980;4:727-736.

33. Powers WJ, Raichle ME. Positron emission tomography and its application to the study of cerebrovascular disease in man. *Stroke* 1985;16:361-376.

34. Lebrun-Grandie P, Baron JC, Soussaline F, et al. Coupling between regional blood flow and oxygen utilization in the normal human brain. A study with positron tomography and oxygen-15. *Arch Neurol* 1983;40:230-236.

35. Powers WJ. Hemodynamics and metabolism in ischemic cerebrovascular disease. *Neurologic Clinics* 1992;10:31-48.

36. Rapela CE, Green HD: Autoregulation of canine cerebral blood flow. *Circ Res* 1964;15:I205-I211.

37. Harper AM, Glass HI. Effect of alterations in the arterial carbon dioxide tension on the blood flow through the cerebral cortex at normal and low arterial blood pressures. *J Neurol Neurosurg Psychiatry* 1965;28:449-452.

38. Grubb RL Jr, Phelps ME, Raichle ME, et al. The effects of arterial blood pressure on the regional cerebral blood volume by X-ray fluorescence. *Stroke* 1973;4:390-399.

39. Grubb RL Jr, Raichle ME, Phelps ME, et al. Effects of increased intracranial pressure on cerebral blood volume, blood flow, and oxygen utilization in monkeys. *J Neurosurg* 1975;43:385-398.

40. Eklof B, MacMillan V, Siesjo BK. Cerebral energy state and cerebral venous pO$_2$ in experimental hypotension caused by bleeding. *Acta Physiol Scand* 1972;86:515-527.

41. Finnerty FA Jr, Witkin L, Fazekas JF. Cerebral hemodynamics during cerebral ischemia induced by acute hypotension. *J Clin Invest* 1954;33:1227-1232.

42. Kety SS, King BD, Horvath SM, et al. The effects of an acute reduction in blood pressure by means of differential spinal sympathetic block on the cerebral circulation of hypertensive patients. *J Clin Invest* 1950;29:402-407.

43. Lennox WG, Gibbs FA, Gibbs EL. Relationship of unconsciousness to cerebral blood flow and to anoxemia. *Arch Neurol Psych* 1935;34:1001-1013.

44. Frackowiak RS. The pathophysiology of human cerebral ischaemia: A new perspective obtained with positron tomography. *Q J Med* 1985;57:713-727.

45. Cordes M, Henkes H, Roll D, et al. Subacute and chronic cerebral infarctions: SPECT and gadolinium MR imaging. *J Comput Assist Tomogr* 1989;13:567-571.

46. Nemoto E, Snyder JV, Carroll RG, et al. Global ischemia in dogs: Cerebrovascular CO$_2$ reactivity and autoregulation. *Stroke* 1975;6:425-431.

47. Hakim AM, Pokrupa RP, Villanueva J, et al. The effect of spontaneous reperfusion on metabolic function in early human cerebral infarcts. *Ann Neurol* 1987;21:279-289.

48. Rogg J, Rutigliano M, Yonas H, et al. The acetazolamide challenge: Imaging techniques designed to evaluate cerebral blood flow reserve. *AJR* 1989;153:605-612.

49. Chollet F, Celsis P, Clanet M, et al. SPECT study of cerebral blood flow reactivity after acetazolamide in patients with transient ischemia attacks. *Stroke* 1989;20:458-464.

50. Bishop CCR, Burnarel KG, Brown M, et al. Reduced response of cerebral blood flow to hypercapnia: restoration by extracranial-intracranial bypass. *Brit J Surg* 1987;74:802-804.

51. Levine RL, Lagreze HL, Dobkin JA, et al. Cerebral vasocapacitance and TIAs. *Neurology* 1989;39:25-29.

52. Kanno I, Uemura K, Higano S, et al. Oxygen extraction fraction at maximally vasodilated tissue in ischemic brain estimated from regional CO$_2$ responsiveness measured by positron emission tomography. *J Cereb Blood Flow Metab* 1988;8:227-235.

53. Powers WJ. Positron emission tomography in cerebrovascular disease: Clinical applications. In Liss AR (ed): *Clinical Neuroimaging* (Frontiers of Clinical Neuroscience Series, Vol. 4), New York, Alan R. Liss, Inc. 1988:49-74.

54. Herold S, Brown MM, Frackowiak RSJ, et al. Assessment of cerebral haemodynamic reserve: Correlation between PET and CO$_2$ reactivity measured by the intravenous 133 xenon injection technique. *J Neurol Neurosurg Psychiatry* 1988;51:1045-1050.

55. Ringelstein EB, Sievers C, Ecker S, et al. Non-invasive assessment of CO$_2$-induced cerebral vasomotor response in normal individuals and patients with internal carotid artery occlusions. *Stroke* 1988;19:963-969.

56. Karnik R, Valentin A, Winkler W, et al. Sex-related differences in acetazolamide-induced cerebral vasomotor reactivity. *Stroke* 1996;27:56-58.

57. Ehrenreich DL, Burns RA, Alman RW, et al. Influence of acetazolamide on cerebral blood flow. *Arch Neurol* 1961;5:227-232.

58. Piepgras A, Schmiedek P, Leinsinger G, et al. A simple test to assess cerebrovascular reserve capacity using transcranial Doppler sonography and acetazolamide. *Stroke* 1990;21:1306-1311.

59. Kleiser B, Widder B. Course of carotid artery occlusions with impaired cerebrovascular reactivity. *Stroke* 1992;23:171-174.

60. Silvestrini M, Troisi E, Cupini LM, et al. Transcranial Doppler assessment of the functional effects of symptomatic carotid stenosis. *Neurology* 1994;44:1910-1914.

61. Detre JA, Alsop DC, Vives LR, et al. Noninvasive MRI evaluation of cerebral blood flow in cerebrovascular disease. *Neurology* 1998;50:663-641.

62. Kazumata K, Tanaka N, Ishikawa T, et al. Dissociation of vasoreactivity to acetazolamide and hypercapnia. Comparative study in patients with chronic occlusive major cerebral artery disease. *Stroke* 1996, 27:2052-2058.

63. Liu H-M, Tu Y-K, Yip P-K, et al. Cerebral blood flow and cerebrovascular reactive capacity in patients with bilateral high-grade carotid artery stenosis. *Acta Neurol Scand* 1996;166 (Suppl):90-92.

64. Nighoghossian N, Trouillas P, Philippon B, et al. Cerebral blood flow reserve assessment in symptomatic vs. asymptomatic high-grade internal carotid artery stenosis. *Stroke* 1994;25:1010-1013.

65. Dahl A, Russell D, Rootwelt K, et al. Cerebral vasoreactivity assessed with transcranial Doppler and regional cerebral blood flow measurements. *J Cereb Blood Flow Metab* 1994;14:974-981.

66. Sette G, Baron JC, Mazoyer B, et al. Local brain hemodynamics and oxygen metabolism in cerebrovascular disease. *Brain* 1989;112:931-951.

67. Gibbs JM, Wise RJS, Leenders KL, et al. Evaluation of cerebral perfusion reserve in patients with carotid artery occlusion. *Lancet* 1984;1:310-314.

68. Powers WJ, Grubb RL Jr, Raichle ME: Physiological responses to focal cerebral ischemia in humans. *Ann Neurol* 1984;16:546-552.

69. Powers WJ. Is the ratio of cerebral blood volume to cerebral blood flow a reliable indicator of cerebral perfusion pressure? *J Cereb Blood Flow Metab* 1993;13(Supp 1):5325.

70. Knapp WA, Von Klummer R, Kubler W: Imaging of cerebral blood flow-to-volume distribution using SPECT. *J Nucl Med* 1986;27:465-470.

71. DiPiero V, Peran D, Savi A, et al. Sequential assessment of regional cerebral blood flow, regional cerebral blood volume, and blood-brain barrier in focal cerebral ischemia case report. *J Cereb Blood Flow Metab* 1986;6:379-384.

72. Hirano T, Minematsu K, Hasegawa Y, et al. Acetazolamide reactivity on 123 I-IMP single photon emission computed tomography in patients with major cerebral artery occlusive disease; correlation with positron emission tomography parameters. *J Cereb Blood Flow Metab* 1994;14:763-770.

73. Hayashida K, Hirose Y, Tanaka Y, et al. Stratification of severity by cerebral blood flow, oxygen metabolism, and acetazolamide reactivity in patients with cerebrovascular disease. In Ishii Y, et al. (eds): *Recent Advances in Biomedical Imaging*. Elsevier Science B.V., 1997:113-119.

74. Sugimori H, Ibayashi S, Fujii K, et al. Can transcranial Doppler really detect reduced cerebral perfusion states? *Stroke* 1995;26:2053-2060.

75. Nariai T, Suzuki R, Hirakawa K, et al. Vascular reserve in chronic cerebral ischemia measured by the acetazolamide challenge test: Comparison with positron emission tomography. *Am J Neuroradiol* 1995;16:563-570.

76. Widder B, Kleiser B, Krapf H. Course of cerebrovascular reactivity in patients with carotid artery occlusions. *Stroke* 1994;25:1963-1967.

77. Ringelstein EB, Otis SM. Physiological testing of vasomotor reserve. In Newell DW, Aeslid R (eds): *Transcranial Doppler*. New York, Raven Press, 1992:83-89.

78. Hasegawa Y, Yamaguchi T, Tsuchiya T, et al. Sequential change of hemodynamic reserve in patients with major cerebral artery occlusions or severe stenosis. *Neuroradiology* 1992;34:15-21.

79. Yokota C, Hasegawa Y, Minematsu K, et al. Effect of acetazolamide reactivity and long-term outcome in patients with major cerebral artery occlusive diseases. *Stroke* 29:640-644, 1998.

80. DeLey G, Nshimyumuremy JB, Leusen J. Hemispheric blood flow in the rat after unilateral common carotid occlusion: Evaluation with time. *Stroke* 1985;16:69-73.

81. Coyle P, Panzenbeck MJ. Collateral development after carotid artery occlusion in Fischer 344 rats. *Stroke* 1990;21:316-321.

82. Webster MW, Makaroun MS, Steed DL, et al. Compromised cerebral blood flow reactivity is a predictor of stroke in patients with symptomatic carotid artery occlusive disease. *J Vasc Surg* 1995;21:338-345.

83. Bornstein NM, Norris JW: Benign outcome of carotid occlusion. *Neurology* 1989;39:6-8.

84. Yamaguchi H, Fukuyama Y, Nagahama Y, et al. Evidence of misery perfusion and risk for recurrent stroke in major cerebral arterial occlusive diseases from PET. *J Neurol Neurosurg Psychiatry* 1996;61:18-25.

85. Grubb RL Jr, Derdeyn CP, Fritsch SM, et al. Importance of hemodynamic factors in the prognosis of symptomatic carotid occlusion. *JAMA* 1998;280(12):1055-1060.

86. Mintun MA, Raichle ME, Martin WRW, et al. Brain oxygen utilization measured with O-15 radiotracers and positron emission tomography. *J Nucl Med* 1984;25:177-187.

87. Videen TO, Perlmutter JS, Herscovitch P, et al. Brain blood volume, blood flow, and oxygen utilization measured with 0-15 radiotracers and positron emission tomography: Revised metabolic computations. *J Cereb Blood Flow Metab* 1987;7:513-516.

88. Powers WJ, Grubb RL Jr, Darriet D, et al. Cerebral blood flow and cerebral metabolic rate of oxygen requirements for cerebral function and viability in humans. *J Cereb Blood Flow Metab* 1985;5:600-608.

89. Powers WJ, Martin WR, Herscovitch P, et al. Extracranial-intracranial bypass surgery: Hemodynamic and metabolic effects. *Neurology* 1984;34:1168-1174.

90. Grubb RL Jr. Management of the patient with carotid occlusion and a single ischemic event. *Clin Neurosurg* 1986;33:251-260.

91. Samson Y, Baron JC, Rousser MG, et al. Effects of extra-intracranial arterial bypass on cerebral blood flow and oxygen metabolism in humans. *Stroke* 16:609-616, 1985.

92. Gibbs JM, Wise RJ, Thomas DJ, et al. Cerebral haemodynamic changes after extracranial-intracranial bypass surgery. *J Neurol Neurosurg Psychiatry* 1987;50:140-150.

93. Baron JC, Bousser MG, Rey A, et al. Reversal of focal "misery-perfusion syndrome" by extra-intracranial arterial bypass in hemodynamic cerebral ischemia. *Stroke* 1981;12:454-459.

94. Baron JC, Rey A, Guillard A, et al. Non-invasive tomographic imaging of cerebral blood flow (CBF) and oxygen extraction fraction (OEF) in superficial temporal artery to middle cerebral artery (STA-MCA) anastomosis. In Meyer JS, Lechner H, Reivich M, Ott EO (eds): *Cerebral Vascular Disease*. Amsterdam, Excerpta Medica, 1981:58-64.

95. Leblanc R, Tyler JL, Mohr G, et al. Hemodynamic and metabolic effects of cerebral revascularization. *J Neurosurg* 1987;66:529-535.

96. Kawamura S, Sayama I, Yasui N, et al. Haemodynamic and metabolic changes following extra-intracranial bypass surgery. *Acta Neurochir* 1994;126:135-139.

97. Vorstrup S, Brun B, Lassen NA: Evaluation of the cerebral vasodilatory capacity by the acetazolamide test before EC-IC bypass surgery in patients with occlusion of the internal carotid artery. *Stroke* 1986;17:1291-1298.

98. Batjer H, Devous MD, Purdy PD, et al. Improvement in regional cerebral blood flow and cerebral vasoreactivity after extracranial-intracranial arterial bypass. *Neurosurgery* 1988;22:913-919.

99. Karnik R, Valentin A, Ammerer HP, et al. Evaluation of vasomotor reactivity by transcranial Doppler and acetazolamide test before and after extracranial-intracranial bypass in patients with internal carotid artery occlusions. *Stroke* 1992;23:812-817.

100. Anderson DE, McLane MP, Reichman OH, et al. Improved cerebral blood flow and CO_2 reactivity after microvascular anastomosis in patients at high risk for recurrent stroke. *Neurosurgery* 1992;31:26-34.

101. Widder B, Kornhuber HH: Extra-intracranial bypass surgery in carotid artery occlusions: Who benefits? *Neurol Psychiat Brain Res* 1994;2:126-131.

Chapter 3

Extracranial-Intracranial Bypass: Surgical Considerations

Marc R. Mayberg, MD

Introduction

C. Miller Fisher first conceived a potential benefit for extracranial-intracranial (EC/IC) bypass grafting in 1951: "Someday vascular surgery will find a way to bypass the occluded portion of the artery during the period of ominous fleeting symptoms. Anastomosis of the external carotid artery or one of its branches with the internal carotid artery above the area of narrowing should be feasible."[1] At that time, the concept of cerebral revascularization seemed logical and desirable, as vascular bypass surgery elsewhere in the body was becoming a standard therapy to prevent or reverse local tissue ischemia. On the other hand, little was known at that time regarding the processes by which the craniocervical circulation ensures adequate blood flow to the brain, including mechanisms such as collateral flow, autoregulation and angiogenesis, all of which were undiscovered or poorly understood. Thus, the impetus for developing surgical techniques to revascularize the brain was founded in a genuine belief that augmentation of flow through major conducting arteries to the brain could prevent or possibly reverse cerebral ischemia. These concepts became a technical reality in the 1960s with the development of advanced microsurgical techniques (see below). In that process, several surgical procedures were developed and were widely adopted as potential therapeutic alterna-

From: Choi D, Dacey RG, Hsu CY, Powers WJ. *Cerebrovascular Disease: Momentum at the End of the Second Millennium.* Armonk, NY: Futura Publishing Company, Inc., © 2002.

tives for a variety of disorders attributed to cerebrovascular pathology. However, the publication of the EC/IC bypass trial[2] in 1985 showed that superficial temporal artery to middle cerebral artery (STA-MCA) bypass was ineffective over a broad range of clinical conditions. The EC/IC bypass trial was a well-constructed and scientifically valid study which had widespread ramifications in the practice of medicine. Most directly, the number of EC/IC bypass procedures for cerebral revascularization dropped substantially, reimbursement for these procedures was reduced or eliminated, and the exposure of neurosurgical residents to these procedures over a several year period was markedly diminished. During this interval, several large prospective multi-center randomized trials showed benefit for another cerebral revascularization procedure, carotid endarterectomy, in reducing stroke for patients with symptomatic[3-5] and asymptomatic[6,7] carotid stenosis. In addition, accumulating retrospective[8,9] and prospective[10] data have suggested that there may, in fact, be a subgroup of patients with occlusive cerebral vascular disease at higher risk for stroke who would benefit from EC/IC bypass. Moreover, indications for EC/IC bypass in conditions other than occlusive cerebral vascular disease (e.g. aneurysm trapping,[11,12] skull base tumors,[13] and Moya-Moya disease[14-16]) have persisted, and surgical technology has progressed since the era of the EC/IC bypass trial. This chapter will describe the basic surgical considerations related to cerebral revascularization in light of historical aspects, various categories of EC/IC bypass procedures, surgical techniques, indications for surgery, complications and relative indications for each procedure.

History of Cerebral Revascularization

The concept of cerebral revascularization actually predated Miller Fisher's prophetic statement in 1951. As early as 1939, German and Taffel[17] performed direct apposition of the temporalis muscle to the primate brain (encephalomyosynangiosis) in an attempt to increase cerebral blood flow. This procedure was subsequently applied to humans in 1942.[18] In 1949, Beck[19] attempted a carotid-jugular fistula with the goal of increasing oxygenation in the cerebral venous system. The first EC/IC bypass was attempted in 1951 by Pool[20] who performed a superficial temporal to anterior cerebral artery bypass using plastic tubing (which was occluded on the postoperative angiogram). The first extracranial carotid to intracranial saphenous vein graft was performed in 1963.[21] The major breakthrough in bypass procedures to revascularize the brain was coincident with the development of the operating microscope, which enabled microvascular anatomosis for small (< 2 mm) vessels. In Donaghy's laboratory in Vermont, the STA-MCA anastomosis was perfected,[22] and the first human STA-MCA bypass was performed in 1967.[23] Lougheed[24] and Tew[25] were among several authors describing the initial experience with saphenous vein interposition EC/IC bypass grafts. Revascularization of the posterior circulation became feasible in the late 1970s.[25,27] In the early 1980s a number of single center, retrospective reports were published regarding EC/IC bypass documenting excellent patency rates, low complications and improved clinical outcome for a variety of cerebral vascular disorders.[11,12,28-42]

Cerebral Revascularization Procedures

In the broadest sense, cerebral revascularization includes any interventional procedure which is designed to increase blood flow through craniocephalic vessels serving the brain. Endarterectomy and surgical reconstruction of the carotid and vertebral arteries at the aortic arch has been described elsewhere[43] and will not be discussed in this context. *Extracranial* to *extracranial* bypass procedures have been advocated for both anterior circulation and posterior circulation lesions,[34] although no controlled trials have been performed to demonstrate efficacy. Endarterectomy has been applied to a variety of sites in the cranial cervical circulation, including common carotid, internal carotid, extracranial and intracranial vertebral, and middle cerebral arteries.[44] Except for cervical internal carotid artery endarterectomy, there has been no scientific evidence showing efficacy for these procedures. Although several trials[3-7] have shown a benefit for carotid endarterectomy in preventing stroke, it is not clear that the prophylactic benefit is derived from direct hemodynamic effects as opposed to eliminating a source of emboli. More recently, several retrospective studies have suggested benefit for angioplasty and stenting at various sites and the craniocervical circulation, including cervical[45-47] and intracranial[48] arteries. The efficacy of these procedures has yet to be shown.

STA-MCA Bypass

Superficial temporal to middle cerebral artery anastomosis has traditionally been the most common procedure used for cerebral revascularization. The procedure is relatively straightforward, only moderately invasive for the patient, and can be performed by most experienced surgeons with excellent patency rates and low complications. The technique for STA-MCA bypass has been described in detail elsewhere.[27,34] Patients with appropriate indications for STA-MCA bypass

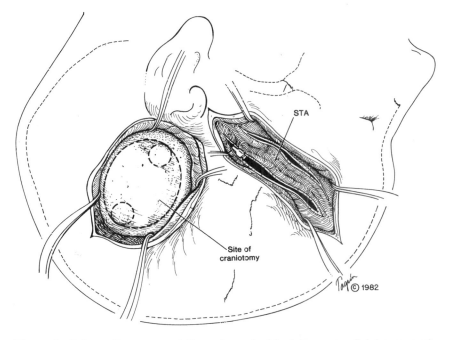

Figure 1. Schematic representation of surgical incision, superficial temporal artery and craniotomy site for STA-MCA anastomosis. (Reprinted from Ojemann RL and Crowell RM: **Surgical Management of Cerebrovascular Disease,**[34] with permission.)

(see below) usually have preoperative angiography performed. An essential requirement for this procedure is the presence of one or two large (> 1.5 mm internal diameter) superficial temporal artery branches ipsilateral to the lesion being treated. In most cases, the larger anterior branch is used as donor vessel, although the posterior branch or both branches may be used. A distal parietal branch of the middle cerebral artery in the Sylvian fissure can often be identified from the angiogram as the recipient site, although the actual identification occurs at the time of surgery.

Under general anesthesia, the course of the superficial temporal artery is mapped on the scalp surface prior to incision. A curvilinear incision is made to encompass both the donor STA branch and the craniotomy site, which overlies the posterior aspect of the Sylvian fissure above the ear (Figure 1). The superficial temporal artery is then dissected from the adjacent fascia with an investing cuff of fascial tissue and mobilized over a 6–10 cm segment. After a craniotomy is fashioned, the dura is opened and the Sylvian fissure divided to identify a 1.5–2 mm vessel. The recipient MCA vessel is clamped and the donor STA is attached by end-to-side anatomosis using multiple fine interrupted

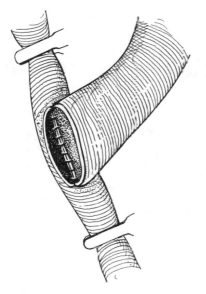

Figure 2. End-to-side anastomosis of superficial temporal artery to parietal branch of middle cerebral artery in the Sylvian fissure. (Reprinted from Ojemann RL and Crowell RM: **Surgical Management of Cerebrovascular Disease,**[34] with permission.)

sutures (Figure 2). In certain settings, two STA branches can be used for a double end-to-end anatomosis to a single recipient artery. The clips are removed and flow through the anastomosis is measured by Doppler. After allowing adequate space for the passage of the STA donor artery through the craniectomy site and dura. the bone is replaced. In experienced hands, the entire procedure takes about 2–3 hours and the postoperative recovery is rapid due to the minimal brain dissection or retraction. Graft patency is monitored in the postoperative period by bedside Doppler of the superficial temporal artery, and generally a postoperative angiogram is performed to assess the degree of cerebral revascularization (Figure 3). Typically, both angiographic and measured flow through the bypass graft increase over the first 6–8 weeks after the procedure with maturation of the graft.

Alternative Bypass Grafts Using External Carotid Artery Branches

In various settings, it may be advantageous to utilize branches of the external carotid artery other than STA to perform an EC/IC bypass. When the STA is small or otherwise unsuitable for bypass grafting (e.g. prior cranial surgery), an occipital artery-MCA anastomosis can be

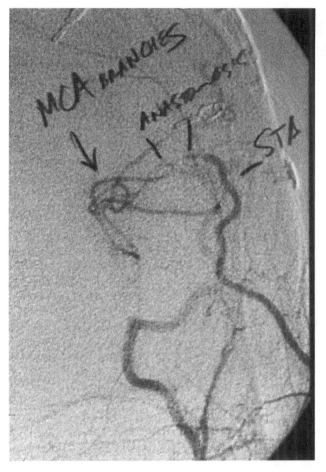

Figure 3. Post-operative angiogram showing retrograde filling of parietal MCA branches through a patent STA-MCA bypass.

substituted.[49] In the posterior circulation, occipital to posterior inferior cerebellar artery (PICA) or occipital to anterior inferior cerebellar artery (AICA) bypass procedures have been described.[26,50] In either case, the procedure is similar to that performed for STA-MCA, with the exception of a suboccipital craniotomy and the utilization of a distal PICA or AICA branch as the recipient site. In certain patients with lesions affecting the mid-portion of the basilar artery (e.g. fusiform basilar aneurysm), an STA to superior cerebellar artery or STA-to-posterior cerebellar artery anastomosis is indicated.[26,27,51] In both of these procedures, a longer segment of STA must be mobilized to achieve an anastomosis at depth adjacent to the basilar bifurcation. Nevertheless, revascularization of the posterior circulation with retrograde flow through the basilar artery can provide excellent cerebral blood flow to the brainstem and cerebellum, enabling proximal ligation of one or both vertebral arteries.

Interposition Saphenous Vein Grafts

As discussed below, a major disadvantage of the STA-MCA anastomosis is the relatively limited blood flow at the immediate completion of the procedure. Although flows through the graft increase over time, they are often not immediately sufficient to provide adequate regional cerebral blood flow, especially in the setting of associated vessel ligation. Thus, in several clinical situations it may be appropriate to consider EC/IC bypass using a high flow interposition saphenous vein graft.

In 1974, Tew[25] described cervical carotid to supraclinoid ICA bypass to provide high anterograde flow to the intracranial cerebral circulation. Several subsequent reports[40,52-55] have elaborated a variety of techniques utilizing interposition vein grafts. In brief, the saphenous vein is removed from a separate incision in the lower leg. The proximal anastomosis can originate from the subclavian artery,[54] common carotid artery[56] external carotid artery[52] or the stump of an occluded internal carotid artery (ICA).[40] The vein graft is then tunneled subcutaneously into the temporal region, where it is anastomosed with a proximal ICA, MCA, posterior cerebral artery or other appropriate sites (Figures 4 and 5). A variation of this approach uses a petrous ICA to supraclinoid ICA interposition vein graft to bypass the cavernous segment of the ICA, as in the example of a giant intracavernous aneurysm. Some authors have suggested the utilization of autologous radial artery[57] or synthetic graft[58] as the interposition vascular conduit.

The indications for saphenous vein interposition graft are generally related to the necessity to establish immediate high flow through the bypass. Whereas STA-MCA may provide only 25 to 50 cc/min immediately after bypass,[55,59,60] a saphenous vein graft to the proximal ICA may provide flows in excess of 100 cc/min (Figure 6).[61] Such a high flow bypass may be necessary in the setting of planned elective vascular ligation, eg, trapping of an aneurysm or resection of a skull base tumor involving the petrous or cavernous ICA. In general, preoperative temporary balloon occlusion by endovascular technique may determine whether a patient will tolerate major vessel occlusion, or whether a high flow bypass is necessary.[13,62-64] Some groups[65] have advocated additional evocative testing of cerebral hemodynamic reserve to determine the need for bypass associated with elective vascular occlusion. Other indications for using saphenous vein graft include an atretic or absent STA or vasculopathy affecting the donor vessel. De-

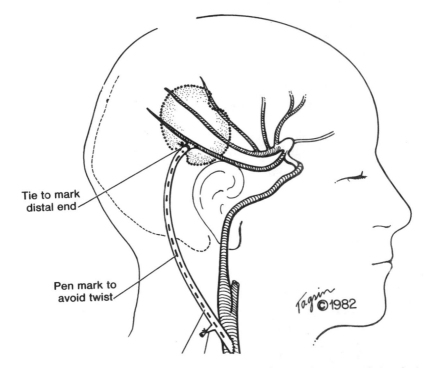

Tie to mark
distal end

Pen mark to
avoid twist

Tagrin ©1982

Figure 4. Schematic representation of interposition saphenous vein graft. In this case, the graft extends from the cervical common carotid artery to a parietal branch of the middle cerebral artery. (Reprinted from Ojemann RL and Crowell RM: **Surgical Management of Cerebrovascular Disease,**[34] with permission.)

spite its utility in certain clinical settings, there are several disadvantages associated with a saphenous vein interposition bypass graft. First, although patency rates of 90% or better have been reported,[40,52,54,66] in general the patency rates are better with direct arterial-arterial anastomoses. The need for two anastomoses in an interposition graft increases the likelihood of technical failure. In addition, manipulation of the graft during harvesting, the subcutaneous tunneling procedure, and the potential for postoperative kinking of the graft due to neck movement likely contribute to the lower patency rates for vein bypass compared to STA-MCA.

Pedicle Grafts

In certain conditions, it may be difficult or impossible to perform direct anastomosis of extracranial to intracranial vessels. This may be due to small size for both donor and recipient vessels (eg, children),

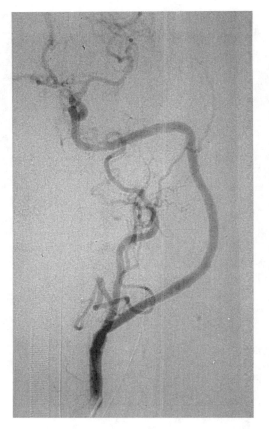

Figure 5. Angiogram demonstrating left cervical common carotid to petrous internal carotid artery saphenous vein bypass. Note the angiographic filling of the left hemisphere circulation through the bypass.

or due to vasculopathy affecting either donor or recipient vessel which makes anastomosis impossible. In these settings, several types of pedicle grafts have been developed. In fact, the earliest EC/IC bypass involved placing the temporalis muscle directly on the surface of the brain, as described above.[18] This procedure, encephalomyosinangiosis, has largely been replaced by a similar procedure known as encephalo-duroangiosynangiosis (EDAS).[14,15,67.68] In EDAS, the superficial temporal artery and adjacent fascia is dissected along its length and brought through an opening in skull and dura to lie in direct apposition along the frontal or parietal cortical surface. In both types of procedure, there is no immediate increase in blood flow through the pedicle graft. However, over time, angiogenesis occurs with the development of a rich vascular network from the pedicle onto the brain surface. A similar procedure has been described using a vascularized segment of omentum, which is brought through a subcutaneous tunnel to the brain

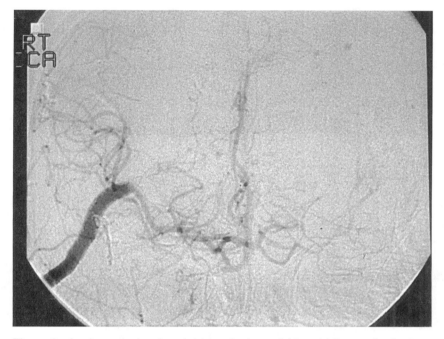

Figure 6. Angiogram showing right cervical carotid to middle cerebral artery saphenous vein bypass graft in a patient with bilateral carotid occlusions. Note that flow through the bypass fills both hemispheres.

surface.[15,69] The major indication for pedicle graft bypass to the brain is Moya-Moya disease, especially in children.[14,15,67,70]

Indications for EC/IC Bypass

Prior to the EC/IC bypass trial,[2] a wide variety of indications for EC/IC bypass procedure were described (Table 1). These included cervical ICA trauma[71-73] or dissection,[52,74,75] adjunct to elective surgical intracranial vascular ligation for aneurysm[11,12,76-79] or skull base tumor,[13,80] MCA occlusion,[81-86] cervical or intracranial ICA occlusion,[75,87,88] inoperable ICA stenosis,[75,83] ischemic retinopathy,[39,83] acute stroke,[30,89] multi-infarct dementia[90,91]or Moya-Moya disease.[15,16,67,92-94] As discussed elsewhere in this volume, the EC/IC bypass trial[2] clearly demonstrated no benefit in preventing stroke among a group of patients with ICA or MCA occlusion, or surgically inaccessible lesions of the ICA. The immediate result of the EC/IC bypass trial was substantial decrease in the frequency of these procedures being performed, and a dramatic limitation in the indications for the procedure.

Table I: Indications for EC/IC Bypass

(Prior to 1985)

Internal Carotid Artery Trauma
Internal Carotid Artery Dissection
Elective Major Vessel Ligation
  – Aneurysm
  – Tumor
Middle Cerebral Artery Occlusion
Internal Carotid Artery Occlusion
Inoperable Internal Carotid Artery Stenosis
Ischemic Retinopathy
Acute Stroke
Multi-Infarct Dementia
Moya-Moya Disease

In the intervening 13 years since the publication of the EC/IC Bypass Trial, controvery has persisted about the appropriateness, specific indications, and cost-effectiveness of cerebral revascularization procedures. As discussed elsewhere in this volume, several reports[10,95-99] have suggested that there may exist a subgroup of patients with cerebral occlusive disease at risk for stroke who might benefit from EC/IC bypass. In addition, compared to 20 years ago, advances in imaging, assessment of cerebral hemodynamic and surgical and anesthetic techniques provide a new setting in which to study these procedures.

References

1. Fisher CM. Occlusion of the internal carotid artery. *Arch Neurol Psych* 1951;65:346-377.
2. The EC/IC Bypass Study Group. Failure of extracranial-intracranial arterial bypass to reduce the risk of ischemic stroke. Results of an international randomized trial. *N Engl J Med* 1985;313:1191.
3. European Carotid Surgery Trialists" Group. MRC European carotid surgery trial. *Lancet* 1991;337:1235-1243.
4. Mayberg M, Wilson E, Yatsu F, et al. Carotid endarterectomy and prevention of cerebral ischemia in symptomatic carotid stenosis. *JAMA* 1991;266:3289-3294.
5. North American Symptomatic Carotid Endarterectomy Trial Collaborators. Beneficial effect of carotid endarterectomy in symptomatic patients with high-grade carotid stenosis. *N Engl J Med* 1991;325:445-453.
6. Executive Committee for the Asymptomatic Carotid Atherosclerosis Study. Endarterectomy for asymptomatic carotid artery stenosis. *JAMA* 1995;273:1421-1428.

7. Hobson RI, Weiss D, Fields W, et al. Efficacy of carotid endarterectomy for asymptomatic carotid stenosis. *N Engl J Med* 1993;328:221-227.

8. Furlan AJ, Whisnant JP, Baker HLJ. Long-term prognosis after carotid artery occlusion. *Neurology* 1980;30:986.

9. Powers WJ, Martin WR, Herscovitch P, et al. Extracranial-intracranial bypass surgery: Hemodynamic and metabolic effects. *Neurology* 1984;34(9):1168-1174.

10. Grubb R, Powers W, Derdeyn C, et al. Increased oxygen extraction fraction in symptomatic patients with complete carotid artery occlusion predicts a subsequent increased incidence of ipsilateral ischemic stroke. Proceedings of the 66th Annual Meeting of the American Association of Neurological Surgeons. Philadelphia, PA: American Association of Neurological Surgeons, 1998.

11. Ausman JI, Diaz FG, Sadasivan B, et al. Giant intracranial aneurysm surgery: The role of microvascular reconstruction. *Surg Neurol* 1990;34(1):8-15.

12. Spetzler RF, Owen MP. Extracranial-intracranial arterial bypass to a single branch of the middle cerebral artery in the management of a traumatic aneurysm. *Neurosurgery* 1979;4(4):334-337.

13. McIvor NP, Willinsky RA, TerBrugge KG, et al. Validity of test occlusion studies prior to internal carotid artery sacrifice. *Head Neck* 1994;16(1):11-16.

14. Matsushima T, Inoue T, Suzuki SO, et al. Surgical treatment of moyamoya disease in pediatric patients--comparison between the results of indirect and direct revascularization procedures. *Neurosurgery* 1992;31(3):401-405.

15. Fukui M. Current state of study on moyamoya disease in Japan. *Surg Neurol* 1997;47(2):138-143.

16. Karasawa J, Touho H, Ohnishi H, et al. Long-term follow-up study after extracranial-intracranial bypass surgery for anterior circulation ischemia in childhood moyamoya disease. *J Neurosurg* 1992;77(1):84-89.

17. German WJ, Taffel M. Surgical production of collateral intracranial circulation. *Proc Soc Exp Biol Med* 1939;42:349-353.

18. Kredel FE. Collateral cerebral circulation by muscle graft. Technique of operation with report of 3 cases. *Southern Surgeon* 1942;10:235-244.

19. Beck CS, McKhann FC, Belnap WD. Revascularization of the brain through establishment of a cervical arteriovenous fistula. *J Pediatr* 1949;35:317-329.

20. Pool JL, Potts DG. Aneurysms and arteriovenous anomalies of the brain. New York: Hoeber, 1964.

21. Woringer E, Kunlin J. Anastomose entre la carotide preimitive et la carotide intra-cranienne ou la sylvienne par greffon selon la technique de la suture suspendue. *Neurochirurgie* 1963;9:181-188.

22. Jacobson JH, Suarez E. Microsurgery in anastomosis of small vessels. *Surg Forum* 1960;11:243-245.

23. Yasargil MG. Diagnosis and indications for operations in cerebrovascular oclusive disease. In Yasargil MG (ed): Microsurgery Applied To Neurosurgery. New York, London, Stuttgart,: Georg Thieme Verlag, Academic Press, 1969.

24. Lougheed WM, Marshall BM, Hunter M, et al. Common carotid to intracranial internal carotid bypass venous graft. Technical note. *J Neurosurg* 1971;34(1):114-118.

25. Tew JM. Reconstructive intracranial vascular surgery for prevention of stroke. *Clin Neurosurg* 1975;22:264-280.

26. Ausman JI, Diaz FG, Vacca DF, et al. Superficial temporal and occipital artery bypass pedicles to superior, anterior inferior, and posterior inferior cerebellar arteries for vertebrobasilar insufficiency. *J Neurosurg* 1990;72(4):554-558.

27. Sundt TMJ, Whisnant JP, Piepgras DG, et al. Intracranial bypass grafts for vertebral-basilar ischemia. *Mayo Clin Proc* 1978;53(1):12-18.

28. Awad I, Furlan AJ, Little JR. Changes in intracranial stenotic lesions after extracranial-intracranial bypass surgery. *J Neurosurg* 1984;60(4):771-776.

29. Chater N. Neurosurgical extracranial-intracranial bypass for stroke: With 400 cases. *Neurol Res* 1983;5(2):1-9.

30. Crowell RM, Olsson Y. Effect of extracranial-intracranial vascular bypass graft on experimental acute stroke in dogs. *J Neurosurg* 1973;38(1):26-31.

31. Day AL. Extracranial-intracranial bypass grafting in the surgical treatment of bacterial aneurysms: report of two cases. *Neurosurgery* 1981;9(5):583-588.

32. Hopkins LN, Grand W. Extracranial-intracranial arterial bypass in the treatment of aneurysms of the carotid and middle cerebral arteries. *Neurosurgery* 1979.

33. Kobayashi H, Hayashi M, Kawano H, et al. Evaluation of extracranial-to-intracranial bypass surgery using iodine 123 iodoamphetamine single-photon emission computed tomography. *Surg Neurol* 1991;35(6):436-440.

34. Ojemann R, Crowell R. Surgical Management of Cerebrovascular Disease. Baltimore: Williams & Wilkins, 1983.

35. Peerless SJ, Ferguson GG, Drake CG. Extracranial-intracranial (EC/IC) bypass in the treatment of giant intracranial aneurysms. *Neurosurg Rev* 1982;5(3):77-81.

36. Popp AJ, Chater N. Extracranial to intracranial vascular anastomosis for occlusive cerebrovascular disease: Experience in 110 patients. *Surgery* 1977;82(5):648-654.

37. Reinmuth OM. Intracranial bypass surgery for cerebral arterial disease and the responsibility of the practicing physician. *Stroke* 1979;10(3):344-347.

38. Samson DS, Boone S. Extracranial-intracranial (EC-IC) arterial bypass: Past performance and current concepts. *Neurosurgery* 1978;3(1):79-86.

39. Shibuya M, Suzuki Y, Takayasu M, et al. Effects of STA-MCA anastomosis for ischaemic oculopathy due to occlusion of the internal carotid artery. *Acta Neurochir Wien* 1990;103(1-2):71-75.

40. Sundt TMJ, Piepgras DG, Houser OW, et al. Interposition saphenous vein grafts for advanced occlusive disease and large aneurysms in the posterior circulation. *J Neurosurg* 1982;56(2):205-215.

41. Whisnant JP. Extracranial-intracranial arterial bypass. *Neurology* 1978;28(3):209-210.

42. Yasargil MG, Yonekawa Y. Results of microsurgical extra-intracranial arterial bypass in the treatment of cerebral ischemia. *Neurosurgery* 1977;1(1):22-24.

43. Moore WS. Surgery for Cerebrovascular Disease: Second Edition. Philadelphia, W.B. Saunders, 1996.

44. Mayberg MR. Extracranial occlusive disease of the carotid artery. (4th Edition ed.) Philadelphia, W.B. Saunders, 1996.

45. Yadav JS, Roubin GS, Iyer S, et al. Elective stenting of the extracranial carotid arteries. *Circulation* 1997;95(2):376-381.

46. Storey GS, Marks MP, Dake M, et al. Vertebral artery stenting following percutaneous transluminal angioplasty. Technical note. *J Neurosurg* 1996;84(5):883-887.

47. Crawley F, Clifton A, Markus H, Brown MM. Delayed improvement in carotid artery diameter after carotid angioplasty. *Stroke* 1997;28(3):574-579.

48. Rostomily RC, Mayberg MR, Eskridge J, et al. Resolution of petrous internal carotid artery stenosis after transluminal angioplasty. *J Neurosurg* 1992;76:520-523.

49. Spetzler R, Chater N. Occipital artery-middle cerebral anastomosis for cerebral artery occlusive disease. *Surg Neurol* 1974;2:235-238.

50. Sundt TMJ, Whisnant JP, Piepgras DG, et al. Intracranial bypass grafts for vertebral-basilar ischemia. *Mayo Clin Proc* 1978;53(1):12-18.

51. Hopkins LN, Bundy JL, Castellani D. Extracranial-intracranial arterial bypass and basilar artery ligation in the treatment of giant basilar artery aneurysms. *Neurosurgery* 1983;13(2):189-194.

52. Morgan MK, Sekhon LH. Extracranial-intracranial saphenous vein bypass for carotid or vertebral artery dissections: A report of six cases. *J Neurosurg* 1994;80(2):237-246.

53. Schmidt JH, Witsberger TA. Treatment of giant intracranial aneurysm with carotid ligation, saphenous vein bypass graft. *W V J Med* 1992:346-347.

54. Spetzler RF, Rhodes RS, Roski RA, et al. Subclavian to middle cerebral artery saphenous vein bypass graft. *J Neurosurg* 1980;53(4):465-469.

55. Zarins CK, DelBeccaro EJ, Johns L, et al. Increased cerebral blood flow after external carotid artery revascularization. *Surgery* 1981;89(6):730-734.

56. Moeller E. Cervical common carotid to supraclinoid intracranial internal carotid artery saphenous vein bypass. *J Neurosurg Nurs* 1974;6(2):132-136.

57. Hadeishi H, Yasui N, Okamoto Y. Extracranial-intracranial high-flow bypass using the radial artery between the vertebral and middle cerebral arteries. Technical note. *J Neurosurg* 1996;85(5):976-979.

58. Okada Y, Shima T, Nishida M, et al. Retroauricular subcutaneous Dacron tunnel for extracranial-intracranial autologous vein bypass graft. Technical note. *J Neurosurg* 1994;81(5):800-802.

59. Carter LP, Crowell RM, Sonntag VK, et al. Cortical blood flow during extracranial-intracranial bypass surgery. *Stroke* 1984;15(5):836-9.

60. Schmiedek P, Gratzl O, Steinhoff H. Regional blood flow measurement in extra-intracranial anastomoses for cerebral ischemia. Methodologic aspects. *Acta Radiol Suppl Stockh* 1976;347:247-251.

61. Samson DS, Hodosh RM, Clark WK. Microsurgical treatment of transient cerebral ischemia. Preliminary results in 50 patients. *JAMA* 1979;241(4):376-378.

62. Barnett DW, Barrow DL, Joseph GJ. Combined extracranial-intracranial bypass and intraoperative balloon occlusion for the treatment of intracavernous and proximal carotid artery aneurysms. *Neurosurgery* 1994;35(1):92-97.

63. Standard SC, Ahuja A, Guterman LR, et al. Balloon test occlusion of the internal carotid artery with hypotensive challenge. *Am J Neuroradiol* 1995;16(7):1453-1458.

64. Walker BS, Mathews D, Batjer H, et al. Detection of cerebral hypoperfusion during trial carotid occlusion with reversal following extracranial-intracranial bypass prior to permanent occlusion. *Clin Nucl Med* 1994;19(6): 499-503.

65. Yonas H, Kaufmann A. Combined extracranial-intracranial bypass and intraoperative balloon occlusion for the treatment of intracavernous and proximal carotid artery aneurysms [letter; comment]. *Neurosurgery* 1995;36(6):1234.

66. Regli L, Piepgras DG, Hansen KK. Late patency of long saphenous vein bypass grafts to the anterior and posterior cerebral circulation. *J Neurosurg* 1995;83(5):806-811.

67. Tenjin H, Ueda S. Multiple EDAS (encephalo-duro-arterio-synangiosis). *Childs Nerv Syst* 1997;13(4):220-224.

68. George BD, Neville BG, Lumley JS. Transcranial revascularisation in childhood and adolescence. *Dev Med Child Neurol* 1993;35(8):675-682.

69. Havlik RJ, Fried I, Chyatte D, et al. Encephalo-omental synangiosis in the management of moyamoya disease. *Surgery* 1992;111(2):156-162.

70. Kuroda S, Houkin K, Kamiyama H, et al. Regional cerebral hemodynamics in childhood moyamoya disease. *Childs Nerv Syst* 1995;11(10):584-590.

71. D'Alise MD, Vardiman AB, Kopitnik TAJ, et al. External carotid-to-middle cerebral bypass in the treatment of complex internal carotid injury. *J Trauma* 1996;40(3):452-455.

72. Gewertz BL, Samson DS, Ditmore QM, et al. Management of penetrating injuries of the internal carotid artery at the base of the skull utilizing extracranial-intracranial bypass. *J Trauma* 1980;20(5):365-369.

73. Hunt JL, Snyder WH. Late false aneurysm of the carotid artery: repair with extra-intracranial arterial bypass. *J Trauma* 1979;19(3):198-200.

74. Pozzati E, Giuliani G, Acciarri N, et al. Long-term follow-up of occlusive cervical carotid dissection. *Stroke* 1990;21(4):528-531.

75. Heros RC, Sekhar LN. Diagnostic and therapeutic alternatives in patients with symptomatic "carotid occlusion" referred for extracranial-intracranial bypass surgery. *J Neurosurg* 1981;54(6):790-796.

76. Drake CG, Peerless SJ, Ferguson GG. Hunterian proximal arterial occlusion for giant aneurysms of the carotid circulation. *J Neurosurg* 1994;81(5): 656-665.

77. Heros RC, Nelson PB, Ojemann RG, et al. Large and giant paraclinoid aneurysms: Surgical techniques, complications, and results. *Neurosurgery* 1983;12(2):153-163.

78. Larson JJ, Tew JMJ, Tomsick TA, et al. Treatment of aneurysms of the internal carotid artery by intravascular balloon occlusion: Long-term follow-up of 58 patients. *Neurosurgery* 1995;36(1):26-30.

79. Spetzler RF, Roski RA, Schuster H, et al. The role of EC-IC in the treatment of giant intracranial aneurysms. *Neurol Res* 1980;2(3-4):345-359.

80. Moritake K, Handa H, Yamashita J, et al. STA-MCA anastomosis in patients with skull base tumours involving the internal carotid artery--Haemodynamic assessment by ultrasonic Doppler flowmeter. *Acta Neurochir Wien* 1984;72(1-2):95-110.

81. Ueda S, Fujitsu K, Inomori S, et al. Thrombotic occlusion of the middle cerebral artery. *Stroke* 1992;23(12):1761-1766.

82. Yoshimoto Y, Kwak S. Superficial temporal artery--middle cerebral artery anastomosis for acute cerebral ischemia: The effect of small augmentation of blood flow. *Acta Neurochir Wien* 1995;137(3-4):128-137.

83. Kawaguchi S, Sakaki T, Kamada K, et al. Effects of superficial temporal to middle cerebral artery bypass for ischaemic retinopathy due to internal carotid artery occlusion/stenosis. *Acta Neurochir Wien* 1994;129(3-4):166-170.

84. Lawner PM, Simeone FA. Treatment of intraoperative middle cerebral artery occlusion with pentobarbital and extracranial-intracranial bypass. Case report. *J Neurosurg* 1979;51(5):710-712.

85. Sundt TMJ, Siekert RG, Piepgras DG, et al. Bypass surgery for vascular disease of the carotid system. *Mayo Clin Proc* 1976;51(11):677-692.

86. Samson DS, Neuwelt EA, Beyer CW, et al. Failure of extracranial-intracranial arterial bypass in acute middle cerebral artery occlusion: Case report. *Neurosurgery* 1980;6(2):185-188.

87. Cote R, Barnett HJ, Taylor DW. Internal carotid occlusion: A prospective study. *Stroke* 1983;14(6):898-902.

88. Spetzler RF, Schuster H, Roski RA. Elective extracranial-intracranial arterial bypass in the treatment of inoperable giant aneurysms of the internal carotid artery. *J Neurosurg* 1980;53(1):22-27.

89. Lawner PM, Laurent JP, Simeone FA, et al. Effect of extracranial-intracranial bypass and pentobarbital on acute stroke in dogs. *J Neurosurg* 1982;56(1):92-96.

90. Tatemichi TK, Desmond DW, Prohovnik I, et al. Dementia associated with bilateral carotid occlusions: Neuropsychological and haemodynamic course after extracranial to intracranial bypass surgery. *J Neurol Neurosurg Psychiatry* 1995;58(5):633-636.

91. Tsuda Y, Yamada K, Hayakawa T, et al. Cortical blood flow and cognition after extracranial-intracranial bypass in a patient with severe carotid occlusive lesions. A three-year follow-up study. *Acta Neurochir Wien* 1994;129(3-4):198-204.

92. Houkin K, Kamiyama H, Takahashi A, et al. Combined revascularization surgery for childhood moyamoya disease: STA-MCA and encephalo-duro-arterio-myo-synangiosis. *Childs Nerv Syst* 1997;13(1):24-29.

93. Kobayashi H, Hayashi M, Handa Y, et al. EC-IC bypass for adult patients with moyamoya disease. Neurol Res 1991;13(2):113-116.

94. Suzuki Y, Negoro M, Shibuya M, et al. Surgical treatment for pediatric moyamoya disease: Use of the superficial temporal artery for both areas supplied by the anterior and middle cerebral arteries. *Neurosurgery* 1997;40(2):324-329.

95. Touho H, Karasawa J, Shishido H, et al. Hemodynamic evaluation in patients with superficial temporal artery-middle cerebral artery anastomosis--stable xenon CT-CBF study and acetazolamide. *Neurol Med Chir Tokyo* 1990;30(13):1003-1010.

96. Holzschuh M, Brawanski A, Ullrich W, et al. Cerebral blood flow and cerebrovascular reserve 5 years after EC-IC bypass. *Neurosurg Rev* 1991;14(4):275-278.

97. Ishikawa T, Houkin K, Abe H, et al. Cerebral haemodynamics and long-term prognosis after extracranial-intracranial bypass surgery. *J Neurol Neurosurg Psychiatry* 1995;59(6):625-628.

98. Touho H, Karasawa J, Shishido H, et al. Hemodynamic evaluation before and after the STA-MCA anastomosis--with special reference to measurement of regional transit time with intra-arterial digital subtraction angiography. *Neurol Med Chir Tokyo* 1990;30(9):663-669.

99. Yamashita T, Kashiwagi S, Nakano S, et al. The effect of EC-IC bypass surgery on resting cerebral blood flow and cerebrovascular reserve capacity studied with stable XE-CT and acetazolamide test. *Neuroradiology* 1991;33(3):217-222.

Chapter 4

Extracranial-Intracranial Surgery for Patients with Proven Hemodynamic Compromise:
Is There Sufficient Evidence for a Second-Phase EC/IC Trial?

Henry J.M. Barnett, MD

Introduction

The concept of adding new blood to a brain with compromised circulation from occluded arteries appeared to be a rational addition to stroke prevention measures and even to stroke treatment. The perfection of techniques of microvascular surgery stimulated pioneering neurosurgeons to make preliminary observations. The results were sufficiently encouraging that a randomized international trial was launched in 1977 and reported in 1985.[1] To the disappointment of the investigators, the study was negative. For some of the investigators, and many surgeons who had mastered the difficult technique, the disappointment was tinged with annoyance. Some were angry.[2-5] Reflecting upon the outbursts which appeared on public platforms, in Letters to Editors and even in Editorials, the public outcry comes to mind which erupted when the British public felt that Lord Clive had mishandled his tenure as Viceroy of India in England's colonial days. Macaulay described "a tempest of execration and derision alike to the outbreak of public feeling against the Puritans at the time of the Restoration.[6] Methodists and libertines, philosophers, and buffoons were for once on the same

From: Choi D, Dacey RG, Hsu CY, Powers WJ. *Cerebrovascular Disease: Momentum at the End of the Second Millennium.* Armonk, NY: Futura Publishing Company, Inc., © 2002.

side." Others took a more positive attitude and diligently persisted with studies designed to identify patients with evidence of hemodynamic insufficiency who might form a subgroup in which surgical results might prove beneficial. This work, pursued in several centers, but most encouragingly in St. Louis, has given rise to this present segment of the Princeton Conference.[7]

Brief Resumé of the Extracranial/ Intracranial Bypass Trial

Because the question is being raised about the possible need for another extracranial-intracranial (EC/IC) trial, a brief resumé of the first trial may help to put things in perspective.

The primary question posed was: "Does STA-MCA [superficial temporal artery-middle cerebral artery] anastomosis, despite perioperative risk of stroke and death, reduce the rate of subsequent stroke and stroke-related death in the patients studied?" The answer which derived from 1,377 patients randomized in 71 centers established clearly that fatal and non-fatal strokes occurred earlier and more frequently in patients randomized to EC/IC bypass.[1]

The procedure carried a 12.2% perioperative rate of fatal and non-fatal strokes. In the intention-to-treat analysis, out of 663 patients assigned to surgical treatment, 30 (4.5%) had disabling stroke, including fatal events in 1.1%. Because 10 strokes occurred between randomization and surgery, and these patients were not subjected to bypass, an efficacy analysis was conducted; the disabling stroke rate was found to be 2.5% plus the 0.6% who experienced fatal stroke. The conclusion must be that the procedure did not fail because of surgical incompetence. These morbidity and mortality figures were comparable or superior to the large published uncontrolled case-series.

Predetermined, clinically interesting subgroups, as listed in Table 1, were examined and benefit was not present in any of them. Patients with continuing symptoms despite known occlusion of the carotid artery, with severe (> 70%) MCA stenosis, and with bilateral carotid occlusions were found to have the worst prognosis. The experience of carotid endarterectomy in the North American Symptomatic Carotid Endarterectomy Trial (NASCET) was that the patients with the greatest risk for stroke benefited most from endarterectomy. This increased benefit from surgical intervention in the highest risk patients was not realized with bypass anastomosis.[8] Of 808 patients (30%) in the EC/ IC trial with unilateral internal carotid artery (ICA) occlusion followed for an average of 58 months, 244 experienced strokes both fatal and

Table 1.

Fatal and Nonfatal Stroke Among Clinically Interesting Subgroups.*

Patients†	Medical Group			Surgical Group			Mantel-Haenszel Chi-Square
	No.	Observed	Expected *number of patients*	No.	Observed	Expected	
All patients	714	205	218.3	663	205	191.7	1.72
Excluding those with ICA occlusion, no symptoms‡	438	133	148.0	418	148	133.0	3.23
ICA occlusion, no symptoms‡	276	72	69.9	245	57	59.1	0.13
ICA occlusion, symptoms§	147	51	61.7	140	64	53.3	4.04
ICA stenosis (≥70%)	72	26	27.1	77	29	27.9	0.10
MCA stenosis (≥70%)	59	14	20.5	50	22	15.5	4.74
Bilateral carotid occlusion	43	17	17.4	31	14	13.6	0.02
MCA occlusion	79	18	16.9	80	16	17.1	0.15
First TIA within 3 mo. of entry and total TIAs >3	87	27	31.5	109	41	36.5	1.32

*Values listed under the heading "Observed" indicate the observed number of patients in each treatment group who had a stroke. Those listed under "Expected" indicate the number of patients in each treatment group who would be expected to have a stroke if surgery had no effect, taking into account differences in sample size and duration of follow-up.
† ICA denotes internal carotid artery, MCA middle cerebral artery, and TIA transient ischemic attack.
‡ No symptoms were experienced between angiographic demonstration of the occlusion and randomization.
§ Symptoms were experienced between angiographic demonstration of the occlusion and randomization.
This table has been reproduced with permission from the *New England Journal of Medicine.*[1]

nonfatal. This gives an annual risk of stroke of 6%. No benefit from EC/IC surgery was found.

Compared to patients with a low vascular risk profile, a high risk profile added to the seriousness of the outlook for patients in the individual radiological sub-groups (Figures 1A and 1B). However, benefit was not detectable in either of these risk profile groupings.

Frequent (more than 6) transient ischemic attacks (TIAs) in the 90 days before by-pass were reported in 266 patients. Randomization allotted 128 of these patients to medical and 138 to bypass surgery. The survival analyses were identical in the two groups (chi-square 0.00). Recentness of events produced results slightly in favor of medical therapy, both for the 741 patients whose last event was within 30 days, and for the 636 patients whose last event occurred beyond 30 days but prior to 90 days.

Bilateral carotid occlusion has been of special interest because of the assumption that it can be perceived as more likely to impair cerebral hemodynamics by denying to the brain the use of potentially compensatory channels. The EC/IC Study included and reported upon 74 patients with this finding.[9] As an indication of the effectiveness of the Circle of Willis, it was noted at the time of entry into the trial that 40% of these patients were still employed and without significant disability. Only ten of them had symptoms which might have been considered at the bedside to have a hemodynamic basis for the recurrent symptoms. Had the study not included a control group it would have been easy to attribute the cessation of these events to the procedure because EC/IC surgery was performed in five patients and their symptoms immediately ceased. However, four of the five assigned to medical therapy also stopped having the events when questioned at the time of their second follow-up; one had died of a non-cerebral cause. It was possible to conclude that bilateral occlusion of the carotid arteries was compatible with useful survival but not to establish that EC/IC anastomosis improved upon the outlook for these patients.

Prospective Follow-Up of Patients with Unilateral ICA Occlusion

As well as the patients in the EC/IC Trial, two other prospective studies of therapy under the author's direction have afforded the opportunity to determine the outlook for patients with single ICA occlusions. In the Canadian Aspirin Trial, 47 patients with ICA occlusion were followed by participating neurologists for an average of 3 years.[10] Eleven strokes occurred (23%) of which 7 were ipsilateral (15%). The annual ipsilateral stroke rate was 5%. In the 2,887 patients studied in

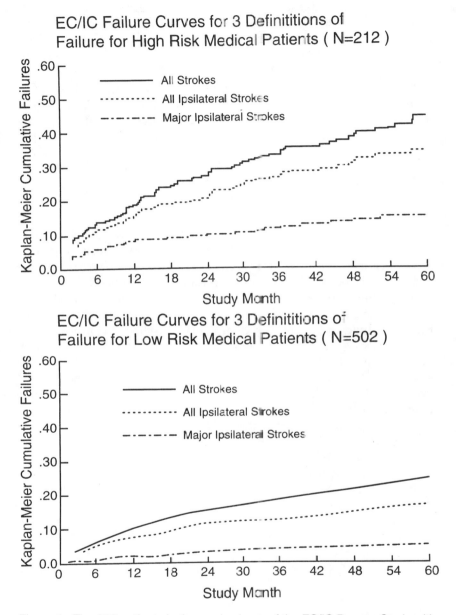

Figure 1. The 212 patients in the medical arm of the EC/IC Bypass Study with a high vascular risk profile (A) experienced more outcome events over time in 3 definitions of failure than did the 502 patients (B) with lower vascular risk profiles (unpublished data from EC/IC Bypass Study).

NASCET, 155 were found at the time of randomization to have occlusion of the artery contralateral to the randomized lesion (NASCET – unpublished data 1998). Ischemic events appropriate to the occlusion occurred 12 times, but 5 of these were at the time of surgery. Thus 7 occurred spontaneously for an annual ipsilateral stroke rate of 0.9%. Of these 7, only one retained a Rankin score at or above 3. The others improved to a better level of function. In 3 of the 12, a cardiac source was entertained as the probable cause of the stroke.

Putative Causes of Symptoms with ICA Occlusion

Symptoms of a type that can reasonably be assigned to poor perfusion (so-called "misery perfusion") occasionally were recognized clinically in patients with bilateral carotid occlusion. These phenomena are noted less frequently in patients with unilateral occlusion. When they occur in either situation, they may be exercise-induced, orthostatically-induced, and even light-induced, resulting in episodes of amaurosis-fugax. A clinical phenomenon of aggravated ischemic symptoms was observed by Caplan and Sergay, in patients in the early post-infarction period who were subjected prematurely to the erect position in a bedside chair.[11] Presumably, the auto-regulation interfered with by the cerebral infarction had not yet become re-established in an adequate manner.

Failure of cerebral circulatory mechanisms such as seen in vasovagal syncope, serious gastro-intestinal bleeding, iatrogenic hypotension and serious heart block, will lead to hemodynamic insufficiency. It may be aggravated and be focal instead of diffuse in the presence of ICA occlusion. The requirement for these patients is correction of the central mechanism, not the restoration of carotid blood flow.

No good figures are available but at the present time it is reasonable to state that the majority of the frequent instances of focal ischemia in the presence of ICA occlusion, are of thrombogenic origin. Emboli from the distal "white-tail" of a thrombus in an occluded artery, emboli from a diseased companion external carotid artery, emboli from the stump of the carotid artery, probably emboli from the recently-described and now identifiable symptomatic aortic arch ulcerative atheroma, or coincidental cardiac embologenic conditions constitute the common potential reasons for the ischemia. Two examples have been brought to the author's attention of large white platelet emboli passing through MCA cortical branches at craniotomy to effect bypass in patients with ICA occlusion. One is illustrated here (Figure 2) and one has been previously published.[12]

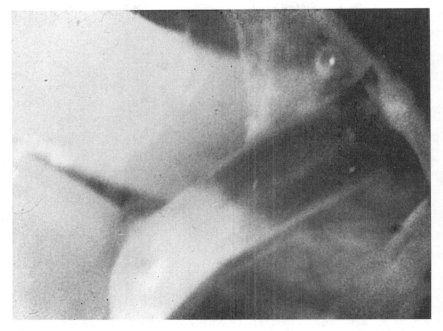

Figure 2. A cortical branch of the middle cerebral artery exposed during a middle cerebral artery – superficial temporary artery anastomosis. The left hand portion of the artery is filled with white (platelet-fibrin) thrombo-emobolic material. The patient had an ipsilateral internal carotid artery occlusion. *Reproduced with permission of Dr. N. Hopkins.*

Why Did the EC/IC Trial
Fail to Show Benefit?

Failure was not due to participation in the trial of incompetent surgeons. A low disabling and fatal stroke rate and an achievement of a 96% patency rate in the postoperative angiograms attest to this. It was not because of inadequate anastomoses of the type performed during the trial. The stroke-free survival was compared in 200 patients with the worst postoperative angiograms and in the 225 with the best angiograms. Each was measured for the size of anastomosing vessels, branches were counted and each patient assigned a multifactorial score. No modern perfusion studies were done. Patients with the most luxuriant anastomoses experienced worse outlooks than did those with evidence of poor anastomoses (Figure 3).

Failure of the EC/IC procedure may best be explained by the presumption that, in most instances, the original and recurrent ischemic events were due to thromboembolism and not to hemodynamic failure. Because of the difficulty posed by the exactness with which this distinc-

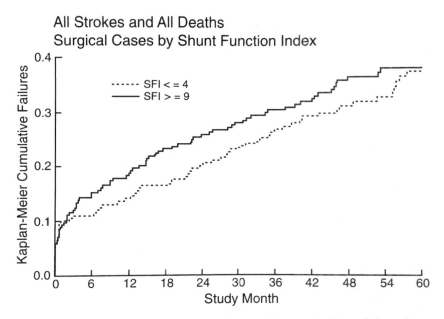

Figure 3. An inverse correlation was observed for surgical benefit in patients who had a well-defined anastomosis of generous size and multiple cortical branches (a high "shunt function index") compared to those who had more meager angiographic evidence of an adequate anastomosis.

tion can be made in individual patients, it has to be conceded that this is only informed speculation. An interesting observation was made by J.M. Orgogozo exploring the EC/IC data-base: five instances were encountered in which a good anastomosis was observed in subsequent angiograms to be obstructed by a lesion with features of embolic obstruction. These patients came to attention in a study of carotid stumps in angiograms exhibiting what were interpreted as thrombi in the stumps (Figures 4A and 4B). (Orgogozo, J.M., unpublished EC/IC Study data, 1986)

Should there be Another EC/IC Bypass Study?

Occasional uncontrolled case-series have appeared claiming benefit for standard or new methods of EC/IC anastomosis. Frequently quoted in this context is a report by McCormick et al. from Ausman's department.[13] Seventeen patients were stated to have a poorly-defined entity called "disabling transient ischemic attacks," and were subjected to five different types of anastomoses. Perioperative stroke, periopera-

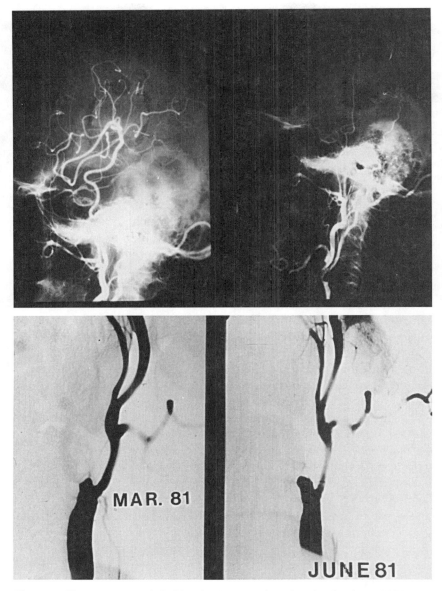

Figure 4. The anastomosis in March 1981 was luxuriant but by June 1981 was obstructed and no longer functioning (A). The stump of the internal carotid artery in March 1981 had a concave distal end which had become longer and rounder by June 1981 (B). The assumption is reasonable that thrombus had been present in the top of the stump in March and had passed into the external carotid artery by June 1981, abruptly obstructing the anastomosis.

tive death, failure to achieve a patent anastomosis or failure to prevent recurrent symptoms were reported in 9 of the 17 patients. Despite this 52% failure rate, the authors concluded that "disabling TIA responds to surgical revascularization and that surgery in an effective therapeutic alternative." They went on to state that "the disabled condition of these patients represents an ethical barrier to a natural history study." The writer of this review disagrees and in the absence of controls shown to have a worse outlook, regards this claim with skepticism.

There are much more compelling reasons for contemplating a second EC/IC Bypass Study. There is much better data available on measurements of hemodynamic compromise. Using these measures as surrogate outcomes raises hopes that the clinical responses may parallel these observations.[14] Possibly new surgical techniques may deliver larger volumes of blood.[15] If the new study can be justified and is to be done, it cannot be delayed too long because many of the large cadre of surgeons who became skilled at this procedure have not been practicing this skill for a decade.

The biggest concern is to identify how many patients who are threatening stroke in our communities have hemodynamic compromise. Can they be identified if positron-emission tomography (PET) scans are not available? The correct patients for the study will be those who have the marked hemodynamic compromise associated with increased oxygen extraction fraction in the PET scan. They must be submitted to a well-defined and uniform operative procedure carried out with an acceptable perioperative complication rate and a high success rate in effecting patency. The sample-size must be adequate to be reasonably certain of answering the question. The centers with the appropriate skills need to be fully committed and to follow a scrupulously defined methodology. An energetic committed and relentless leadership is a sine qua non. Built into such a trial must be careful gathering of data about cost-effectiveness and quality of life benefits.

The sample size, dependent on the perceived number of outcomes for a population of patients with ICA occlusion and proven hemodynamic compromise, and counting upon a reasonable surgical skill, will vary between 200 to 2200 patients divided into medical and surgical cohorts (Table 2). As is often the case in this situation the truth may lie in the middle range. If the patients with a hemodynamic compromise have a stroke risk at the highest levels found with ICA occlusion, and the surgeons are of exceptional competence, the lower figure for the sample size may prove to be adequate to give a credible result. It may be necessary to recalculate the sample-size based on the first year or two of trial experience, and to use the data from the first part of the study as an internal pilot study.

Table 2.

Sample Size: Medical vs. EC/IC for ICA Occlusion.

Risk Ipsilateral Stroke at 5 yrs Medical	EC/IC	RRR	Total Study Size
15%	9%	40%	920
25%	9%	64%	172
15%	11%	27%	2218
25%	11%	56%	236

80% Power at 5% Significance Level
Assumptions: Ipsilateral Stroke Risk Medical = 3% or 5% per year
Ipsilateral Stroke Risk Surgical = 4% or 6% perioperative + per year
Note: A higher stroke risk for patients with proven hemodynamic compromise (increased Oxygen Extraction Fraction by Pet scanning or its equivalent) will reduce the sample-size provided the surgical risk stays the same.

Conclusion

A case can be made for a rigorously-conducted new trial. Only patients with ICA occlusion proven to have hemodynamic compromise should be studied. Prevention of stroke should be the goal. It will be reasonable to conduct such a trial confined to centers with PET scans. It will not be reasonable, even if efficacy can be shown, to expect that the procedure will be efficacious if a less demanding technology than PET scanning is not developed and put into use if the rigorous study shows benefit. Then it will be possible to generalize the results of the trial. It will be wrong to extrapolate the results of this study to patients without proven perfusion deficiency, and probably in the long run there will be no more than a small number of suitable candidates detectable in any stroke center. Cost-effectiveness, including quality of life, will need to be carefully scrutinized.

References

1. The EC/IC Bypass Study Group. Failure of extracranial-intracranial arterial bypas to reduce the risk of ischemic stroke. Results of an international randomized trial. *N Engl J Med* 1985;313:1191-1200.
2. Sundt TM Jr. Was the international randomized trial of extracranial-intracranial arterial bypass representative of the population at risk? *N Engl J Med* 1987;316(13):814-816.
3. Ausman JI, Diaz FG. Critique of the extracranial-intracranial bypass study. *Surg Neurol* 1986;26:218-221.
4. Day AL, Rhoton AL, Little JR. The extracranial-intracranial bypass study. *Surg Neurol* 1986;26:222-226.

5. Relman AS. The extracranial-intracranial arterial bypass study. What have we learned? *N Engl J Med* 1987;316(13):809-810.

6. Macaulay L. "Lord Clive." In Gross J (ed): The Oxford Book of Essays. Oxford, UK: Oxford University Press, 1991:149-163

7. Grubb R, Derdeyn C, Fritsch S, et al. Cerebral hemodynamics and stroke risk. Presentation at the 21st Princeton Conference on Cerebrovascular Disease: Momentum at the End of the Millennium, Friday May 8, 1998.

8. North American Symptomatic Carotid Endarterectomy Trial Collaborators. Beneficial effect of carotid endarterectomy in symptomatic patients with high-grade stenosis. *N Engl J Med* 1991;325:445-453.

9. Wade JPH, Wong W, Barnett HJM, et al. Bilateral occlusion of the internal carotid arteries. *Brain* 1987;110:667-682.

10. Coté R, Barnett HJM, Taylor DW. Internal carotid occlusion: A prospective study. *Stroke* 1983;14:898-902.

11. Caplan LR, Sergay S. Positional cerebral ischaemia. *J Neurol Neurosurg Psychiatry* 1976;39:385-391.

12. Barnett HJM, Eliasziw M, Meldrum HE. Drugs and surgery in the prevention of ischemic stroke. *N Engl J Med* 1995;332:238-248.

13. McCormick PW, Tomecek FJ, McKinney J, et al. Disabling cerebral transient ischemic attacks. *J Neurosurg* 1991;75:891-901.

14. Barnett HJM. Hemodynamic cerebral ischemia. An appeal for systematic data gathering prior to a new EC/IC trial. *Stroke* 1997;28:1857-1860.

15. Klijn CJM, Kappelle LJ, Tulleken CAF, et al. Symptomatic carotid artery occlusion. A reappraisal of hemodynamic factors. *Stroke* 1997;28:2084-2093.

Mediators and Modulators of Ischemic Injury: Hot Topics

Chapter 5

Poly(ADP-ribose) Polymerase in Ischemia-Reperfusion Injury

Valina L. Dawson, PhD and
Ted M. Dawson, MD, PhD

Introduction

Ischemic injury can trigger deoxyribonucleic acid (DNA) strand damage and breakage. In part, this DNA damage is mediated by peroxynitrite, a cytotoxin formed by the reaction of nitric oxide (NO) with superoxide anion. DNA knicks and breaks induce rapid activation of the nuclear enzyme, poly(ADP-ribose) polymerase (PARP). PARP catalyzes the transfer of adenosine diphosphate (ADP) ribose from nicotinamide adenine dinucleotide (NAD) to itself and other nuclear proteins. Under conditions of severe injury, activation of PARP can lead to dramatic decreases in intracellular NAD. A decrease in NAD will slow the rate of glycolysis, electron transport and subsequently ATP formation. For every mol of NAD consumed, four free energy equivalents of ATP are required to regenerate cellular concentrations of NAD. In the setting of peroxynitrite formation mitochondrial respiratory enzymes (complex I in particular) are damaged, further inhibiting ATP formation and subsequent NAD regeneration. Ischemic injury can lead to excessive activation of PARP and energy impairment leading to cell death. Inhibition of PARP pharmacologically or genetic knockout of PARP confers dramatic protection against ischemic and excitotoxic injury.

From: Choi D, Dacey RG, Hsu CY, Powers WJ. *Cerebrovascular Disease: Momentum at the End of the Second Millennium.* Armonk, NY: Futura Publishing Company, Inc., © 2002.

ADP-ribosylation

ADP-ribosylation of proteins is a signaling mechanism which can elicit a wide variety of biologic responses. ADP-ribosylation reactions were initially discovered in an attempt to understand how bacterial toxins cause disease.[1] Diphtheria toxin inhibits mammalian protein synthesis through inhibition of elongation factor-2 by ADP-ribosylation.[2] Subsequently, cholera toxin and pertussis toxin were also identified as ADP-ribosylating toxins with G-proteins as their substrate. Although ribosylation events induced by bacterial toxins have been an area of intense investigation for over 30 years, other ribosylation signaling pathways have also been described. Cyclization of the ADP-ribose yields cyclic ADP-ribose, a ligand for the ryanodine receptor.[3] Cyclic ADP-ribose is important in the regulation of intracellular calcium levels in many cells including neurons.[4-6] Nitric oxide may contribute to regulation of intracellular calcium levels by activating GTP cyclase which in turn activates ribosocyclase resulting in increased cyclic ADP-ribose and subsequent release of intracellular calcium via the ryanodine receptor.[7,8] Nitric oxide may also signal through ADP-ribosylation via mono-ADP-ribosylation of the various proteins.[9-11] Recently a family of arginine mono-ADP-ribosyl transferases has been cloned and expression localized to muscle, lymphatic tissues, testis, bone marrow, and erythroblasts. Intriguingly, these enzymes are predicted to be secretory or membrane proteins suggesting that mono-ADP-ribosyl transferases might be part of the signaling mechanism for cell attachment or cell-cell contact.[12,13]

In addition to cyclic ADP-ribose and mono-ADP-ribosylation reactions, poly-ADP-ribosylation is elicited by the enzyme poly(ADP-ribose) polymerase (EC2.4.2.30) (PARP).[14,15] PARP is also termed poly(-ADP-ribose) synthetase (PARS) or poly(ADP-ribose) transferase (pADPRT). PARP is a nuclear protein with a complex enzymology.[16-18] PARP appears to be responsible for catalyzing essentially three different chemical reactions.[19] First, it adds an ADP-ribose residue from NAD to an accessor amino acid. Second, it adds sucessive additional ADP-ribose residues to the 2-hydroxyl of the adenine ribose. Third, it can catalyze branching by adding an ADP-ribose residue to the 2-hydroxyl of the nicotinamide ribose. All of these reactions appear to be mediated by the one protein.[19] In fact, PARP is the only known enzyme which catalyzes poly-ADP-ribosylation. PARP is a large, 116 kilodalton (Kd) protein with three main functional domains. The end terminal domain contains the nuclear localization signal, two unusual zinc finger structures and a DNA binding domain. The zinc fingers are essential for DNA binding and sensing of single and double strand knicks and breaks. The mid portion of the enzyme contains the auto-modification site in which PARP catalyzes self-ADP-ribosylation.[20] The C-terminal fragment binds NAD and mediates the enzymatic activity of PARP.[16-18] While the C-terminal fragment alone can carry out all the enzymatic activities of PARP, it has only 0.2% of the activity of the complete protein.[17] From deletion and mutation studies it appears that the DNA binding domains and the zinc fingers not only recognize the DNA knicks and breaks but also somehow activate the enzyme perhaps through a conformational change in the protein which increases its kinetic abilities.[21]

PARP in DNA Repair

The exact role of PARP in DNA repair is still under investigation. PARP is activated by free DNA ends, either single strand or double strand breaks.[16,18] Studies with pharmacologic inhibitors have demonstrated that cytotoxicity induced by DNA damage from ultraviolet irradiation or chemical agents increased in the presence of PARP inhibitors indicating a critical role for PARP in the cellular response to DNA damage.[22] However, other studies have suggested a suicide role for PARP and observe cytoprotection with PARP inhibitors following DNA damage.[23,24] A new role for PARP has been proposed. It is suggested local poly(ADP-ribose) synthesis in the vicinity of a DNA strand breaks results in negative charge repulsion (Figure 1), and this may function to prevent biologically inappropriate homologous recombination events within tandem repeat DNA sequences.[25,26] This implicates PARP in maintaining genomic stability. This hypothesis would indicate that PARP participates in DNA repair but is not a necessary component of the basic process of DNA repair. PARP then, is important in correct and efficient DNA repair. Its role in cytotoxicity is likely dependent on the type of insult, severity of insult and the cell-type under stress.

The physiologic outcome of poly-ADP-ribosylation in PARP activation is still under investigation. Poly-ADP-ribosylation has been implicated in the regulation of gene expression and gene amplification, cell differentiation, malignant transformation, mitosis as well as necrotic and apoptotic death.[1,20] To place this wide variety of biologic activities in context, it is important to note that many of these results were obtained using non-specific, pharmacologic inhibitors of PARP at relatively high concentrations. Additionally, many of these observations are stimulus and cell-type dependent and are not easily replicated in different cell models or with different stimuli. The recent generation of PARP null mice provides an important opportunity to understand

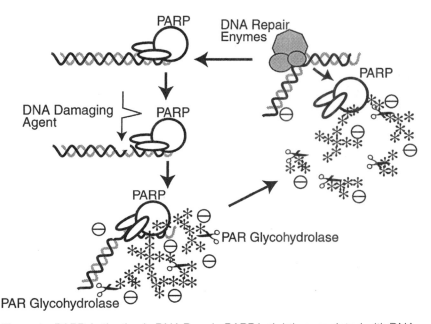

Figure 1. PARP Activation in DNA Repair. PARP is tightly associated with DNA. Upon damage to DNA resulting in either single strand or double strand breaks, PARP senses the free DNA ends and is activated to synthesize and attach polymers of ADP-ribose to nuclear proteins, including PARP itself. This local poly(ADP-ribose) (PAR) synthesis in the vicinity of a DNA strand breaks results in negative charge repulsion, which may function to prevent biologically inappropriate homologous recombination events within tandem repeat DNA sequences. At the same time PARP is activated, PAR glycohydrolase is activated to degrade the polymers. PAR glycohydrolase clips the polymer first into large pieces and over time degrades the polymer into smaller units. Once ribosylated, PARP dissociates from the DNA allowing DNA repair enzymes access to the damaged DNA. This model suggests that PARP is necessary for efficient and accurate DNA repair but that it is not a necessary component of the basic process of DNA repair.

the physiologic role of PARP.[27] Cells from PARP null animals have normal DNA repair, albeit slower, in response to radiation injury[28] and undergo normal apoptosis in response to treatment with anti-Fas, tumor neurosis factor alpha, gamma- irradiation, and dexamethasone, indicating (as others have observed[29]) that PARP is dispensable in apoptosis. However, when the intensity of the radiation insult is markedly increased, DNA repair is impaired in PARP null tissue and the cells undergo apoptotic cell death.[30] A role for maintaining genomic stability has been confirmed in the PARP null mice as tissues from these mice exhibit high levels of sister chromatid exchange, indicative of elevated recombination rates.[31] PARP, along with DNA dependent protein kinase, is critically important in maintaining genomic stability and PARP null mice have increased variable diversity joining (VDJ) recombination events.[28,31]

The Suicide Theory of PARP Activation

NAD is important in the regulation of a variety of cellular processes. NAD is a co-factor for glycolysis and thus, contributes to the generation of adenosine triphosphate (ATP) for most cellular activities. NAD is also the precursor of NADPH, a co-factor for the pentoshunt, for bio-reductive synthetic pathways as well as the maintenance of reduced glutathione pools. The observation that activation of PARP can lead to an acute depletion of cellular NAD levels has led to the proposal that NAD consumption following DNA damage and activation of PARP can adversely affect cellular energetics leading to cell death.[23,24,32,33] The proposal suggests cells which have incurred significant DNA damage should be prevented from undergoing further cell division, and excessive activation of PARP could lead to appropriate suicide of these severely damaged cells. The majority of these studies were performed in fibroblasts and tumor cell lines, and the cytotoxic triggers were alkalining agents, radiation, and hydrogen peroxide.[23,24,32]

The discovery that NO could mediate a component of glutamate neurotoxicity[34,35] led investigators to explore the various signaling complexes induced by production of NO. Since NO could regulate the activity of GAPDH through mono-ADP-riboxylation,[9-11] the potential for other ADP-riboxylation events was investigated. Zhang and colleagues[33] discovered that NO, and more importantly, peroxynitrite, could efficiently trigger PARP activation and poly(ADP-ribose) formation (Figure 2). Neuronal damage following ischemic insult is thought to be elicited in large part by activation of the N-methyl-D-aspartate (NMDA), a subtype of glutamate receptors.[36,37] NMDA antagonists block neuronal damage induced by ischemic insult both *in vitro* and *in vivo* in a variety of animal species. Neurotoxicity elicited by activation of the NMDA receptors is mediated in large part by NO formation as well as increased superoxide anion formation.[34,35,38] The reaction of NO and superoxide anion yields a potent oxidant, peroxynitrite.[39] Neurotoxicity induced by NMDA or ischemic insult can be significantly inhibited with inhibitors of NO synthase.[40-42] Additionally, targeted disruption of the neuronal isoform of NO synthase results in decreased infarct volume following vascular stroke.[43] Cultures from nNOS null mice are resistant to NMDA and ischemic injury.[38]

Since NO and peroxynitrite could activate poly(ADP-ribose) polymerase a role for PARP activation in excitotoxicity and ischemic reper-

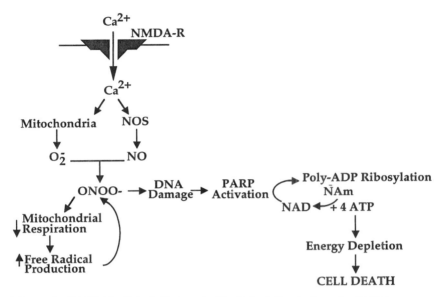

Figure 2. PARP Mediated Glutamate Excitotoxicity. Acting via NMDA receptors, glutamate triggers an influx of Ca^{2+} activating mitochondria and in nNOS neurons inducing the production of NO. Mitochondrial activation results in an increase in superoxide anion ($O_2\bullet^-$) production. NO is a diffusible molecule which combines with superoxide to form peroxynitrite (OONO-). Peroxynitrite damages mitochondrial enzymes decreasing mitochondrial respiration and the production of ATP and, peroxynitrite damages MnSOD further increasing the production of superoxide anion. Peroxynitrite has limited diffusion across membranes and can leave the mitochondria and enter the nucleus where it damages DNA. Nicks and fragments of DNA activate PARP. Massive activation of PARP leads to ADP-ribosylation and depletion of NAD. ATP is depleted in an effort to resynthesize NAD. In the setting of impaired energy generation due to mitochondrial dysfunction this loss of NAD and ATP leads to cell death.

fusion injury has been investigated.[33,44] Ischemia-reperfusion injury can be modeled *in vitro* by exposing primary neuronal cultures to combined oxygen-glucose deprivation, exposure to glutamate, NMDA, or NO donors. Several classes of PARP inhibitors are neuroprotective in these models in a dose-dependent manner. The rank order of potency of the different classes of PARP inhibitors correlates with the degree of neuroprotection, implicating the inhibition of PARP is neuroprotective.[33] Confirmation of the role of PARP in eliciting neuronal cell death is provided by observations that primary neuronal cultures from PARP null mice are resistant to toxicity elicited by combined oxygen-glucose deprivation or by neurotoxic concentrations of NMDA or NO generators.[44] The physiologic relevance of these *in vitro* studies is supported by the observation of reduced infarct volume following transient middle cerebral artery occlusion in PARP null mice.[44,45] A contribution to reduction in infarct volume by genetic background in these genetically engineered mice is unlikely, as the PARP null mice are on a congenic 129 background and littermate controls were used.[44] Further support that PARP is important in neuronal injury following ischemic insult is provided by a similar reduction in infarct volume following transient middle cerebral artery occlusion in a PARP null line on a mixed genetic background of 129/C57B6 mice.[45] Therefore, the reduction in infarct volume in these two separate lines of PARP null mice is likely due to the absence of PARP rather than other genetic variables. Histologic examination reveals that ADP-ribose formation is increased and NAD levels are decreased following focal ischemic insult in wild-type tissue ipsilateral but not contralateral to the insult. In the PARP null mice no ADP-ribose formation is observed and NAD levels are spared.[44,45] Pharmacologic inhibition with a novel PARP inhibitor, 3,4-dihydro-5-[4-1(1-piperidynil) buthoxy]-1(2H)-isoquinolinone, reduces infarct volume following transient middle cerebral artery occlusion in rats.[46] The dramatic neuroprotection observed in the PARP null mice following transient middle cerebral artery occlusion exceeds the degree of protection observed for any other genetically engineered mouse model including transgenic superoxide dismutase mice and neuronal NOS knockout mice. This suggests that multiple toxic insults may converge on PARP activation to result in neuronal cell death (Figure 3).

Although PARP mediates a major component of excitotoxicity in forebrain neurons both *in vitro* and *in vivo*, in cerebellar granule cell cultures it has been reported that glutamate and NO toxicity is PARP-independent but caspase dependent.[47] These results highlight the importance of examining excitotoxic mechanisms in the cell type of interest and further indicate that PARP-dependent and PARP-independent pathways will likely be regional and cell-type specific as well as dependent on the neurotoxic stimulus. In the forebrain areas susceptible to damage in stroke, the dramatic reduction in neuronal damage both *in vitro* and *in vivo* by pharmacologic inhibition and genetic knockout of PARP implicates a major role for PARP activation and the genesis of neurotoxicity and suggests PARP activation and ischemic injury may be a chokepoint at which several neurotoxic pathways converge.

Reperfusion Injury in Other Organs

PARP activation in reperfusion injury is not confined to the brain. Recent reports indicate that inhibition of PARP is cytoprotective in the reperfused gut, skeletal muscle, reina and heart.[32] In the heart inhibition of PARP reduces infarct size and plasma creatinine phosphokinase activity as well as improving the metabolic status in the histologic

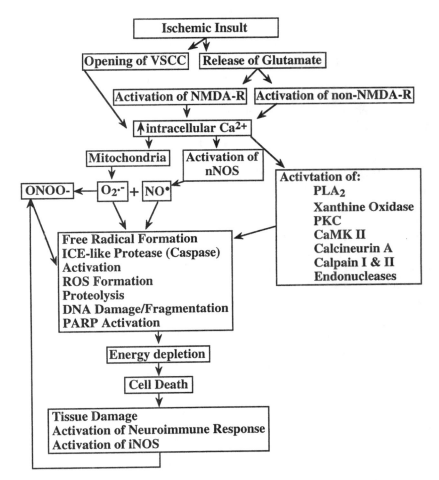

Figure 3. A simple model of PARP activation in ischemia/reperfusion injury. Blood vessel occlusion induces a multitude of cellular events. Ischemia results in the reduction of the resting membrane potential of glia and neurons in the brain. Potassium leaks out of cells and depolarizes neurons leading to a massive release of glutamate resulting in pathologic increases in intracellular calcium. Acting via NMDA receptors, glutamate triggers a release of NO which combines with superoxide to form peroxynitrite. Peroxynitrite damages DNA whose fragments activate PARP. Massive activation of PARP leads to ADP-ribosylation and depletion of NAD. ATP is depleted in an effort to resynthesize NAD leading to cell death by energy depletion. It is possible that other calcium-dependent processes and free radical mediated injury pathways feed into the PARP pathway. Abbreviations: CBF, cerebral blood flow; VSCC, voltage dependent calcium channels; NMDA-R, N-methyl-D-aspartate receptor; $O_2\bullet^-$, superoxide anion; nNOS, neuronal nitric oxide synthase; PLA$_2$, phospholipase A$_2$; PKC, protein kinase C; ROS, reactive oxygen species, PARP, poly (ADP)ribose polymerase; ICE, interleukin-1ß converting enzyme.

outcome of the reperfused myocardium.[48,49] Additionally, the reduction in cardiac myeloperoxidase activity after PARP inhibition indicates a reduction in infiltration of neutrophil granulocytes into the reperfused myocardium.[49] Surprisingly, although PARP inhibitors are not direct scavengers of peroxynitrite and do not directly inhibit NOS activity, PARP inhibitors can reduce the amount of peroxynitrite in reperfused myocardium.[49] It is likely that inhibition of PARP interrupts a positive feed forward cycle in which cellular injury induces neutrophil recruitment leading to peroxynitrite formation and subsequent further endothelial injury and upregulation of adhesion factors leading to more neutrophil recruitment. Since PARP inhibitors will decrease the level of endothelial injury,[50] fewer neutrophils are recruited and less peroxynitrite is generated. Consistent with this notion, direct measurements by intravital microscopy of perfused mesenteries demonstrate a reduction of adherent neutrophils into inflamed tissue following inhibition of PARP.[51]

PARP and Apoptosis

Apoptosis (programmed cell death) can be induced in a variety of cell types by numerous different molecules including cytokines, chemotherapy agents, toxins, as well as growth factor deprivation. Apoptosis is morphologically characterized by cell shrinkage and blebbing of plasma membranes by nuclear condensation, by formation of apoptotic bodies.[52,53] The executioners of this cell death pathway, which contributes significantly to the morphologic changes, are a series of proteases termed caspases.[54] PARP is cleaved by caspase-3 in the nuclear localization domain between aspartate ASP-214 and Gly-215 into a classic 29 and 85 Kd fragments.[54] PARP cleavage has become a biochemical hallmark of apoptosis and is a commonly used biochemical marker for caspase-3 activation and apoptotic processes. Since PARP is commonly cleaved in many different cell types stimulated by a variey of insults to undergo apoptosis, the question has arisen what role PARP plays in the apoptotic process. One group suggests that PARP plays a key role in apoptotic processes perhaps through poly(ADP-ribosyl)ation-induced inhibition of pro-apoptotic proteins.[55] Theoretically, cleavage of PARP during the apoptotic process would prevent further poly(ADP-ribosyl)ation leading to activation of subsequent secondary apoptotic processes. Additionally, since NAD and ATP are required for apoptosis to continue to completion, cleavage of PARP would prevent depletion of these energy substrates by activation of PARP following intranuclear somal degradation and generation of free DNA ends. However, several studies have observed that the absence of PARP or

PARP mutations lacking the caspase-3 cleavage site do not affect the progression of apoptotic processes.[28,29,31] The question of whether cleavage of PARP is important in the apoptotic process has not been rigorously tested yet. There are two consecutive caspase cleavage sites in the nuclear localization domain. Most studies have only mutated the caspase-3 cleavage site. Furthermore, the experiments using this mutation were performed in cell free extracts and only address the question of whether DNA fragmentation would still occur in the presence of uncleavable PARP.[29] These studies do not address the question whether the rate of cellular apoptosis could be altered by the inability to cleave to PARP. It would seem reasonable that PARP would be an early target for caspase cleavage for apoptosis to occur. Apoptosis is an energy-requiring process and for the program to be completed, sufficient concentrations of NAD and ATP are required. If PARP were activated by free DNA ends following DNA fragmentation and subsequently began to consume NAD and ATP, there may not be sufficient energy equivalents to complete the apoptotic program. This latter hypothesis awaits investigation with the genetically engineered PARP knock-in animals in which the PARP caspase-3 cleavage sites have been mutated and the gene knocked back into the PARP null transgenic mice.

Summary

PARP is a large multi-functional protein that has been thought to function predominantly as a DNA integrity sensor and participate in DNA repair. Its potential role in participating in selective cell death has only recently been appreciated. The profound cytoprotection afforded either by PARP inhibition or PARP knockout in both the brain and the heart emphasizes the importance of the activity of this protein in ischemia and reperfusion injury. The development of more potent and selective agents is a highly promising area for potential therapeutic intervention against ischemic damage. Particularly because PARP activation appears to be a downstream event from early cell death triggers such as glutamate release and NO formation, and due to the potential for numerous toxic networks to converge on PARP activation, the generation of nontoxic and selective agents shows great promise for the future therapy of stroke as well as cardiac infarction. Additionally, the role of PARP activation and inflammation is just being studied and investigated. In several models of inflammation PARP inhibitors are dramatically protective and have the ability to reduce inflammatory responses.[51,56,57] This additional activity of PARP inhibition may also contribute to the pronounced neuroprotection and cardiac protection following ischemic insult and reperfusion. More detailed studies are required to fully understand the biologic consequences of PARP activation in both ischemic injury and inflammation, however, this area of investigation may provide clinically useful therapeutic strategies for the treatment of ischemic injury.

References

1. Shall S. ADP-ribosylation reactions. *Biochimie* 1995;77:313-318.
2. Collier RJ. Effect of diphtheria toxin on protein synthesis: Inactivation of one of the transfer factors. *J Mol Biol* 1967;25:83-98.
3. Lee HC, Walseth TF, Bratt GT, et al. Structural determination of a cyclic metabolite of NAD+ with intracellular Ca2+-mobilizing activity. *J Biol Chem* 1989;264:1608-1615.
4. Empson RM, Galione A. Cyclic ADP-ribose enhances coupling between voltage-gated Ca2+ entry and intracellular Ca2+ release. *J Biol Chem* 1997;272:20967-20970.
5. Petersen OH. Inositol trisphosphate and cyclic ADP ribose as long range messengers generating local subcellular calcium signals. *J Physiol Paris* 1995;89:125-127.
6. Mothet JP, Fossier P, Meunier FM, et al. Cyclic ADP-ribose and calcium-induced calcium release regulate neurotransmitter release at a cholinergic synapse of Aplysia. *J Physiol (Lond)* 1998;507:405-414.
7. Clementi E. Role of nitric oxide and its intracellular signalling pathways in the control of Ca2+ homeostasis. *Biochem Pharmacol* 1998;55:713-718.
8. Lee HC. Mechanisms of calcium signaling by cyclic ADP-ribose and NAADP. *Physiol Rev* 1997;77:1133-1164.
9. Dimmeler S, Lottspeich F, Brune B. Nitric oxide causes ADP-ribosylation and inhibition of glyceraldehyde-3- phosphate dehydrogenase. *J Biol Chem* 1992;267:16771-16774.
10. Zhang J, Snyder SH. Nitric oxide stimulates auto-ADP-ribosylation of glyceraldehyde-3- phosphate dehydrogenase. *Proc Natl Acad Sci USA* 1992;89:9382-9385.
11. Molina y Vedia L, McDonald B, Reep B, et al. Nitric oxide-induced S-nitrosylation of glyceraldehyde-3-phosphate dehydrogenase inhibits enzymatic activity and increases endogenous ADP- ribosylation. *J Biol Chem* 1992;267:24929-24932.
12. Moss J, Zolkiewska A, Okazaki I. ADP-ribosylarginine hydrolases and ADP-ribosyltransferases. Partners in ADP-ribosylation cycles. *Adv Exp Med Biol* 1997;419:25-33.
13. Koch-Nolte F, Haag F. Mono(ADP-ribosyl) transferases and related enzymes in animal tissues. Emerging gene families. *Adv Exp Med Biol* 1997;419:1-13.
14. Chambon P, Weil JD, Doly J, et al. On the formation of a novel adenylic compound by enzymatic extracts of liver nuclei. *Biochem Biophys Res Commun* 1966;25:638-643.
15. Tsopanakis C, McLaren EA, Shall S. Purification of poly(adenosine diphosphate ribose) polymerase from pig thymus. *Biochem Soc Trans* 1976;4:774-777.

16. Lautier D, Lagueux J, Thibodeau J, et al. Molecular and biochemical features of poly (ADP-ribose) metabolism. *Mol Cell Biochem* 1993;122:171-193.

17. de Murcia G, Schreiber V, Molinete M, et al. Structure and function of poly(ADP-ribose) polymerase. *Mol Cell Biochem* 1994;138:15-24.

18. de Murcia G, Menissier de Murcia J. Poly(ADP-ribose) polymerase: A molecular nick-sensor. *Trends Biochem Sci* 1994;19:172-176.

19. Ruf A, Rolli V, de Murcia G, et al. The mechanism of the elongation and branching reaction of poly(ADP- ribose) polymerase as derived from crystal structures and mutagenesis. *J Mol Biol* 1998;278:57-65.

20. Lindahl T, Satoh MS, Poirier GG, et al. Post-translational modification of poly(ADP-ribose) polymerase induced by DNA strand breaks. *Trends Biochem Sci* 1995;20:405-411.

21. Trucco C, Flatter E, Fribourg S, et al. Mutations in the amino-terminal domain of the human poly(ADP-ribose) polymerase that affect its catalytic activity but not its DNA binding capacity. *FEBS Lett* 1996;399:313-316.

22. Griffin RJ, Curtin NJ, Newell DR, et al. The role of inhibitors of poly(ADP-ribose) polymerase as resistance- modifying agents in cancer therapy. *Biochimie* 1995;77:408-422.

23. Berger NA. Poly(ADP-ribose) in the cellular response to DNA damage. *Radiat Res* 1985;101:4-15.

24. Nagele A. Poly(ADP-ribosyl)ation as a fail-safe, transcription-independent, suicide mechanism in acutely DNA-damaged cells: A hypothesis. *Radiat Environ Biophys* 1995;34:251-254.

25. Satoh MS, Poirier GG, Lindahl T. Dual function for poly(ADP-ribose) synthesis in response to DNA strand breakage. *Biochemistry* 1994;33:7099-7106.

26. Satoh MS, Lindahl T. Role of poly(ADP-ribose) formation in DNA repair. *Nature* 1992;356:356-358.

27. Wang ZQ, Auer B, Stingl L, et al. Mice lacking ADPRT and poly(ADP-ribosyl)ation develop normally but are susceptible to skin disease. *Genes Dev* 1995;9:509-520.

28. Wang ZQ, Stingl L, Morrison C, et al. PARP is important for genomic stability but dispensable in apoptosis. *Genes Dev* 1997;11:2347-2358.

29. Liu X, Zou H, Slaughter C, et al. DFF, a heterodimeric protein that functions downstream of caspase-3 to trigger DNA fragmentation during apoptosis. *Cell* 1997;89:175-184.

30. de Murcia JM, Niedergang C, Trucco C, et al. Requirement of poly(ADP-ribose) polymerase in recovery from DNA damage in mice and in cells. *Proc Natl Acad Sci USA* 1997;94:7303-7307.

31. Morrison C, Smith GC, Stingl L, et al. Genetic interaction between PARP and DNA-PK in V(D)J recombination and tumorigenesis. *Nat Genet* 1997;17:479-482.

32. Szabo C, Dawson VL. Role of poly (ADP-ribose) synthetase in inflammation and reperfusion injury. *Trends in Pharmacol Sci* 1998;19(7):287-298. 33. Zhang J, Dawson VL, Dawson TM, et al. Nitric oxide activation of poly(ADP-ribose) synthetase in neurotoxicity. *Science* 1994;263:687-689.

34. Dawson VL, Dawson TM, London ED, et al. Nitric oxide mediates glutamate neurotoxicity in primary cortical cultures. *Proc Natl Acad Sci USA* 1991;88:6368-6371.

35. Dawson VL, Dawson TM, Bartley DA, et al. Mechanisms of nitric oxide-mediated neurotoxicity in primary brain cultures. *J Neurosci* 1993;13:2651-2661.

36. Choi DW. Cerebral hypoxia: Some new approaches and unanswered questions. *J Neurosci* 1990;10:2493-2501.

37. Meldrum B, Garthwaite J. Excitatory amino acid neurotoxicity and neurodegenerative disease. *Trends Pharmacol Sci* 1990;11:379-387.

38. Dawson VL, Kizushi VM, Huang PL, et al. Resistance to neurotoxicity in cortical cultures from neuronal nitric oxide synthase deficient mice. *J Neurosci* 1996;16:2479-2487.

39. Beckman JS, Crow JP. Pathological implications of nitric oxide, superoxide and peroxynitrite formation. *Biochem Soc Trans* 1993;21:330-334.

40. Nowicki JP, Duval D, Poignet H, et al. Nitric oxide mediates neuronal death after focal cerebral ischemia in the mouse. *Eur J Pharmacol* 1991;204:339-340.

41. Dawson TM, Dawson VL. Protection of the Brain from Ischemia. In Batjer HH (ed): *Cerebrovascular Disease*. Philadelphia, PA: Lippincott-Raven Publishers 1997:319-325

42. Dawson TM, Snyder SH. Gases as biological messengers: Nitric oxide and carbon monoxide in the brain. *J Neurosci* 1994;14:5147-5159.

43. Huang Z, Huang PL, Panahian N, et al. Effects of cerebral ischemia in mice deficient in neuronal nitric oxide synthase. *Science* 1994;265:1883-1885.

44. Eliasson MJL, Sampei K, Mandir AS, et al. Poly(ADP-Ribose) Polymerase Gene Disruption Renders Mice Resistant to Cerebral Ischemia. *Nat Med* 1997;3:1-8.

45. Endres M, Wang ZQ, Namura S, et al. Ischemic brain injury is mediated by the activation of poly(ADP- ribose)polymerase [In Process Citation]. *J Cereb Blood Flow Metab* 1997;17:1143-1151.

46. Takahashi K, Greenberg JH, Jackson P, et al. Neuroprotective effects of inhibiting poly(ADP-ribose) synthetase on focal cerebral ischemia in rats. *J Cereb Blood Flow Metab* 1997;17:1137-1142.

47. Leist M, Single B, Kunstle G, et al. Apoptosis in the absence of poly-(ADP-ribose) polymerase. *Biochem Biophys Res Commun* 1997;233:518-522.

48. Thiemermann C, Bowes J, Myint FP, et al. Inhibition of the activity of poly(ADP ribose) synthetase reduces ischemia-reperfusion injury in the heart and skeletal muscle. *Proc Natl Acad Sci USA* 1997;94:679-683.

49. Zingarelli B, Cuzzocrea S, Zsengeller Z, et al. Protection against myocardial ischemia and reperfusion injury by 3- aminobenzamide, an inhibitor of poly (ADP-ribose) synthetase. *Cardiovasc Res* 1997;36:205-215.

50. Szabo C, Cuzzocrea S, Zingarelli B, et al. Endothelial dysfunction in a rat model of endotoxic shock. Importance of the activation of poly (ADP-ribose) synthetase by peroxynitrite. *J Clin Invest* 1997;100:723-735.

51. Szabo C, Lim LH, Cuzzocrea S, et al. Inhibition of poly (ADP-ribose) synthetase attenuates neutrophil recruitment and exerts antiinflammatory effects. *J Exp Med* 1997;186:1041-1049.

52. Raff MC. Social controls on cell survival and cell death. *Nature* 1992;356:397-400.

53. Raff MC, Barres BA, Burne JF, et al. Programmed cell death and the control of cell survival: Lessons from the nervous system. *Science* 1993;262:695-700.

54. Villa P, Kaufmann SH, Earnshaw WC. Caspases and caspase inhibitors. *Trends Biochem Sci* 1997;22:388-393.

55. Simbulan-Rosenthal CM, Rosenthal DS, Iyer S, et al. Transient poly(ADP-ribosyl)ation of nuclear proteins and role of poly(ADP-ribose) polymerase in the early stages of apoptosis. *J Biol Chem* 1998;273:13703-13712.

56. Cuzzocrea S, Zingarelli B, Gilad E, et al. Protective effects of 3-aminobenz-amide, an inhibitor of poly (ADP- ribose) synthase in a carrageenan-induced model of local inflammation. *Eur J Pharmacol* 1998;342:67-76.

57. Szabo C, Virag L, Cuzzocrea S, et al. Protection against peroxynitrite-induced fibroblast injury and arthritis development by inhibition of poly-(ADP-ribose) synthase. *Proc Natl Acad Sci USA* 1998;95:3867-3872.

Chapter 6

Superoxide Dismutase in Cerebral Ischemia

Pak H. Chan, PhD

Oxygen free radicals, or oxidants, have been implicated in the development of many neurological disorders and brain dysfunctions.[1-5] A role that oxygen free radicals may play in brain injury appears to involve reperfusion after cerebral ischemia. In either global or focal cerebral ischemia, cerebral blood flow (CBF) is significantly reduced in the brain regions that are supplied with oxygen by the occluded vessel. Reoxygenation during reperfusion provides oxygen to sustain neuronal viability and also provides oxygen as a substrate for numerous enzymatic oxidation reactions that produce reactive oxidants. In addition, reflow after occlusion often causes an increase in oxygen to levels that cannot be utilized by mitochondria under normal physiological flow conditions. It has been demonstrated that about 2%–5% of the electron flow in isolated brain mitochondria produces superoxide ($O_2\bullet^-$) and hydrogen (H_2O_2).[6] These constantly produced oxygen radicals are scavenged, respectively, by superoxide dismutases (SODs) and by glutathione peroxidases (GSHPx), and catalase. Other antioxidants, including glutathione (GSH), ascorbic acid, and vitamin E, are also likely to be involved in the detoxification of free radicals. During reperfusion, it is likely that these antioxidative defense mechanisms are perturbed as a result of the overproduction of oxygen radicals, inactivation of detoxification systems, consumption of antioxidants, and the failure to adequately replenish them in ischemic brain tissue. Due to technical difficulties, the level of oxygen free radicals in

This work was supported by National Institutes of Health grants, NS14543, NS25372, NS36147, AG08938 and NO1 NS52334, and contract NO1 NS82386.

From: Choi D, Dacey RG, Hsu CY, Powers WJ. *Cerebrovascular Disease: Momentum at the End of the Second Millennium.* Armonk, NY: Futura Publishing Company, Inc., © 2002.

brain tissue ischemia is generally assessed by indirect methods, including lipid peroxidation,[7,8] protein oxidation,[9] and DNA damage.[10,11] Recent advances in methodologies have allowed investigators to measure hydroxyl radicals by salicylate hydroxylation[12] and nitric oxide (NO) radicals (NO•) by a porphyrinic microsensor[13] and by electron paramagnetic resonance spin trapping[14] in ischemic brain tissue. In addition, several chemical and biochemical methods have been developed to measure superoxide radicals in neurons that undergo oxidative stress.[15-20] Despite these useful measurements for O_2•$^-$, hydroxyl (•OH) and NO• radicals, establishment of the causative role of oxygen radicals in ischemic brain injury remains a difficult task for stroke researchers and neuroscientists. One strategy is the molecular genetic approaches using transgenic (Tg) and knockout mutant mice to dissect out the molecular and cellular mechanisms involving oxygen radicals in ischemic brain damage.

Antioxidant Enzyme SODs and Cerebral Ischemia

Several enzymes, including SOD, GSHPx, glutathione reductase and catalase are endogenous antioxidants that process specific free radical scavenging properties. Superoxide dismutases, in particular, have been used extensively to reduce superoxide radical-associated ischemic brain damage (Table 1). Based on the metal ion requirements and the anatomical distribution, three types of SODs exist in brain cells. CuZn-SOD is a cytosolic enzyme that requires both copper and zinc ions as co-factors. It is a dimeric protein that is coded by the human CuZn-SOD transgene (*SOD*-1) on chromosome 21 in human cells. Manganese (Mn-SOD) is a mitochondrial enzyme with requirements for Mn^{2+}.[21] It is a tetrameric protein that is coded by the *SOD*-2 gene in chromosome 4 in human cells. Both CuZn-SOD and Mn-SOD from various sources have been fully characterized biochemically and the cDNAs of both human enzymes have been successfully cloned.[22,23] A copper-containing SOD (*SOD*-3) has been identified in the extracellular space and its gene successfully cloned (Table 1).[24] As specified, for superoxide radicals, CuZn-SOD has been used extensively to reduce brain injury induced by ischemia and reperfusion. Unfortunately, investigators have obtained varying degrees of success and failure when free, non-modified SOD was used to ameliorate ischemic brain injury.[25] The extremely short half-life of CuZn-SOD (6 minutes) in circulating blood and its failure to pass the blood-brain barrier (BBB) make it difficult to use enzyme therapy in cerebral ischemia. However, a modified enzyme with an increased half-life, such as polyethylene glycol-

Table 1.

Mammalian Superoxide Dismutases.

	CuZn-SOD	Mn-SOD	EC-SOD
Location	Cytosol	Mitochondria	Extracellular space
Mw	32,000	88,000	120,000
Structure	Dimer	Tetramer	Tetramer
Metals (g-atoms/subunit)	Cu 1, Zn 1	Mn 1	Cu 1, Zn 1
KSOD (M^{-1} sec $^{-1}$)	1.2×10^9	1.3×10^9	1×10^9
Chromosome	21 (human) 17 (Mouse)	6 (Human) 16 (Mouse)	? ?
Gene designation	SOD-1	SOD-2	SOD-3
Disease	Amyotrophic lateral sclerosis (familial)	?	?

SOD = superoxide dismutase; Mw = molecular weight (in kilodaltons); KSOD = reaction constant.

conjugated SOD (PEG-SOD), has been successfully used to reduce infarct volume in rats that have been subjected to focal cerebral ischemia.[26,27] Liposome-entrapped SOD has an increased half-life (4.2 hours), BBB permeability, and cellular uptake, and it has also proven to be an effective treatment in reducing the severity of traumatic and focal ischemic brain injuries.[28,29] Yet, in some instances, modified SOD (ie, PEG-SOD) has been used with conflicting results.[25] The fact that the results are mixed makes it imperative to use other experimental strategies so that the role of SOD can be fully established in cerebral ischemia.

SOD Tg and Knockout Mutant Mice as Useful Tools to Study the Role of Oxidants in Ischemic Brain Injury

One strategy to study the role of oxidants in ischemic brain injury is to use Tg/knockout technology to alter the levels of pro-oxidants, antioxidants and oxidant-related enzymes or proteins and to study the role of a specific antioxidant in ischemic brain injury.

Using the Tg technology, several mice strains with various genotypes that relate to oxidant/antioxidant enzymes/proteins have been successfully developed. Most of these Tg and knockout mutant animals have been used in the study of the role of oxidants in ischemic brain injury (Table 2).

In the studies using Tg mice that overexpress *SOD*-1, two models of focal cerebral ischemia are used. One model is achieved by permanent occlusion of the left middle cerebral artery (MCA) just proximal to the piriform branch in the anesthetized mouse. Immediately following occlusion of the MCA, the left common carotid artery (CCA) is permanently ligated and the right CCA is temporarily occluded for 1 hour followed by additional reperfusion for 24 hours. The total infarct volume (mm^3) is reduced by 36% in *SOD*-1 Tg mice as compared to nontransgenic (nTg) mice. Brain edema is also reduced in both the MCA territory and the anterior cerebral artery area, a region that corresponds to the "ischemic penumbra." Antioxidants GSH and ascorbic acid are maintained at higher levels in the penumbra area than in the same anatomical regions in nTg mouse brains.[30] In another study that involved the use of *SOD*-1 Tg mice, MCA occlusion was achieved with a 5–0 rounded nylon suture placed within the internal cerebral artery followed by withdrawal of the suture to allow reperfusion. The infarct volume was reduced by 26% in *SOD*-1 Tg mice at 3 hours of reperfusion after 3 hours of ischemia[31] and by 40% in *SOD-1* Tg mice at 24 hours

Table 2.

Transgenic and Knockout Mutant Mice in the Study of the Role of Oxidants in Ischemic Brain Injury.

Gene	Enzyme/Protein	Transgene/Knockout	Study	Effect	Reference
SOD-1	CuZn-superoxide dismutase	Human transgene	Focal cererbral ischemia	+	44
SOD-1	CuZn-superoxide dismutase	Human transgene	Transient focal cerrebral ischemia	+	31
SOD-1	CuZn-superoxide dismutase	Human transgene	Transient global cerebral ischemia	+	55
SOD-1	CuZn-superoxide dismutase	Human transgene	Permanent focal cerebral ischemia	NP	33
BCL-2	BCL-2 protein	Human transgene neuronal-specific	Permanent focal cerebral ischemia	+	45
bFGF	Basic fibroblast growth factor	Human transgene	Hypoxia/ischemia	+	46
GSHPx	Glutathione peroxidase	Human transgene	Transient focal cerebral ischemia	+	47
nNOS	Neuronal nitric oxide synthase	Homozygous (-/-) knockout	Permanent focal cerebral ischemia	–	48
nNOS	Neuronal nitric oxide synthase	Homozygous (-/-) knockout	Transient focal cerebral ischemia	+	56
nNOS	Neuronal nitric oxide synthase	Homozygous (-/-) knockout	Transient global cerebral ischemia	+	57
eNOS	Endothelial nitric oxide synthase	Homozygous (-/-) knockout	Permanent focal cerebral ischemia	–	49,50
iNOS	Inducible nitric oxide synthase	Homozygous (-/-) knockout	Transient focal cerebral ischemia	+	51
p53	p53 protein	Homozygous (-/-) knockout	Permanent focal cerebral iscchemia	+	52
sod-1	CuZn-superoxide dismutase	Homozygous (-/-); Heterozgous (+/-)	Transient focal cerebral ischemia	–	53
sod-2	Mn superoxide dismutase	Heterozygous (+/-)	Trunsient focal cerebral ischemia	–	54
sod-2	Mn-superoxide dismutase	Heterozygous (+/-)	Permanent focal cerebral ischemia	–	20
APP	Amyloid precursor protein	Human transgene	Transient focal cerebral ischemia	–	58
COX-2 (PGHS 2)	Cyclo-oxygnase 2	Homozygous (-/-) knockout	Transient focal cerebral ischemia	+	59

+ = neuronal protection; NP = no protection; – = exacerbates ischemic infarction.

after 1 hour of MCA occlusion, as compared to nTg mice.[32] The decrease in the infarct volume in *SOD*-1 Tg mice clearly parallels the reduction of neurological deficits and is not related to the changes in CBF. On the other hand, infarct volume produced in *SOD*-1 Tg mice that are subjected to 24 hours of permanent MCA occlusion using intraluminal suture blockade is not different from that of nTg mice,[33] suggesting that the increased ischemic severity resulting from prolonged cerebral ischemia will limit the protective role of CuZn-SOD against neuronal injury.

Transient global ischemia has been one of the most interesting pathological conditions in stroke studies, and has been investigated in great detail because of unclearly understood mechanisms of selective vulnerability and delayed neuronal cell death in several regions of the brain, including the hippocampal CA_1 subregion, cortical layers 1 and 3, and the striatum. In rats, global ischemia can be induced by bilateral common carotid artery (BCCA) occlusion with hemorrhagic hypotension,[34] 4-vessel occlusion (BCCAs and vertebral arteries),[35] and 3-vessel occlusion (BCCAs and artery).[36] Gerbils have been used for global ischemia studies because of their unique and convenient vascular anatomy. Since gerbils lack the posterior communicating artery (PcomA) connecting between anterior and posterior circulation of the brain, and because of their anatomy, global ischemia is induced by simple BCCA occlusion. On the other hand, global ischemia cannot be induced by BCCA occlusion in rats or mice because of the existence of the PcomA. The PcomA supplies blood flow from posterior circulation as collateral blood flow, when bilateral carotid arteries are occluded. Although attempts have been made by us to apply those rat global ischemia models to mice, because of high mortality and frequent complications such as convulsive seizures after ischemia, success has been difficult to accomplish.

A new mouse model of global ischemia has recently been developed based on the relationship of plasticity of the PcomA, ischemia duration, and neuronal injury following global ischemia in this model.[37]

Injured neurons in the hippocampus showed various levels of severity after global ischemia. The hemisphere with the hypoplastic PcomA was therefore used to normalize the anatomic background which could affect the ischemic condition induced by BCCA occlusion. Several types of damaged neurons were observed in the hippocampal injury. Some of those neurons displayed a slightly condensed nucleus. The most frequently observed neurons in the injured hippocampus had an oval-shaped or triangular-shaped nucleus. In particular, the neurons with an oval-shaped nucleus occasionally displayed small particles that appeared to be apoptotic bodies in the cytosol. These compact neurons were observed in the same lesion of the hippocampus.

The hippocampal neurons with different morphological features had swollen cell bodies or cell lysis.

The hippocampal injury with hypoplastic PcomA in the ipsilateral hemisphere was evaluated at 5 and 10 minutes of ischemia followed by reperfusion at 1 and 3 days. These data demonstrate that hippocampal injury was reduced in Tg mice as compared with nTg mice (Figure 1A). In the 5-minute ischemia group, hippocampal injury progressed from 1–3 days after ischemia, although a statistical difference was not seen between 1 and 3 days. No significant difference was seen between the nTg and Tg mice at 1 day. At 3 days, however, the hippocampal injury in the Tg mice was significantly lower than that in the nTg mice (Figure 1A).

In the 10-minute ischemia group, hippocampal injury was reduced in the Tg mice. The hippocampal injury at 1 day was significantly more severe in the nTg mice than the Tg mice, and was likely to progress only in the Tg mice and to maximize at 1 day in the nTg animals, although the statistical significance was not obtained (Figure 1A).

On the basis of these biochemical and morphological features of ischemic neurons in the hippocampal CA_1 subregion, we used the TUNEL (terminal deoxynucleotidyl transferase-mediated uridine 5′-triphosphate-biotin nick end labeling) method to determine the ratio of neurons that were positively stained among the total ischemic neurons at 1 or 3 days after global ischemia. In the 5-minute ischemia group, the ratio was significantly lower in the nTg and compared with the Tg mice at 1 day. These TUNEL-positive neurons were 21.9% and 44.2% of the total injured neurons in nTg and Tg mice, respectively. At 3 days after 5 minutes of ischemia, this ratio was 34.1% in the nTg mice and 42.5% in the Tg mice. In the 10-minute group, the ratio was 38.6% in the nTg animals and 35.0% in the Tg mice at 1 day, and 38.2% in the nTg mice and 31.1% in the Tg mice at 3 days.

The hippocampal injury with a PcomA patency in the ipsilateral hemisphere was evaluated in *Sod1* -/- knockout mutant mice. Unlike in the *SOD1* Tg mice, the hippocampal injury was exacerbated in the *Sod1* -/- mice at 3 days after 5 minutes of ischemia compared to wild-type mice. No significant difference in the hippocampal injury was observed between the *Sod1* -/- mutants and wild-type mice at 1 day following 5 minutes of ischemia (Figure 1B).

Conclusion

The present study demonstrates that endogenously overexpressed CuZnSOD (SOD1) plays a protective role in the development of neu-

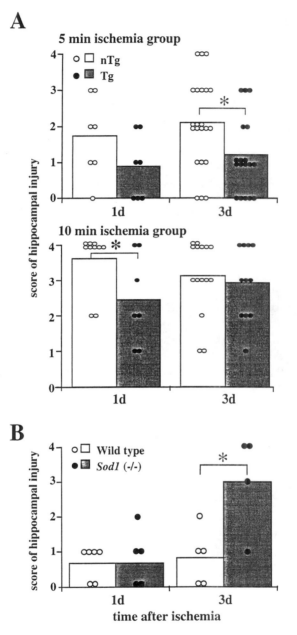

Figure 1. **A.** Qualitative analysis of neuronal damage of the hippocampal injury in nTg and Tg mice at 1 and 3 days after global ischemia. White and black dots show the score of the injury in the hemisphere used in nTg and Tg mice, respectively, and each column shows mean score of the hippocampal injury of each group. * $P < 0.05$, Mann-Whitney U test. Hippocampal injury was

(continued)

ronal necrosis and apoptosis after transient focal cerebral ischemia and the reduction of hippocampal injury after transient global ischemia. In the case of transient global ischemia, the protective role was obtained in both acute injury after relatively intense ischemia and in delayed-progress injury after relatively mild ischemia. *In situ* detection of DNA fragmentation by TUNEL staining demonstrated that apoptotic neuronal death partly contributes to hippocampal injury after transient global ischemia in mice. Furthermore, neuroprotective action by over-expressed CuZnSOD (SOD1) is also involved in the apoptotic process after global ischemia.

In the study of global, as well as focal ischemia, both physiological and anatomical backgrounds are important factors affecting the outcome of neuronal injury, especially in the experiments where genetically different animals were used. In this study, physiological conditions, including mean arterial blood pressure and arterial blood gas, were not significantly different among nTg mice, Tg mice and knockout mutants. Other factors, including the patency of the PcomA, are probably the most important components of the anatomic background affecting the outcome in global ischemia.[38]

Recent studies have demonstrated that apoptosis, in addition to necrosis, is involved in hippocampal injury after global ischemia.[39,40] It has been demonstrated that DNA fragmentation contributes to hippocampal injury after global ischemia in mice. The hippocampal injury displayed several types of morphological features in ischemic neurons. These neurons were observed in both ischemia groups in both groups of mice. Not all of the neurons displaying the morphological features of apoptosis were labeled by TUNEL staining. In the 5-minute ischemia group, the percent of TUNEL-positive neurons was increased at 1 day

---

Figure 1. *(continued)* ameliorated in Tg mice, in the 5- and 10-minute ischemia groups, and at both 1 and 3 days. The tendency of delayed development of the hippocampal injury was demonstrated in the 5-minute group, and the injury was significantly milder in Tg than nTg mice at 3 days. However, this injury was near the peak at 1 day after 10 minutes of ischemia in nTg mice, although it progressed at 3 days in Tg mice. In the 10-minute group, a significant difference was obtained at 1 day rather than 3 days. **B.** Qualitative analysis of neuronal damage of the hippocampus in *Sod1 -/-* mutant and wild-type mice at 1 and 3 days after global ischemia. Open and closed circles show the scores for the injury in the hemisphere used in the wild-type and *Sod1 -/-* mice, and each column shows the mean scores of the hippocampal injury in each group. *$P < 0.05$, Mann-Whitney U test. The hippocampal injury was exacerbated in the *Sod1 -/-* mice at 3 days after 5 minutes of ischemia compared to the wild-type mice. No significant difference in hippocampal injury was observed between *Sod1 -/-* mutant mice and wild-type mice 1 day after 5 minutes of ischemia.

in the Tg mice compared to the nTg mice, although the total injury to the hippocampus was reduced in the Tg mice. However, in the 10-minute ischemia group, this ratio was almost the same between the nTg and Tg mice. This discrepancy in the ratio of TUNEL-positive neurons between the 5- and 10-minute ischemia groups might result from a difference of intensity of the ischemic insult. A decrease of TUNEL-positive neurons means that TUNEL-negative cells, which might also include necrotic cells, increased in the nTg mice after 5 minutes of ischemia. Thus, the increased TUNEL-positive neurons in the Tg mice following 5 minutes of ischemia may reflect more TUNEL-positive neurons that were unmasked by necrotic neurons. It has been demonstrated that excitotoxicity mediated by the N-methyl-d-aspartate receptor induces calcium overload and generates superoxide anions, causing neuronal injury, and two distinct pathways to neuronal death, apoptosis or necrosis, have been demonstrated depending on the intensity of the insult.[41] We have demonstrated that oxygen deprivation alone, but not combined with a substrate, induces DNA degradation in cortical neurons.[42] Considering these findings together with the present results, overexpressed CuZnSOD effectively detoxifies abnormally overproduced superoxide anions and reduces oxidative stress to neurons, which might also alter the pathways of neuronal death, apoptosis or necrosis in Tg mice. On the other hand, after intense ischemia by 10 minutes of BCCA occlusion, the ratio was not altered in Tg mice that overexpress CuZnSOD, while oxidative stress might be partly detoxified by overexpressed CuZnSOD and hippocampal injury as shown in the histological analysis.

It is now clear that oxidants play a major role in brain damage in cerebrovascular diseases. The successful making of SOD-1 Tg mice as well as knockout mutants of sod-1, sod-2, neuronal nitric oxide synthase (NOS), endothelial NOS, inducible NOS, cyclo-oxygenase 2, and many other Tg and knockout mutant mice has allowed stroke researchers and neuroscientists a unique opportunity to study the oxidative mechanisms underlying the complex neuronal responses to ischemic insults (Table 2). It is clear that these genetically modified mice could also be useful for the study of neurodegenerative diseases and neurological disorders other than cerebrovascular diseases. Despite these successful beginnings, there are obvious advantages to using larger animal species (ie, rats) for Tg animals and knockout mutants since many models for stroke and cerebrovascular disease have been mainly developed in rats.[43] The successful creation of Tg and knockout mutant rats will be an invaluable addition to the study of the mechanisms underlying ischemic brain damage in the well-established focal, thrombolytic and global ischemia models.

References

1. Chan PH. Antioxidant-dependent amelioration of brain injury: Role of CuZn-superoxide dismutase. *J Neurotrauma* 1992;2 S417-S423.

2. Chan PH. The role of oxygen radicals in brain injury and edema. In Chow CK (ed): *Cellular Antioxidant Defense Mechanisms*. Boca Raton, FL: CRC Press; 1988:89-109.

3. Hall ED, Braughler JM. Central nervous system trauma and stroke. II. Physiological and pharmacological evidence for involvement of oxygen radicals and lipid peroxidation. *Free Radic Biol Med* 1989;6:303-313.

4. Kontos HA. Oxygen radicals in cerebral vascular injury. *Circ Res* 1985;57:508-516.

5. Siesjö BK, Agardh CD, Bengtsson F. Free radicals and brain damage. *Cerebrovasc Brain Metab Rev* 1989;1:165-211.

6. Boveris A, Chance B. The mitochondrial generation of hydrogen peroxide. *Biochem J* 1973;134:707-716.

7. Meister A. Glutathione metabolism and its selective modification. *J Biol Chem* 1988;263:17205-17208.

8. Watson BD, Busto R, Goldberg WJ, et al. Lipid peroxidation in vivo induced by reversible global ischemia in rat brain. *J Neurochem* 1984;42:268-274.

9. Carney JM, Starke-Reed PE, Oliver CN, et al. Reversal of age-related increase in brain protein oxidation decrease in enzyme activity, and loss in temporal and spatial memory by chronic administration of the spin-trapping compound N-tert-butyl-L-phenylnitrone. *Proc Natl Acad Sci USA* 1991;88:3633-3636.

10. Cathcart R, Schwiers E, Saul RL, et al. Thymine glycol and thymidine glycol in human and rat urine: A possible assay for oxidative DNA damage. *Proc Natl Acad Sci USA* 1984;81:5633-5637.

11. Huang TT, Carlson EJ, Leadon SA, et al. Relationship of resistance to oxygen free radicals to CuZn-superoxide dismutase activity in transgenic, transfected and trisomic cells. *FASEB J* 1992;6:903-910.

12. Oliver CN, Starke-Reed PE, Stadtman ER, et al. Oxidative damage to brain proteins, loss of glutamine synthetase activity and production of free radicals during ischemia/reperfusion-induced injury to gerbil brain. *Proc Natl Acad Sci USA* 1990;87:5144-5147.

13. Malinski T, Bailey F, Zhang ZG, et al. Nitric oxide measured by a porphyrinic microsensor in rat brain after transient middle cerebral artery occlusion. *J Cereb Blood Flow Metab* 1993;13:355-358.

14. Tominaga T, Sato S, Ohnishi J, et al. Potentiation of nitric oxide formation following bilateral carotid occlusion and focal cerebral ischemia in the rat: In vivo detection of the nitric oxide radical by electron paramagnetic resonance spin trapping. *Brain Res* 1993;614:342-346.

15. Bindokas VP, Jordán J, Lee CC, et al. 1993;1996; Superoxide production in rat hippocampal neurons: Selective imaging with hydroethidine. *J Neurosci* 1993;16:1324-1336.

16. Dugan LL, Sensi SL, Canzoniero LMT, et al. Mitochondrial production of reactive oxygen species in cortical neurons following exposure to N-methyl-d-aspartate. *J Neurosci* 1995;15:6377-6388.

17. Fabian RH, DeWitt DS, Kent TA. In vivo detection of superoxide anion production by the brain using a cytochrome C electrode. *J Cereb Blood Flow Metab* 1995;15:242-247.

18. Lafon-Cazal M, Pietri S, Culcasi M, et al. NMDA-dependent superoxide production and neurotoxicity. *Nature* 1993;364:535-537.

19. Patel M, Day BJ, Crapo JD, et al. Requirement for superoxide in excitotoxic cell death. *Neuron* 1996;16:345-355.

20. Murakami K, Kondo T, Kawase M, et al. Mitochondrial susceptibility to oxidative stress exacerbates cerebral infarction that follows permanent focal cerebral ischemia in mutant mice with manganese superoxide dismutase deficiency. *J Neurosci* 1998;18:205-213.

21. Oberley LW. *Superoxide Dismutase*. Vol. 1. Boca Raton, FL: CRC Press; 1982:1-141.

22. Levanon D, Lieman-Hurwitz J, Dafni N, et al. Architecture and anatomy of the chromosomal locus in human chromosome 21 encoding in the Cu/Zn superoxide dismutase. *EMBO J* 1985;4:77-84.

23. Lieman-Hurwitz J, Dafni N, Lavie V, et al. Human cytoplasmic superoxide dismutase cDNA clone: A probe for studying the molecular biology of Down syndrome. *Proc Natl Acad Sci USA* 1982;79:2808-2811.

24. Marklund SL. Human copper-containing superoxide dismutase of high molecular weight. *Proc Natl Acad Sci USA* 1982;79:7634-7638.

25. Chan PH, Epstein CJ, Kinouchi H, et al. Role of superoxide dismutase in ischemic brain injury: Reduction of edema and infarction in transgenic mice following focal cerebral ischemia. *Prog Brain Res* 1993;96:97-104.

26. He YY, Hsu CY, Ezrin AM, et al. Polyethylene glycol-conjugated superoxide dismutase in focal cerebral ischemia-reperfusion. *Am J Physiol* 1993;265:H252-H256.

27. Liu TH, Beckman JS, Freeman BA, et al. Polyethylene glycol-conjugated superoxide dismutase and catalase reduce ischemic brain injury. *Am J Physiol* 1989;256:H589-H593.

28. Imaizumi S, Woolworth V, Fishman RA, et al. Liposome-entrapped superoxide dismutase reduces cerebral infarction in cerebral ischemia in rats. *Stroke* 1990;21:1312-1317.

29. Chan PH, Longar S, Fishman RA. Protective effects of liposome-entrapped superoxide dismutase on post-traumatic brain edema. *Ann Neurol* 1987;21:540-547.

30. Kinouchi H, Epstein CJ, Mizui T, et al. Attenuation of focal cerebral ischemic injury in transgenic mice overexpressing CuZn superoxide dismutase. *Proc Natl Acad Sci USA* 1991;88:11158-11162.

31. Yang G, Chan PH, Chen J, et al. Human copper-zinc superoxide dismutase transgenic mice are highly resistant to reperfusion injury after focal cerebral ischemia. *Stroke* 1994;25:165-170.

32. Kamii H, Kinouchi H, Chen SF, et al. SOD-1 transgenic mice: An application to the study of ischemic brain injury. In: Ohnishi ST (ed): *Membrane-Linked Diseases*. Vol. 4. Boca Raton, FL: CRC Press; 1995:423-431.

33. Chan PH, Kamii H, Yang G, et al. Brain infarction is not reduced in SOD-1 transgenic mice after a permanent focal cerebral ischemia. *Neuroreport* 1993;5:293-296.

34. Smith ML, Bendek G, Dahlgren N, et al. Models for studying long-term recovery following forebrain ischemia in the rat. 2. A 2-vessel occlusion model. *Acta Neurol Scand* 1984;69:385-401.

35. Pulsinelli WA, Brierley JB, Plum F. Temporal profile of neuronal damage in a model of transient forebrain ischemia. *Ann Neurol* 1982; 1:491-498.

36. Kameyama M, Suzuki J, Shirane R, et al. A new model of bilateral hemispheric ischemia in the rat—three vessel occlusion model. *Stroke* 1985;16:489-493.

37. Murakami K, Kondo T, Kawase M, et al. The development of a new mouse model of global ischemia: Focus on the relationships between ischemia duration, anesthesia, cerebral vasculature, and neuronal injury following global ischemia in mice. *Brain Res* 1998;780:304-310.

38. Barone FC, Knudsen DJ, Nelson AH, et al. Mouse strain differences in susceptibility to cerebral ischemia are related to cerebral vascular anatomy. *J Cereb Blood Flow Metab* 1993;13:683-692.

39. MacManus JP, Buchan AM, Hill IE, et al. Global ischemia can cause DNA fragmentation indicative of apoptosis in rat brain. *Neurosci Lett* 1993;164:89-92.

40. Nitatori T, Sato N, Waguri S, et al. Delayed neuronal death in the CA1 pyramidal cell layer of the gerbil hippocampus following transient ischemia is apoptosis. *J Neurosci* 1995;15:1001-1011.

41. Bonfoco E, Krainc D, Ankarcrona M, et al. Apoptosis and necrosis: Two distinct events induced, respectively, by mild and intense insults with N-methyl-d-aspartate or nitric oxide/superoxide in cortical cell cultures. *Proc Natl Acad Sci USA* 1995;92:7162-7166.

42. Copin J-C, Reola LF, Chan TYY, et al. Oxygen deprivation but not a combination of oxygen, glucose, and serum deprivation induces DNA degradation in mouse cortical neurons *in vitro:* Attenuation by transgenic overexpressing of CuZn-superoxide dismutase. *J Neurotrauma* 1996;13:233-244.

43. Ginsberg MD. Models of cerebral ischemia in the rodent. In Schurr A, Rigor BM (eds): *Cerebral Ischemia and Resuscitation.* Boca Raton, FL: CRC Press; 1990:1-15.

44. Kinouchi H, Mizui T, Carlson EJ, et al. Alteration of cerebral infarction and antioxidant levels in focal cerebral ischemia in transgenic mice overexpressing CuZn-SOD. First International Neurotrauma Symposium, May 14-17, 1991, Fukushima City, Japan.

45. Martinou JC, Dubois-Dauphin M, Staple JK, et al. Overexpression of BCL-2 in transgenic mice protects neurons from naturally occurring cell death and experimental ischemia. *Neuron* 1994;13:1017-1030.

46. MacMillan V, Judge D, Wiseman A, et al. Mice expressing a bovine basic fibroblast growth factor transgene in the brain show increased resistance to hypoxemic-ischemic cerebral damage. *Stroke* 1993;24:1735-1739.

47. Weisbrot-Lefkowitz M, Reuhl K, Perry B, et al. Overexpression of human glutathione peroxidase protects transgenic mice against focal cerebral ischemia/reperfusion damage. *Mol Brain Res* 1998;53:333-338.

48. Huang Z, Huang PL, Panahian N, et al. Effects of cerebral ischemia in mice deficient in neuronal nitric oxide synthase. *Science* 1994;265:1883-1885.

49. Huang PL, Huang Z, Mashimo H, et al. Hypertension in mice lacking the gene for endothelial nitric oxide synthase. *Nature* 1995;377:239-242.

50. Huang Z, Huang PL, Fishman MC, et al. Focal cerebral ischemia in mice deficient in either endothelial (eNOS) or neuronal nitric oxide (nNOS) synthase. *Stroke* 1996;27:173 (Abstract).

51. Iadecola C, Zhang F, Casey R, et al. Delayed reduction of ischemic brain injury and neurological deficits in mice lacking the inducible nitric oxide synthase gene. *J Neurosci* 1997;17:9157-9164.

52. Crumrine RC, Thomas AL, Morgan PF. Attenuation of p53 expression protects against focal ischemic damage in transgenic mice. *J Cereb Blood Flow Metab* 1994;14:887-891.

53. Kondo T, Reaume AG, Huang T-T, et al. Reduction of CuZn-superoxide dismutase activity exacerbates neuronal cell injury and edema formation after transient focal cerebral ischemia. *J Neurosci* 1997;17:4180-4189.

54. Mikawa S, Li Y, Huang TT, et al. Cerebral infarction is exacerbated in mitochondrial manganese superoxide dismutase (Sod-2) knockout mutant mice after focal cerebral ischemia and reperfusion. *Soc Neurosci Abstr* 1995;21:1268.

55. Murakami K, Kondo T, Epstein CJ, et al. Overexpression of CuZn-superoxide dismutase reduces hippocampal injury after global ischemia in transgenic mice. *Stroke* 1996;28:1797-1804.

56. Hara H, Huang PL, Panahian N, et al. Reduced brain edema and infarction volume in mice lacking the neuronal isoform of nitric oxide synthase after transient MCA occlusion. *J Cereb Blood Flow Metab* 1996;16:605-611.

57. Panahian N, Yoshida T, Huang PL, et al. Attenuated hippocampal damage after global cerebral ischemia in mice mutant in neuronal nitric oxide synthase. *Neuroscience* 1996;72:343-354.

58. Zhang F, Eckman C, Younkin S, et al. Increased susceptibility to ischemic brain damage in transgenic mice overexpressing the amyloid precursor protein. *J Neurosci* 1997;17:7655-7661.

59. Nogawa S, Zhang F, Ross ME, et al. Cyclo-oxygenase-2 gene expression in neurons contributes to ischemic brain damage. *J Neurosci* 1997;17:2746-2755.

Chapter 7

Estrogen as Neuroprotectant in Stroke

*Patricia D. Hurn, PhD, Nabil J. Alkayed,
MD, PhD, Barbara J. Crain, MD, PhD,
Valina L. Dawson PhD, Ted M. Dawson,
MD, PhD, Allen S. Mandir, MD, PhD,
Renata Rusa, MD, Kenji Sampei, MD,
Masahiko Sawada, MD,
Thomas J.K. Toung, MD, and
Richard J. Traystman, PhD*

Introduction

Women are at lower risk than men for stroke. However, cerebral ischemic events do occur in women at all ages and increase in frequency after the menopause, closing this apparent "gender gap." The value of postmenopausal estrogen replacement therapy (ERT) is controversial, with reports of increased,[1] decreased,[2,3] or unchanged[4] stroke risk in ERT users. Most critically, we know little about the comparative vulnerability of females and males to neuronal injury once a vascular incident has occurred or the impact of altering the brain's reproductive steroid milieu on stroke recovery. Estrogen exhibits both vascular[5,6] and nonvascular effects,[7-9] via genomic and nongenomic mechanisms, many of which could confer neuroprotection in the hormone treated brain. Our present studies were designed to determine: 1) if there are inherent

Supported by NIH grants NR33668, NS33668, NS20020

sex-linked injury mechanisms in experimental stroke and 2) if treatment with 17-β estradiol, the principal biologically active estrogen in mammals, can salvage brain tissue after an ischemic event in female or male animals. All animal studies were conducted in accordance with the National Institutes of Health guidelines for the care and use of animals in research. All protocols were approved by our institutional Animal Care and Use Committee. All data are reported as means ± standard error.

Gender Differences in Experimental Stroke

Data from recent animal studies suggest that there are significant gender-specific responses to experimental cerebral ischemia. Female gerbils have lower incidence of and less severe neuronal damage after carotid occlusion than males.[7] Further, thromboembolism induced by carotid artery irradiation produces greater inflammation, but less severe infarcts, in female as compared to male rats.[10] There is also scattered evidence for gender-specific responses to a variety of forms of neuroinjury, including cerebral contusion[11] and hypoxic brain damage.[12] Our studies have used a reversible middle cerebral artery occlusion (MCAO) model to compare differences in histologic outcome among sexually mature, adult males, females and ovariectomized females (OVX). In our animal model, MCAO was accomplished by the intraluminal suture technique for 2 hours of occlusion, followed by removal of the obstructing suture and 22 hours of reperfusion.[13] Laser doppler flowmetry (LDF) was monitored over the parietal cortex to evaluate the ischemic insult throughout the 2 hours of MCAO and immediate reperfusion. Because estrogen is known to be vasoactive, we also measured end-ischemic regional cerebral blood flow (rCBF) using ^{14}C iodoantipyrine autoradiography.[13] Two genetic rat strains were studied at 13-15 weeks of age: non-stroke prone Wistar and spontaneously hypertensive, genetically stroke prone (SHRSP) strain.[13] The purpose was to determine the contribution of blood flow preservation or nonvascular mechanisms to stroke outcome in males, females and OVX. Physiological parameters were controlled and not different among treatment groups. Plasma 17-β estradiol and progesterone levels were determined by radioimmunoassay, as previously described.[14]

Figure 1 summarizes infarction volumes as determined by 2,3,5-triphenyl-tetrazolium chloride (TTC) staining in the cortex and caudate-putamen of Wistar rats. Male and ovariectomized rats sustained larger infarcts than females in both brain regions. Reduction of the LDF signal during MCAO was consistently less in females than in males or OVX (38% ± 3% of baseline in females, as compared to 30% ± 1% and 27%

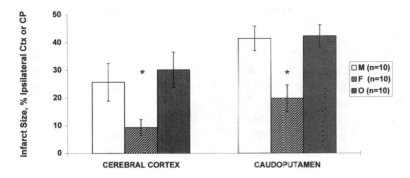

Figure 1. Cerebral infarction after middle cerebral artery occlusion in 3-month-old adult Wistar rats. Infarction volumes were measured at 22 hours of reperfusion by TTC staining and expressed as a percentage of the ipsilateral cortex (Ctx) or caudate-putamen (CP). Values are means ± standard errors for three groups: males (M), females (F), and ovariectomized females (O). * Different from M and O at P ≤ 0.05. Used with permission.[13]

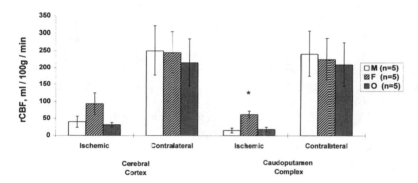

Figure 2. Regional cerebral blood flow (mL/100g/min) as measured by ^{14}C iodoantipyrine autoradiography at 2 hours of middle cerebral artery occlusion. Values are means ± standard errors for three groups of 3-month-old adult Wistar rats: males (M), females (F), and ovariectomized females (O). *Different from M and O at P ≤ 0.05. Used with permission.[13]

± 1% in males and OVX, respectively). Although SHRSP rats had greater infarction size and more severe reduction of the LDF signal during MCAO relative to Wistar rats, the effects of gender and ovariectomy were similar in each strain. Figure 2 shows rCBF at end-ischemia in ischemic regions supplied by the middle cerebral artery and nonischemic, contralateral structures. Females sustained significantly higher rCBF only in the caudate-putamen relative to males or OVX. Mean flow rates in the nonischemic, contralateral tissue were similar among the three groups (eg, in cortex, 246 ± 70 in males, 237 ± 60 in females, and 213 ± 70 ml/100g/min in OVX).

These data suggest that there are significant gender differences in response to focal cerebral ischemia after cerebrovascular occlusion, and that the effect is important in both genetically stroke prone animals and normal Wistars. Loss of female sex steroids eliminated the protection ordinarily enjoyed by the female, and infarction volumes in OVX resembled those of the male animal. It seems likely that estrogen was the major hormonal neuroprotectant in these experiments, because: 1) estrogen levels were reduced in OVX to that of the male, and 2) although progesterone was reduced relative to normal female values, plasma values remained higher than in the male. Lastly, the data indicate that endogenous estrogen likely acts via both flow-mediated and non-vascular mechanisms in ischemic stroke.

Estrogen Replacement Therapy and Stroke in Female Animals

Using the same experimental model, we have determined if estrogen restoration to physiological levels reduces infarction volume after MCAO in ovariectomized Wistar rats.[15,16] Cohorts of ovariectomized females were treated with either 0, 25, or 100 μg 17-β estradiol implants, yielding plasma estradiol levels of 3 ± 2, 20 ± 25, and 38 ± 20 ng/mL in the three respective groups. Plasma progesterone levels were reduced from normal values in all animals, and similar among groups (9 ± 5, 12 ± 7, and 9 ± 4 ng/mL in 0, 25, and 100 μg groups). Both cortical and striatal infarction volumes were reduced in the 25 μg vs 0 μg group (from 12 ± 10 to 3% $\pm$ 8% in cortex and from 31% $\pm$ 20% to 13% $\pm$ 12 % in the caudate-putamen). There was no difference in infarction between the 100 and 0 μg treatment groups. Monitoring of LDF during MCAO indicated that the signal was reduced to approximately 30% of baseline in all animals, regardless of treatment group. Similarly, end-ischemic regional CBF, as measured with ^{14}C iodoantipyrine autoradiography, was not altered in animals treated with the neuroprotective 25 μg estradiol dose. These data suggest that exogenous estrogen treatment can ameliorate injury after vascular occlusion in previously estrogen-deficient female rats. However, estrogen replacement to physiological, rather than supraphysiological levels, appears essential for neuroprotection. Therefore, the therapeutic window in females may be narrow.

Estrogen as Neuroprotectant in the Male Brain

An important question is whether exogenous estrogen can protect the male brain, interacting with tissue not ordinarily exposed to high concentrations of female reproductive steroids. We hypothesized that estrogen treatment to levels considered physiological in females might also be effective in male rats and reduce stroke injury.[17] Further, testosterone was examined, in part, to determine if the steroid's activity could be excluded as an alternative explanation for gender differences in stroke. Like estrogen, testosterone is a vasodilator of some vascular beds.[18,19] possibly by a common mechanism involving vascular smooth muscle potassium channels.[20] Androgen receptors are present in brain regions not associated with reproduction, but their localization in cerebral vessels is unclear.[21] Therefore, we reasoned that exogenous estrogen treatment in males could interact with native testosterone and alter tissue outcome after MCAO.

Male Wistar rats were treated with acute or chronic estrogen administration: Premarin (USP) 1mg/kg IV, immediately prior to MCAO (Acute, n = 13, plasma estradiol = 171 ± 51 pg/mL); 7 days of 25 μg (E25, n = 10, 10 ± 3 pg/mL) or 100 μg 17-β estradiol (E100, n = 12, 69 ± 20 pg/mL) by subcutaneous implant; or saline (SAL, n = 21, 3 ± 1 pg/mL).[17] Cortical infarct volumes were reduced in all estrogen treated groups: acute (21% ± 4% of ipsilateral cortex), E25 (12% ± 5%) and E100 (12% ± 3%) relative to SAL (38% ± 5%). Caudate infarction was similarly decreased: acute (39% ± 7% of ipsilateral striatum), E25 (25% ± 7%) and E100 (34% ± 6%) relative to SAL (63% ± 4%). In a second protocol, rats were castrated to deplete endogenous testosterone then treated with the 25 or 100 μg estradiol implants. Castration did not alter ischemic outcome; cortical and caudate infarction (% of respective ipsilateral regions) were 37% ± 5% and 59% ± 5% in castrated males and 39% ± 7% and 57% ± 5% in noncastrated males. Estrogen replacement reduced infarction volume in castrated animals to the same extent as in noncastrated males. It was also observed via LDF monitoring that the signal was reduced to approximately 25% of baseline in all animals, regardless of treatment group.

These data suggest that both acute and chronic 17-β estradiol treatment protects male brain in experimental stroke. Doses which yield physiological or supraphysiological plasma steroid levels are equally efficacious in the male, unlike the female rat. Because even a single Premarin injection immediately prior to MCAO strongly reduces tissue injury, nongenomic mechanisms of action are likely. Further, testosterone is not deleterious to the ischemic male brain, nor does testosterone availability alter estradiol-mediated tissue salvage after MCAO.

Reproductively Senescent Animals

We have also examined stroke outcomes in 16 month old, reproductively senescent Wistar rats to test the hypothesis that gender differ-

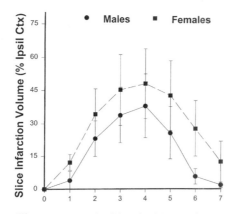

Figure 3. Gender differences are lacking in 16 month, reproductively senescent Wistar rats treated with 2 hours of middle cerebral artery occlusion and 22 hours of reperfusion. Infarction volume was not different between males and females in the cortex or striatum (not shown here). Values are means ± standard errors for 7 brain slices, expressed as a percentage of the ipsilateral cortex.

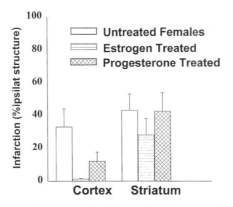

Figure 4. Hormone replacement in 16-month-old, reproductively senescent Wistar female rats. All animals were treated with 2 hours of reversible middle cerebral artery occlusion and 22 hours of reperfusion. See text for details of hormone treatment paradigm. Values are means ± standard errors for each group of five animals, shown as a percentage of the ipsilateral cortex or striatum.

ences are lost as endogenous hormone levels wane.[22] As shown in Figure 3, stroke volume after MCAO (2 hours of occlusion, 22 hours reperfusion) is equivalent in females and males. These observations are consistent with the concept that endogenous ovarian steroids are neuroprotective in stroke and offer an insight into the rise in stroke rates in postmenopausal versus premenopausal human females. When estrogen is restored in females via subcutaneous 17β-estradiol implant (25 μg, 7–10 days duration), infarction size is reduced (Figure 4). The effect is most prominant in cortex. Chronic progesterone treatment (10 mg implant, 7–10 days duration) also reduces cortical injury, but less dramatically. Whether combined estrogen-progestin treatment further protects the brain, or results in a deleterious interaction, remains to be shown. Nevertheless, these unique experiments in aged Wistars demonstrate that the benefit of estrogen replacement is not restricted to young animals, artificially deprived of ovarian steroids. Physiological doses of 17-β estradiol are clearly efficacious in the reproductively senescent rat.

Multiple Mechanisms are Likely

In combination, these studies suggest that endogenous estrogen acts by both flow-mediated and non-vascular mechanisms to reduce tissue injury during MCAO, while pharmacological estrogen preparations activate parenchymal mechanisms. The estrogenic steroids are believed to have both classical genomic actions and less well understood, nongenomic cell membrane-associated activity.[23] Classical estrogen signaling occurs via an intracellular receptor, essentially a ligand-activated transcription factor that binds target DNA and alters gene transcription (Figure 5). Estrogen receptor (ER)-mediated gene transcription is initiated as the protein's binding domain interacts with a hormone responsive element or consensus palindromic DNA sequence. Estrogen receptor antagonists (eg, tamoxifen and the steroid ICI family) block estrogen's actions by inhibiting ER- initiated gene activation in a tissue-specific manner.[24] Because there are estrogen response elements on the genes which regulate rate-limiting enzymes required for biosynthesis of both prostacyclin (PGI_2) and nitric oxide, it is possible that estrogen amplifies vasodilator release.[25] A large literature links estrogen to endothelium-dependent vasodilation in the coronary and uterine circulations, and suggests that estrogen may upregulate nitric oxide synthase (NOS). We have shown that chronic estrogen treatment elevates basal cerebral microvascular cGMP content, although the effect is restricted to high estradiol doses of pure pharmacological relevance.[26]

However, our studies demonstrate that exogenous estrogen significantly reduces stroke volume without altering intra-ischemic CBF. This suggests that the impact on stroke outcome occurs via non-vascular mechanisms within the parenchyma. Estrogen has a widespread group of cellular targets within the brain. Early autoradiographic studies using ^{3}H-estradiol injections demonstrate numerous sites of nuclear accumulation and retention of radioactivity in the brain and spinal cord of both sexes.[27] Further, the steroid has direct and surprisingly rapid effects on neuronal tissue, for example, by altering synaptic plas-

Classical Steroid Receptor Signaling

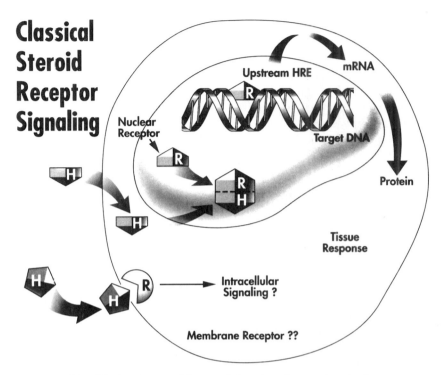

Figure 5. Simplified schema of intracellular signaling pathways for estrogen in hormonally responsive tissue.

ticity. Synaptic density within areas such as the hippocampus fluctuates with the estrous cycle and can be altered in less than 24 hours by exogenous estradiol.[28] Hormone response elements for estrogen are present on numerous genes, including the constituitive isoform of NOS.[29] Nitric oxide synthase activity in cerebellar homogenates has been reported to increase during pregnancy or estrogen treatment.[30] Thus we examined stroke outcomes in female transgenic mice deficient in neuronal NOS (nNOS) to determine if there are gender differences in nNOS-mediated neuroinjury.[31] Age-matched male and female (20–29g) mice were anesthetized with 1%–1.2% halothane and treated with permanent unilateral MCAO by the intraluminal filament insertion technique. After 18 hours of MCAO, the brain was analyzed by TTC staining for infarction volume. Genetic screening to confirm nNOS deletion was performed by PCR from DNA extracted and purified from tail samples. Male nNOS deficient mice were well protected during MCAO as compared to their wild-type counterparts, as has been previously reported.[32] However, female animals appeared indifferent to nNOS deficiency in that infarction volume was not different in any brain region as compared to that sustained by female wild-type animals. These data suggest that estrogen's neuroprotective properties in stroke are not mediated through nitric oxide-associated mechanisms. The overall importance of NO-toxicity in the female brain requires further investigation.

Conclusions

There are significant sex-linked differences in tissue damage after experimental stroke. Endogenous estrogens appear to be neuroprotective by a combination of non-vascular mechanisms and by partial preservation of intra-ischemic rCBF in selected brain regions. In contrast, exogenous 17-β estradiol treatment protects the brain without altering rCBF, likely by direct effect on neurons and/or glia. The cellular and molecular mechanisms are likely multifactorial and not related to nNOS-mediated injury. Lastly, pre-ischemic estrogen treatment is effective in both male and female brain, although the dose and mechanisms may differ between the sexes. Although these findings suggest a plausible and novel clinical utility for estrogen, numerous experiments are needed in the future to determine the steroid's therapeutic window of activity and dose-response relationships in stroke.

References

1. Wilson PWF, Garrison RJ, Castelli W. Postmenopausal estrogen use, cigarette smoking, and cardiovascular morbidity in women over 50. *N Engl J Med* 1985;313:1038-1043.
2. Finucane FF, Madans JH, Bush TL, et al. Decreased risk of stroke among postmenopausal hormone users. *Arch Intern Med* 1993;153:73-79.
3. Paganini-Hill A, Ross RK, Henderson BE. Postmenopausal oestrogen treatment and stroke: A prospective study. *Br Med J* 1988;297:519-522.
4. Petitti DB, Sidney S, Quesenberry CP Jr, et al. Ischemic stroke and use of estrogen and estrogen / progestogen as hormone replacement therapy. *Stroke* 1998;29:23-28.
5. Farhat MY, Lavigne MC, Ramwell PW. The vascular protective effects of estrogen. *FASEB* 1996;10:615-624.
6. Mendelsohn ME, Karas RH. Estrogen and the blood vessel wall. *Curr Opin Cardiol* 1994;9:619-626.
7. Hall ED, Pazara KE, Linseman KL. Sex differences in postischemic neuronal necrosis in gerbils. *J Cereb Blood Flow Metab* 1991;11:292-298.
8. Mermelstein PG, Becker JB, Surmeier DJ. Estradiol reduces calcium currents in rat neostriatal neurons via a membrane receptor. *J Neurosci* 1996;16(2):595-604.
9. Woolley CS, McEwen BS. Estradiol mediates fluctuation in hippocampal synapse density during the estrous cycle in the adult rat. *J Neurosci* 1992;12:2549-2554.

10. Li K, Futrell N, Tovar S, et al. Gender influences the magnitude of the inflammatory response within embolic infarcts in young rats. *Stroke* 1996;27:498-503.

11. Roof RL, Duvdevani R, Stein DG. Gender influences outcome of brain injury: Progesterone plays a protective role. *Brain Res* 1993;607:333-336.

12. Saiyed M, Riker WK. Cholinergic and anticholinergic drug effects on survival during hypoxia: Significant gender differences. *J Pharmacol Exp Ther* 1993;264:1146-1153.

13. Alkayed NJ, Harukuni I, Kimes AS, et al. Gender-linked brain injury in experimental stroke. *Stroke* 1998;29:159-166.

14. Hurn PD, Littleton-Kearney MT, Kirsch JR, et al. Postischemic cerebral blood flow recovery in the female: Effect of 17β-estradiol. *J Cereb Blood Flow Metab* 1995;15:666-672.

15. Rusa R, Crain B, Traystman R, et al. Protective role of estrogen in experimental stroke. *J Cereb Blood Flow Metab* 1997;17:S384.

16. Rusa R, Crain B, Traystman R, et al. Neuroprotective effect of 17β estradiol in experimental stroke. *Stroke* 1998;29:330.

17. Toung TJK, Traystman RJ, Hurn PD. Estrogen-mediated neuroprotection after experimental stroke in males. *Stroke* 1998; 29(8):1666-1670.

18. Yue P, Chatterjee K, Beale C, et al. Testosterone relaxes rabbit coronary arteries and aorta. *Circulation* 1995;91:1154-1160.

19. Chou TM, Sudhir K, Hutchison SJ, et al. Testosterone induces dilation of coronary conductance and resistance arteries in vivo. *Circulation* 1996;94(10):2614-9.

20. White RE, Darkow DJ, Falvo Lang JLF. Estrogen relaxes coronary arteries by opening BKCa channels through a cGMP-dependent mechanism. *Circ Res* 1995;77:936-942.

21. Takeda H, Chodak G, Mutchnik S, et al. Immunohistochemical localization of androgen receptors with mono-and polyclonal antibodies to androgen receptor. *J Endocrinol* 1990;126:17-25.

22. Hurn PD, Alkayed NJ, Crain BJ, et al. Estrogen reduces infarct size after MCA occlusion in postmenopausal rats. *FASEB J* 1998;12;A394.

23. Tischkau SA, Ramirez VD. A specific membrane binding protein for progesterone in rat brain: Sex differences and induction by estrogen. *PNAS* 1993;90:1285-1289.

24. Kangas L. Agonistic and antagonistic effects of antiestrogens in different target organs. *Acta Oncologica* 1992;31:143-146.

25. Mendelsohn ME, Karas RH. Estrogen and the blood vessel wall. *Current Opinion in Cardiol* 1994;9:619-626.

26. Palmon SC, Williams MJ, Littleton-Kearney M, et al. Estrogen increases cGMP in selected brain regions and in cerebral microvessels. *J Cereb Blood Flow Metab* 1998;18(11):1248-1252.

27. Stumpf WE. Estradiol concentrating neurons. *Science* 1986;162:1001-1003.

28. Woolley CS, McEwen BS. Estradiol mediates fluctuation in hippocampal synapse density during the estrous cycle in the adult rat. *J Neurosci* 1992;12:2549-2554.

29. Venema RC, Nishida K, Alexander RW, et al. Orgainzation of the bovine gene encoding endothelial nitric oxide synthase. *Biochim Biophy Acta* 1994;1218:413-420.

30. Weiner CP, Lizasoain I, Baylis SA, et al. Induction of calcium-dependent nitric oxide synthases by sex hormones. *PNAS* 1994;91:5212-5216.
31. Sampei K, Asano Y, Mandir AS, et al. Stroke outcome in antioxidant transgenics: nNOS, Cu-Zn superoxide dismutase and combined mutants. *J Cereb Blood Flow Metab* 1997;17(I):S454.
32. Huang Z, Huang PL, Panahian N, et al. Effects of cerebral ischemia in mice deficient in neuronal nitric oxide synthase. *Science* 1994;265:1882-1885.

Chapter 8

HMG-CoA Reductase Inhibitors Reduce Cerebral Infarct Size by Upregulating Endothelial Nitric Oxide Synthase

Matthias Endres, MD, Ulrich Laufs, MD, James K. Liao, MD, and Michael A. Moskowitz, MD

Introduction

So far, only agents which inhibit thrombocyte aggregation or block the coagulation cascade are used for the prophylactic treatment of ischemic strokes. We demonstrate that the cholesterol-lowering drugs, HMG-CoA reductase inhibitors, decrease stroke damage by a novel mechanism mediated by endothelial nitric oxide synthase (eNOS) upregulation. After chronic treatment of normocholesterolemic mice, HMG-CoA reductase inhibitors augmented cerebral blood flow, reduced cerebral infarct size, and improved neurological function. The upregulation of eNOS by HMG-CoA reductase inhibitors was not associated with changes in serum cholesterol levels, but was reversed by co-treatment with a downstream intermediate, L-mevalonate. HMG-CoA reductase inhibitors had no neuroprotective effects in eNOS-deficient mice,[1] indicating that eNOS upregulation is the predominant, if not the only, mechanism by which HMG-CoA reductase inhibitors

This work was supported by grants from the Deutsche Forschungsgemeinschaft (M.E. and U.L) and the National Institutes of Health (M.A.M and J.K.L.).

From: Choi D, Dacey RG, Hsu CY, Powers WJ. *Cerebrovascular Disease: Momentum at the End of the Second Millennium.* Armonk, NY: Futura Publishing Company, Inc., © 2002.

protect against stroke damage. We suggest that HMG-CoA reductase inhibitors may be used as a novel prophylactic treatment strategy for augmenting cerebral blood flow and reducing brain damage after cerebral ischemia.

Ischemic stroke is a major cause of morbidity and mortality in the elderly population and in patients undergoing cardiovascular surgery.[3] The prophylactic treatment strategies for ischemic strokes are largely limited to decreasing the incidence of ischemic strokes by antiplatelet therapy and do not address the larger issue of reducing stroke size.[2] Although thrombolytic therapy is effective in acutely reducing ischemic stroke size, these agents must be given within a short time after the onset of cerebral ischemia and may cause intracranial hemorrhage.[4] The cholesterol-lowering agents, HMG-CoA reductase inhibitors, have been shown to reduce the incidence of myocardial and cerebral infarctions in hypercholesterolemic individuals.[5,6] Although the beneficial effects are generally believed to be due only to their effects on serum cholesterol levels, recent studies comparing HMG-CoA reductase inhibitors with other cholesterol-lowering drugs have challenged this notion.[7] Since ischemic strokes are not restricted to individuals with hypercholesterolemia, it is important to determine whether these agents can exert neuroprotective effects independent of serum cholesterol levels.

Accordingly, normocholesterolemic, wild-type 129/SV mice were injected subcutaneously daily for 3 or 14 days with simvastatin (Sim, 0.2, 2.0, and 20 mg kg^{-1}). Cerebral infarctions were produced by monofilament occlusion of the left middle cerebral artery (MCA) for 2 hours followed by 22 hours of reperfusion.[8] Pretreatment with Sim for 14 days reduced cerebral infarct size in a concentration-dependent manner by 20%, 25%, and 47% (Figure 1A). The smaller cerebral infarcts in Sim-treated mice persisted for up to 72 hours after MCA occlusion (37% reduction in infarct volume in Sim 2.0 mg kg^{-1} compared to vehicle, $P < 0.01$, n = 9 per group) and corresponded to decreases in neurological motor deficits (Figure 1B).[8] Similar effects of Sim (20 mg kg^{-1}, 14 days) were observed in another strain of wild-type mice (C57BL/6NCrlBR) where cerebral infarct sizes were reduced by 32% compared to untreated animals ($P < 0.05$, n = 8 and 12, respectively). Pretreatment with Sim (2.0 or 20 mg kg^{1}, n = 5-10 per group) for a shorter duration (ie, 3 days) correspondingly produced less neurological benefits (ie, 19% reduction in infarct volume).

To determine whether the neuroprotective effects of Sim were due to changes in cerebral blood flow (CBF), absolute CBF was measured in ventilated mice using an indicator fractionation technique with N-isopropyl-[methyl 1,3 ^{14}C]-*p*-iodoamphetamine.[9] Basal hemispheric CBF was increased by 31% after treatment with Sim (20 mg kg^{-1}) com-

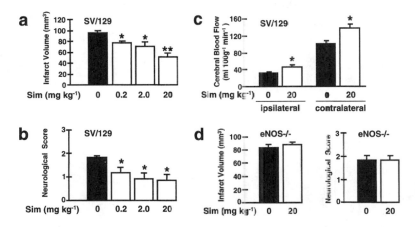

Figure 1. **A.** Treatment with simvastatin (0.2, 2.0 or 20 mg kg^{-1}, subcutaneously daily for 14 days) significantly reduced infarct size after 2 hours of filamentous middle cerebral artery (MCA) occlusion and 22 hours of reperfusion compared to vehicle-injected 129/SV mice. Mean infarct volumes in control groups for each treatment did not vary by more than 5% and are therefore shown as a single group (n = 22). Cerebral infarction volume was determined quantitatively.[8] Smaller infarct sizes were confirmed with an indirect method which corrects for brain swelling.[8] (n = 9–18 per treatment group). *P < 0.05, **P < 0.01. **B.** Sensory-motor deficits were significantly reduced in 129/SV mice treated with simvastatin compared to controls. Mean deficits in control groups for each treatment did not vary by more than 5% and are therefore shown as a single group (n = 22). Deficits were evaluated by a naive observer using a rating system from 0 (no deficit) to 3 (severe).[5] (n = 9–18 per treatment group). *P < 0.05. **C.** Absolute cerebral blood flow (CBF) was increased in simvastatin-treated mice during focal cerebral ischemia. Wild-type 129/SV mice were injected subcutaneously with saline (n = 10) or simvastatin 20 mg kg^{-1} (n=10) for 14 days. Mice were anesthetized and ventilated and absolute CBF was determined 30 min after filamentous occlusion of the left middle cerebral artery in ischemic tissue (ipsilateral) and corresponding tissue from the contralateral hemisphere using an indicator fractionation technique.[9] *P < 0.05 **D.** Effects of simvastatin on infarct volume and neurological deficits in eNOS-deficient mice (eNOS-/-)[2] after MCA occlusion/reperfusion. Unlike wild-type mice, treatment with simvastatin (20 mg kg^{-1} daily for 14 days) had no effect on infarct volumes or neurological motor deficits in eNOS-deficient mice following MCA occlusion/reperfusion. (Modified from Endres et al.[22])

pared to controls (151 ± 5 versus 117 ± 7 mL 100 g^{-1} min^{-1}, P < 0.05, n = 8 per group). Similar increases in resting blood flow were observed in cerebellum and brainstem. Laser-Doppler flow measurements demonstrated equivalent percent reductions in relative CBF during MCA occlusion (Table 1). However, absolute CBF during ischemia was 48% higher in the ischemic (ipsilateral) and 34% higher in the non-ischemic (contralateral) hemispheres of Sim-treated mice (20 mg kg^{-1} for 14 days) (Figure 1C). The neuroprotective effects of Sim are most likely

Table 1.

Physiologic variables at baseline and during ischemia in SV/129 mice

Parameter	control (n=6)	Sim 0.2 mg kg^{-1} (n=6)	Sim 2.0 mg kg^{-1} (n=6)	Sim 20 mg kg^{-1} (n=6)
MABP (mmHg)				
baseline	90.3 ± 4.5	84.5 ± 4.4	86.3 ± 3.8	86.3 ± 4.9
during	88.8 ± 3.0	84.8 ± 2.5	89.8 ± 2.6	73.2 ± 1.7#
after	82.2 ± 4.1	84.0 ± 4.8	84.3 ± 1.9	76.7 ± 5.0
HR (bpm)				
baseline	424 ± 26	427 ± 23	418 ± 12	489 ± 15
during	438 ± 32	416 ± 25	469 ± 31	488 ± 18
after	466 ± 17	416 ± 25	470 ± 23	560 ± 9¶
pH				
baseline	7.31 ± 0.01	7.30 ± 0.03	7.32 ± 0.01	7.31 ± 0.01
after	7.30 ± 0.02	7.28 ± 0.01	7.29 ± 0.01	7.27 ± 0.02
PaO$_2$ (mmHg)				
baseline	147 ± 16	162 ± 9	156 ± 8	150 ± 5
after	139 ± 15	145 ± 7	149 ± 9	134 ± 6
PaCO$_2$ (mmHg)				
baseline	43.0 ± 1.7	40.0 ± 2.7	42.3 ± 1.4	42.9 ± 1.2
after	41.5 ± 1.2	41.4 ± 0.9	40.2 ± 1.3	43.1 ± 1.9
rCBF (%)				
during	17 ± 3	16 ± 4	14 ± 2	15 ± 2
after	94 ± 8	94 ± 7	85 ± 1.2	89 ± 4

Table 1.

(continued)

Parameter	control (n=6)	Sim 0.2 mg kg^{-1} (n=6)	Sim 2.0 mg kg^{-1} (n=6)	Sim 20 mg kg^{-1} (n=6)
Cholesterol (mg dl^{-1})	140 ± 7 (n=12)	n.d.	158 ± 5 (n=8)	120 ± 20 (n=7)
ALT (U l^{-1})	119 ± 29	n.d.	136 ± 45	124 ± 27
Creatinine (mg dl^{-1})	<0.2	n.d.	<0.2	<0.2
Glucose (mg dl^{-1})	128 ± 2	n.d.	n.d.	124 ± 13

Mice were injected subcutaneously with simvastatin (0.2, 2.0 or 20 mg kg^{-1}) or saline (controls) for 14 days and then subjected to 2 h middle cerebral artery occlusion followed by reperfusion.[8] MABP (mean arterial blood pressure), HR (heart rate), and rCBF (regional cerebral blood flow) were measured at baseline, during MCA occlusion, and until 30 min after reperfusion.[8] Fifty microliter of blood were withdrawn twice, before and directly after MCA occlusion for blood gas determination (pH, PaCO$_2$, PaO$_2$). Rectal temperatures were maintained at 36.5 C ± 1 C by a heating blanket and a feedback control unit and did not differ between groups. After 22 h of reperfusion, blood was withdrawn and serum levels of cholesterol, alanine aminotransferase (ALT), creatinine and glucose were determined. Data are presented as mean ± SE. # P < 0.05 vs control, Sim 0.2 and Sim 2.0; ¶ P < 0.05 vs control, Sim 0.2, Sim 2.0 and vs baseline and during MCA occlusion. (modified from Endres et al., *Proc. Natl. Acad. Sci. U.S.A.*, 1998, submitted)

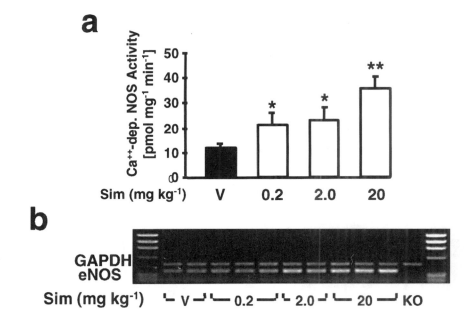

Figure 2. A. NOS catalytic activity was increased in aortas from wild-type 129/SV mice treated with simvastatin (0.2, 2.0 or 20 mg kg^{-1} s.c. for 14 days) compared to vehicle-treated mice. The Ca^{++}-dependent NOS activity was determined by [^{14}C]-arginine to [^{14}C]-citrulline conversion *in vitro*.[2,16] *P < 0.05, **P < 0.01 (n = 5-20 animals per group). **B.** Semi-quantitative RT-PCR demonstrating increases in eNOS mRNA expression after treatment with simvastatin for 14 days in aortas of 129/SV mice. The eNOS-deficient mice (KO) lack eNOS mRNA. Compared to vehicle-treated mice (V), treatment with simvastatin (0.2, 2.0, and 20 mg kg^{-1}) increased eNOS mRNA levels by 31% ± 3% (P < 0.05), 192% ± 7.5% (P < 0.05) and 257% ± 20% (P < 0.01), respectively. Glyceraldehyde 3-phosphate dehydrogenase (GAPDH) mRNA expression was used as an internal standard for comparison. (n = 5 per group). (Modified from Endres et al.[22])

attributed to augmentation of CBF, since Sim had no direct effects on neuronal cells *in vitro* and did not protect human neuroblastoma (SH-SY5Y)[10] or rat pheochromocytoma cell lines (PC-12)[11] from hypoxic injury (data not shown).

Since the endogenous vasodilator, nitric oxide (NO), is an important regulator of blood pressure and blood flow,[1,12-14] we postulated that the neuroprotective effects of HMG-CoA reductase inhibitors may be mediated by endothelium-derived NO. Indeed, mice that are deficient in eNOS exhibit larger cerebral infarcts following MCA occlusion compared to wild-type mice.[15] Treatment with Sim increased Ca^{++}-dependent NOS activity in mice aortas by 1.8- to 3.0-fold, as assayed by [^{14}C]-arginine to [^{14}C]-citrulline conversion (Figure 2A).[1,16] This increase in aortic Ca^{++}-dependent NOS activity by Sim correlated with higher eNOS mRNA levels as measured by semi-quantitative reverse transcription-polymerase chain reaction (Figure 2B). Increased eNOS mRNA levels were also observed in the brains of Sim-treated mice. Neuronal NOS (nNOS) mRNA which was detected in the brain and at low levels in the aorta, was not affected by Sim. Inducible NOS (iNOS) mRNA was not detected under any treatment conditions.

When the cholesterol concentration was clamped *in vitro*, the upregulation of eNOS by Sim was completely reversed in the presence of L-mevalonate, suggesting that increases in eNOS expression *in vivo* are mediated via inhibition of endothelial rather than hepatic HMG-CoA reductase (data not shown). Indeed, by linear regression analyses, there was no correlation between serum cholesterol levels and cerebral infarct sizes (Table 1). Moreover, lovastatin (20 mg kg^{-1} for 14 days), another HMG-CoA reductase inhibitor, also reduced cerebral infarct size by 20% (95 ± 5 to 76 ± 7 mm^3, $P < 0.05$, n = 9 per group) albeit to a lesser extent compared to Sim. Cerebral protection by Sim was not due to changes in arterial blood pressure, heart rate, glucose, PaCO$_2$, PaO$_2$, pH, or temperature (Table 1). In fact, rectal and temporalis muscle temperatures did not differ between groups ($\pm < 0.3°C$: $P > 0.05$) when measured hourly for up to 12 hours after MCA occlusion in vehicle and treated animals (n = 5 per group). At a higher concentration of Sim (ie, 20 mg kg^{-1}), there was a small decrease in arterial blood pressure during ischemia perhaps as a result of higher eNOS activity (Table 1).

To confirm that the upregulation of eNOS mediates the neuroprotective effects of Sim, mutant mice lacking the eNOS gene (eNOS-deficient mice)[1] were treated with Sim (20 mg kg^{-1}) for 14 days. In contrast to wild-type mice, there was no significant reduction in cerebral infarct size or neurological motor deficits in Sim-treated eNOS-deficient mice following MCA occlusion/reperfusion (Figure 1D). The relative CBF during ischemia in Sim- and vehicle-injected eNOS-deficient mice was not different (14% $\pm$ 2% and 15% $\pm$ 3% of baseline, $P > 0.05$). In addition, the cholesterol levels in eNOS-deficient mice were not significantly affected by treatment with Sim (120 $\pm$ 20 vs 140 $\pm$ 7 mg dl^{-1}, $P > 0.05$). The surprising and unique finding, however, is that Sim had no neuroprotective effects in eNOS-deficient mice, suggesting that the upregulation of eNOS is the predominant (if not the only) mechanism by which Sim reduces cerebral infarct size in normocholesterolemic mice. Although we chose to study CBF as an index of eNOS activity, other eNOS-mediated processes such as inhibition of platelet aggregation and monocyte adhesion to the vessel wall may also participate in the neuroprotective mechanism of these drugs.[17]

Since the neuroprotective effects of HMG-CoA reductase inhibitors occurred under normocholesterolemic conditions and in the absence of significant changes in serum cholesterol levels, our findings are distinct from the results of large clinical trials where these agents are found to reduce the incidence of cerebrovascular events in hypercholesterolemic individuals.[5-7] However, we speculate that HMG-CoA reductase inhibitors may decrease the incidence of ischemic stroke, in part, by reducing cerebral infarcts size to levels which are clinically unappreciated. Thus, the results of our study may have wider therapeutic importance since the majority of individuals with ischemic strokes have average cholesterol levels and are not treated with these agents.

Treatment with HMG-CoA reductase inhibitors could also be applicable in other conditions where cerebral ischemia may be encountered such as in patients undergoing elective coronary artery bypass surgery or carotid endarterectomy. By enhancing cerebral blood flow, HMG-CoA reductase inhibitors could also be used in conjuction with other therapeutic drugs to increase drug delivery to the central nervous system. Furthermore, the ability of these agents to upregulate eNOS activity may lead to other therapeutic advantages in the vessel wall. We propose that HMG-CoA reductase inhibitors be considered for the prophylactic treatment of ischemic strokes irrespective of serum cholesterol levels.

Methods

Drugs

HMG-CoA reductase inhibiting drugs (simvastatin and lovastatin, Merck & Co, Inc., Rahway, NJ, USA) were chemically activated by alkaline hydrolysis prior to subcutaneous injection or cell culture treatment as described.[18]

Cell Culture and eNOS Western Blotting

Human endothelial cells from saphenous veins were cultured as described.[19] Human neuroblastoma (SH-SY5Y) and pheochromocytoma cell lines (PC-12) were kindly provided by Gloria Lee, Harvard Medical School. Cells were cultured and differentiated by treatment with 16 nM of 12-0-tetradecanoyl-phorbol-13-acetate (TPA, Sigma) for SH-SY5Y and with 100 ng ml^{-1} of mouse nerve growth factor (Promega) for PC12 as described.[10, 11] Hypoxic conditions and evaluation of survival by trypan blue exclusion were performed as reported.[10] Immunoblotting using a murine monoclonal antibody to human eNOS

(Transduction Laboratories, Lexington, KY) was performed as described.[19]

Animals, Drug Treatment, and Experimental Ischemia

SV/129 and C57BL/6NCrlBR mice (18–22 g, Taconic Farm, Germantown, NY, USA) and eNOS-deficient mice[1] (18–22 g) were injected subcutaneously with 0.1 mL of activated Sim or Lov (0.2–20 mg kg^{-1}) or a corresponding volume of phosphate buffered saline once daily for 3 or 14 days.

Cerebral infarcts were produced by two-hours of MCA occlusion followed by reperfusion.[8] Regional CBF and physiologic parameters were monitored as described.[8] Rectal temperature was maintained at 36.5 ± 1°C with a temperature control unit (FHC, Brunswick, ME, USA) during the monitoring period. In some animals anesthesia was withdrawn after MCA occlusion and normal fluctuations in rectal and temporalis muscle temperature were measured for up to 12 hours. Animals were tested for neurological deficits (from 0 [no deficit] to 3 [severe]) either 22 or 70 hours after reperfusion by a blinded observer.[15] After sacrifice, cerebral infarct sizes were determined on 2,3,5-triphenyltetrazolium chloride-stained 2 mm brain sections (24 hours) or hematoxylin and eosin-stained 20 μm cryostat sections (72 hours) as described.[8] Absolute CBF was measured in anesthetized and ventilated animals under resting conditions or 30 min after filamentous MCA occlusion using an indicator fractionation technique as described.[9] For measurements during ischemia, tissue was obtained and values compared from homologous regions (ischemic and contralateral) enriched with tissue in the middle cerebral artery territory. Serum cholesterol, creatinine, creatinine kinase, and transaminases were determined by Tufts Veterinary Diagnostics Laboratory, Grafton, MA, USA.

Semiquantitative Reverse Transcription-Polymerase Chain Reaction (RT-PCR) and NOS Catalytic Activity

Tissues (aortas or cerebral hemispheres) were quickly isolated and frozen after sacrifice. Total RNA isolation, reverse transcription, and semi-quantitative competitive polymerase chain reaction (PCR) was performed according to standard techniques. The sense (5'-TTCCGGCTGCCACCTGATCCTAA-3') and antisense (5'-AACA-TATGTCC TTGCTCAAGGCA-3') primers for eNOS amplified a 340 bp fragment of murine eNOS which was confirmed by DNA sequencing.[16,20] Primer pairs for nNOS, iNOS and glyceraldehyde 3-phosphate dehydrogenase (GAPDH) were used as described elsewhere.[16,21] Each PCR cycle consisted of denaturing at 94° C for 30 seconds, annealing at 60° C for 30 seconds, and elongation at 72° C for 60 seconds. The linear exponential phases for eNOS and GAPDH PCR were 35 and 22 cycles, respectively. Equal amounts of corresponding NOS and GAPDH RT-PCR products were loaded on 1.5% agarose gels. Optical densities of ethidium-bromide stained DNA bands were quantitated using the NIH Image program[19] and results expressed as NOS/GAPDH ratios. Ca^{++}-dependent NOS catalytic activity was measured by the conversion of $[^{14}C]$-arginine to $[^{14}C]$-citrulline according to standard protocols with modifications as described.[1,16]

Data Analysis

Data are presented as mean ± standard error (SE). Differences between treatment and control groups were compared by paired or unpaired two-tailed student's t-test or by ANOVA followed by Dunnett-test (infarct size), Scheffe-test (physiologic parameters), or Bonferroni-test (absolute CBF). For comparisons of neurological deficits a non-parametric test was used (Mann-Whitney rank sum test). P values of less than 0.05 were considered statistically significant.

Acknowledgment   We thank Christian Waeber for help with the NOS activity assay and Paul L. Huang for providing eNOS knockout mice.

References

1. Huang PL, Huang Z, Mashimo H, et al. Hypertension in mice lacking the gene for endothelial nitric oxide synthase. *Nature* 1995;377:239-242.
2. Patrono C. Aspirin as an antiplatelet drug. *N Engl J Med* 1994;330:1287-1294.
3. Division of Chronic Disease Control and Community. Cardiovascular disease surveillance: Stroke, 1980-1989. Atlanta: Center for Disease Control and Prevention. 1994.
4. The National Insitute of Neurological Disorders and Stroke rt-PA Stroke Study Group. Tissue plasminogen activator for acute ischemic stroke. *N Engl J Med* 1995;333:1581-1587.
5. Scandinavian Simvastatin Survival Study Group. Randomized trial of cholesterol lowering in 4444 patients with coronary heart disease: The scandinavian simvastatin survival study (4S). *Lancet* 1994;344:1383-1389.
6. Cholesterol and Recurrent Events Trial Investigators. The effect of pravastatin on coronary events after myocardial infarction in patients with average cholesterol levels. *N Engl J Med* 1996;335:1001-1009.
7. Packard CJ. Relationship between LDL-cholesterol changes and coronary heart disease event reduction with pravastatin in the West of Scotland Coronary Prevention Study (WOSCOPS). *Circulation* 1997;96 (suppl I):I107.

8. Huang Z, Huang PL, Panahian N, et al. Effects of cerebral ischemia in mice deficient in neuronal nitric oxide synthase. *Science* 1994;265:1883-1885.

9. Fujii M, Hara H, Meng W, et al. Strain-related differences in susceptibility to transient forebrain ischemia in SV-129 and C57Black/6 mice. *Stroke* 1997;28:1805-1811.

10. Pahlman S, Odelstad L, Larson E, et al. Kinetic and concentration effects of TPA-induced differentitaion of cultured human neuroblastoma cells. *Cells Diff* 1983;12:165-170L.

11. Brandt R, Leger J, Lee G. Interaction of tau with the neural plasma membrane mediated by tau's amino-terminal projection domain. *J Cell Biol* 1995;131:1327-1340.

12. Furchgott RF, Zawadzki JV. The obligatory role of endothelial cells in the relaxation of arterial smooth muscle by acetylcholine. *Nature* 1980;288: 373-376.

13. Palmer RMJ, Ferrige AG, Moncada S. Nitric oxide release accounts for the biological activity of endothelium-derived relaxing factor. *Nature* 1987;327:524-526.

14. Ignarro LJ. Biosynthesis and metabolism of endothelium-derived nitric oxide. *Annu Rev Pharmacol Toxicol* 1990;30:535-560.

15. Huang Z, Huang PL, Ma J, et al. Enlarged infarcts in endothelial nitric oxide synthase knockout mice are attenuated by nitro-L-arginine. *J Cereb Blood Flow Metab* 1996;16:981-987.

16. Hara H, Ayata C, Huang PL, et al. (^{3}H)L-NG-Nitroarginine binding after transient focal ischemia and NMDA-induced excitotoxicty in type I and type III nitric oxide synthase null mice. *J Cereb Blood Flow Metab* 1997;17:515-526.

17. Radomski MW, Palmer RM, Moncada S. An L-arginine/nitric oxide pathway present in human platelets regulates aggregation. *Proc Natl Acad Sci USA* 1990;87:5193-5197.

18. Gerson RJ, Mac Donald J, Alberts AW, et al. Animal safety and toxicology of simvastatin and related hydroxy-methylglutaryl-Coenzyme A reductase inhibitors. *Am J Med* 1988;87:28-38.

19. Laufs U, La Fata V, Liao JK. Inhibition of 3-hydroxy-3-methylglutaryl (HMG)-CoA reductase blocks hypoxia-mediated downregulation of endothelial nitric oxide synthase. *J Biol Chem* 1997;172:31725-31729.

20. Nadaud S, Phillipe M, Arnal J-F, et al. Sustained increase in aortic endothelial nitric oxide synthase expression in vivo in a model of chronic high blood flow. *Circ Res* 1996;79:857-863.

21. Haddad EK, Duclos AJ, Lapp WS, et al. Early embryo loss is associated with the prior expression of macrophage activation markers in the decidua. *J Immunol* 1997;158:4886-4892.

22. Endres M, Laufs U, Huang Z, et al. Stroke protection by 3-hydroxy-3-methylglutaryl (HMG)-CoA reductase inhibitors mediated by endothelial nitric oxide synthase. *Proc Natl Acad Sci USA* 1998;95(15):8880-8885.

White Matter Ischemia— Unique Mechanisms of Injury?

Chapter 9

Ischemic Injury to the Cerebral White Matter:
Neuropathology of Human and Experimental Lesions

Leonardo Pantoni, MD and
Julio H. Garcia, MD

Introduction

The study of the responses of the cerebral white matter (WM) to ischemic injury has been neglected possibly because of the assumption that damage to the neuronal perikarya, caused by ischemia, always precedes or occurs simultaneously with the injury to the white matter.

Until the late 1960s diffuse changes affecting the cerebral WM (currently considered as having a possible ischemic origin) were regarded as uncommon. This is explained by the fact that before computerized tomography (CT) could be applied to image the brain, many changes in the structure of the white matter were detectable only at autopsy at a time when the etiology of these white matter changes was extremely difficult to determine. The potential clinical significance of such changes was almost impossible to establish on the basis of retrospective studies that in the past could originate only from postmortem findings.

Interest in understanding mechanisms of WM injury of probable ischemic origin was spurred by the advent of modern neuroimaging techniques that disclose, with increasing frequency, alterations of the

Financial aid for this work was partly provided by USPHS grant NS 31631.

WM that may have either a vascular or an ischemic origin. Also, the prospective evaluation of cognition among persons with white matter abnormalities (visible on CT) uncovered clinical manifestations that could be causally associated with these WM changes. Because of this, more recently attention has been centered on defining, in laboratory models, the effects of hypoxia and ischemia on specific components of the cerebral WM, such as oligodendrocytes and myelinated axons.

Neuropathology of Ischemic Injury to the White Matter: Human Observations

Ischemia can affect the WM in different ways, depending on the severity and duration of the ischemic event. Prolonged occlusion of most large cerebral arteries, for example those involving the middle cerebral artery, cause coagulation necrosis (infarction) of both gray and WM. It is not known whether the consequent neurological deficit depends primarily on the injury to the neuronal perikarya or to the lesions affecting the myelinated axons of the WM bundles. In any event, defining the temporal evolution of WM alterations in human infarcts has received scant attention as exemplified by one recent publication in which the emphasis was placed on describing changes affecting gray matter components.[1] A more recent publication on the histopathology of cerebral ischemia does not mention alterations of the cerebral WM as may occur in human brains injured by either hypoxia or ischemia.[2] However, it is well known that lesions confined to the cerebral WM have been observed in cases of intoxications by either carbon monoxide[3] or cyanide[4] as well as in victims of strangulation and near drowning.[5] Also, cerebral WM lesions etiologically associated with systemic ischemia-hypoxia, have been recorded in neonates under the designation of periventricular leukomalacia.[6] In each of these instances the lesions in the WM have been intuitively attributed to some undefined effects of hypoxia/ ischemia.

At least three types of lesions of vascular (ischemic) origin can affect the cerebral WM: a) small (lacunar) infarcts with a diameter < 15 mm; b) large (diameter >15 mm) infarcts of the centrum semiovale; and c) diffuse subcortical leukoencephalopathy. These diverse type of lesions, which sometimes coexist in the same patient, probably have different pathogenic mechanisms.

Lacunar Infarcts in the White Matter

The corona radiata is a wide band of WM fibers that descends from the cortical mantle to assemble the fibers of the internal capsule.

Both the corona radiata and the internal capsule are common sites of lacunar infarcts. The clinical correlates of lacunar infarcts occurring at this level are varied as a reflection of the confluence, in a small space, of fibers from many kinds of neurons each having very diverse functions.[7]

Lacunar infarcts (lacunes) are brain cavitary lesions; by definition, the widest diameter of a single lacune does not exceed 15 mm. Each lacune is represented by an irregular cavity containing protein-rich fluid and lipid laden macrophages. The numbers of macrophages visible within a lacune vary considerably depending on the age of the lesion. Hemosiderin-laden macrophages can be found less frequently in small brain lesions (lacunes?) that probably represent previous hemorrhages at these sites. The pathogenesis of lacunar infarcts is presumptively linked in most cases to structural alterations in the tunica media of the small (penetrating) blood vessels. Such changes include replacement of the smooth muscle cells by fibro-hyaline material with thickening of the wall and narrowing of the vascular lumen as well as with other structural alterations covered under the generic term of *arteriolosclerosis*.

Arteriolosclerosis is frequently associated with chronic arterial hypertension, diabetes mellitus, and aging.[8-10] In a small percentage of cases, none of these risk factors were detectable in a retrospective clinico-pathologic analysis of a large number of autopsy specimens.[11] The authors suggested that in such cases perhaps an abnormality in the endothelial permeability, of undetermined origin, was responsible for the sclerosing changes visible in the tunica media of the small blood vessels.[11] In addition to arteriolosclerosis, it has been hypothesized that microemboli may occlude small brain vessels and produce lacunar infarcts.[12] A third possible etiology of this kind of lesion is atherosclerosis of the parent vessel causing occlusion of the ostium of the small or penetrating vessel.[13] Lacunar infarcts in the subcortical WM of the centrum semiovale and corona radiata can be found in specimens where the WM parenchyma is otherwise normal but, more frequently, lacunes co-exist with diffuse rarefaction of the WM.[14]

Centrum Semiovale Infarcts

The description of the histopathological features of infarctions involving the cerebral WM has received scant attention. If the process in the WM is similar to that affecting the gray matter, one may assume that shortly after the induction of ischemia a state of spongiosis secondary to the retention of water in the glial compartments, (as well as in the intramyelinic and extracellular spaces) is followed by pyknosis of isolated oligodendrocytes. The eventual necrosis of all glial elements, blood vessels, and myelinated axons (ie, pannecrosis) should be followed by arrival of monocytes/macrophages, ingestion of the cellular debris, and eventual cavitation or formation of a cavity containing lipid-laden macrophages as well as a fluid with a protein content similar to that of plasma. In other words, the features of this WM lesion are thought not to be different from those of a lacune except for the fact that the maximum diameter of the WM lacunae does not exceed 1.5 cm. The presumptive etiology of such areas of pannecrosis in the WM, as in the case with other infarcts, is an ischemic injury of sufficient severity (local CBF values of < 10mL/100gm/min) and of prolonged duration. It is likely that ischemic injuries of moderate severity (local CBF values of 15–20 mL/ 100gm/min) result in structural lesions that are not characterized by pannecrosis/ cavitation but instead by the features of leukoencephalopathy (LE). This type of WM lesion, which in one autopsy series existed in as many as 46% of the cases of Alzheimer disease, has been called by the authors incomplete infarct of the WM, based on their interpretation of the structural and biochemical data derived from these autopsy specimens.[15]

Diffuse Subcortical Leukoencephalopathy

The historical developments of the concept of cerebral LE of possible vascular/ischemic origin have been analyzed separately.[16] In that review, we presented ample evidence to demonstrate that the use of the eponym Binswanger's disease is unjustified and undesirable.[16] Also, we have reported two well documented instances of progressive dementing disorders in patients whose brains, examined at autopsy, did not have the histological features of Alzheimer's disease. Instead, both of these specimens had extensive disease of the cerebral WM and of the small blood vessels of the brain.[17]

The pathogenesis of the diffuse WM changes, frequently detected in elderly patients either by neuroimaging or by pathological examination, is still incompletely elucidated. We completed an extensive review of medical publications dealing with the topic of LE and hypothesized (on the basis of epidemiological data) that some forms of subcortical WM alterations have an ischemic origin;[18] for this reason we include this topic in the present review. Additional and potential mechanisms of LE, such as dysfunction of the blood brain barrier and the effect of chronic brain edema, could concur and contribute to the ischemic injury and to the development of the WM alterations known as subcortical LE.

On neuroimaging, the changes in the WM density, frequently referred to as leukoaraiosis (from the Greek *leuko*= white, and *araiosis*= rarefaction,[19] are seen as either periventricular or subcortical (centrum semiovale) lesions that have either a patchy or a diffuse distribution. These areas of hypodensity on CT or hyperintensity on T_2-weighted magnetic resonance imaging (MRI), are frequently visible in both cerebral hemispheres in an individual subject.

Several studies have attempted to correlate WM alterations (visible on neuroimaging studies) with histologic evaluation of tissue samples. This has been attempted in cases in which CT or MRI showed WM changes (leukoaraiosis) at a time closely related to the autopsy, or in instances in which post-mortem examination of the brain with MRI was completed.

Rarefaction of periventricular white matter correlates with decreased myelin content,[20-27] loss of ependymal cell layer, reactive gliosis (also called granular ependymitis) at the tip of the frontal horns,[20-22,25,26,28] as well as with increased content of periependymal extracellular fluid, and with smaller and fewer number of axons per unit area.[26] Some authors also describe enlarged perivascular spaces at these periventricular locations,[22] but because small lesions in the periventricular WM exist in all age groups,[24,26] many authors do not consider these as being indicative of true pathology.

The histological correlates of subcortical WM changes, detectable by MRI, are even less consistent than those noted for periventricular LE. Tiny focal abnormalities in these studies correspond to enlarged perivascular spaces,[20,25] small cavitary infarcts (or lacunes),[29-31] demyelinating plaques, brain cysts, and congenital diverticuli of the lateral ventricles.[32] MRI methods seem adequate to distinguish between enlarged perivascular Virchow-Robin spaces and lacunar infarcts,[28,32] but in some cases the corresponding pathological abnormality of punctate lesions was undetectable.[27,31-33] The more typical diffuse lesions in the centrum semiovale have been related to myelin *rarefaction* that in most instances spares the U fibers.[20,34] Sometimes these diffuse lesions are accompanied by astrogliosis,[21,33] and diffuse vacuolization of the white matter.[31] The myelin rarefaction does not seem to correspond to true demyelination; among other reasons because eventually the process may also involve destruction of the axons.[34-37] Thickening of the wall of the small vessels (arteriolosclerosis) is commonly found in areas of WM rarefaction.[21,23,27,30,34,37] The radiological-pathological correlation for these diffuse subcortical lesions is not very tight: myelin loss is sometimes present in areas without leuko-araiosis or is more extensive than shown by MRI.[37]

Either structural or functional alterations affecting the small vessels of the brain appear to play a key role in the development of diffuse WM alterations. One of these pathological processes (arteriolosclerosis) eventually leads to marked narrowing of the vessel lumen and loss of the physiological ability to modify the lumen diameter in response to variations in either perfusion pressure or changes in metabolic activity. This loss of autoregulatory mechanisms could cause ischemia in the terminal territories of these vessels (corresponding to the deep borderzone areas).[18] The structural and physiological alterations of small vessels may also be accompanied by a breakdown of the blood-brain barrier. Structural alterations affecting the small (or penetrating) blood vessels of the brain include, in addition to arteriolosclerosis, amyloid angiopathy, CADASIL, and other seemingly genetically transmitted angiopathies.[38] The possible association between cognitive disorders and diseases of the cerebral small blood vessels has been discussed in a separate review.[39]

The effect of ischemia can be either acute, severe and localized, leading to small areas of veritable necrosis (lacunar infarction), or chronic, less severe, and diffuse, leading to the development of histological alterations consistent with the definition of incomplete infarct.[40] Incomplete infarction in the WM is characterized by rarefaction of the myelin sheaths, moderate decrease in the number of oligodendrocytes per unit area, and reactive astrogliosis.[15] Increased water content, and secondary rarefied appearance of the myelinated bundles is another common finding of this type of leukoencephalopathy.

Arteriolosclerosis is mainly associated with long-standing or chronic arterial hypertension. However, structural changes in the WM are found not only in hypertensive patients, but also in the brains of subjects with complex alterations in blood pressure regulation such as a lack of the nocturnal physiological drops[41,42] or wide daily fluctuations.[43] Moreover, the observation that a subgroup of symptomatic patients with WM changes suffers from spontaneous and frequent hypotensive crises[43,44] is consistent with the demonstration of impaired cerebral autoregulation in hypertensive patients who have severe periventricular leukoaraiosis.[45] In patients with arteriolosclerotic vessels, a drop in blood pressure of the type that occurs during cardiac dysrhythmias or as a result of impaired autoregulation could lead to a significant decrease in blood flow in the WM, attributable to the inability of sclerotic vessels to dilate. Autoregulatory limits are shifted upward in hypertensive patients,[46] thus, a rapid reduction of blood pressure, within physiological limits, might markedly reduce cerebral blood flow in the WM of patients with chronic hypertension. Consequently, the cerebral WM of hypertensive patients could become ischemic at blood pressure levels considered normal for normotensive subjects. Moreover, the cerebral autoregulatory mechanisms, in experimental animals, appear to be less efficient in the WM vessels than in the vessels of the gray matter.[47]

Neuropathology of Ischemic Injury to the White Matter: Experimental Observations

Effects of *Global* Cerebral Ischemia

Experimentally induced stenosis of both common carotid arteries in the gerbil induces chronic hypoperfusion of the more rostral portion of the brain; this is because most gerbils lack anastomoses between the carotid and the vertebral arterial systems. Eight to 12 weeks after the application of coiled clips that reduce the flow of blood through the common carotid arteries, gerbils' brains developed areas of rarefaction and gliosis in the WM. These changes were not associated with focal necrosis; and, compared to the injury to the myelin sheaths, the axons in the rarefied regions of the WM were relatively spared.[48] These alterations were not detectable prior to 8 weeks, while their severity increased between 8 and 12 weeks after the ischemic injury. Rarefaction of the WM, in these experiments, was independent of damage to the grey matter and was associated with ventricular dilatation.[48] These findings have been confirmed in similar experiments conducted in other laboratories utilizing gerbils and other animals species.[49,50]

Interestingly, Mongolian gerbils subjected to 15 minutes of bilateral carotid artery occlusion and exposure to 100% normobaric oxygen for the first 3 hours after reperfusion developed more prominent WM lesions than control gerbils breathing room air after reperfusion.[51] The opposite result was true of cortical neurons: fewer injured neuronal perikarya were visible in the brains of gerbils breathing 100% normobaric oxygen compared to the group exposed to transient ischemia and room air. However, mortality was higher in the later group.[51] Histological alterations in the WM in both of these experiments included swelling and fragmentation of myelin sheaths, and decreased stainability with myelin -basic- protein (MBP) antiserum that suggested loss of myelinated sheaths. Macrophages showed intracellular inclusions of MBP positive fragments, while many axons in the same areas appeared structurally intact.[51] These results suggest that hyperoxia, induced immediately after reperfusion, may injure selectively the myelin sheaths. The cause(s) for this remain(s) to be elucidated, but damage to the blood-brain barrier and the consequent development of cerebral edema may account for the increased injury to the WM. The increased susceptibility of the WM to this type of injury (decreased cerebral blood flow secondary to the occlusion of carotid arteries followed by hyperoxia) could be explained by the high content of polyunsaturated fatty acids in the myelinated sheaths. Polyunsaturated fatty acids are particularly prone to undergo peroxidation in the presence of oxygen.[52]

In animals in which an anatomical communication between the anterior (carotid) and posterior (vertebral) arteries is present, chronic cerebral hypoperfusion can be achieved by permanent occlusion of both common carotid arteries. Glial activation and various changes selectively confined to the WM were reported in rats that survived 90 days after this type of injury.[53] Leukocyte infiltration into of the WM was detected beginning 1 hour after the arterial occlusion, and persisted until 90 days. This inflammatory response was followed at 7 days by activation of WM astrocytes as revealed by the presence of an increased number of Glial-Fibrillary-Acidic-Protein positive astrocytes in comparison with control animals. At later intervals, rarefaction of the WM became evident as demonstrated by a myelin staining.[53] Of interest, glial cell activation and reduction of the histologic changes affecting the WM were achieved by the intraperitoneal administration of the immunosuppressant cyclosporin A.[54] These observations suggest that as a result of an ischemic event, an early immunological reaction (partly mediated by leukocytes) could be crucial in the ensuing chronic ischemic damage to the WM.

Effects of *Focal* Cerebral Ischemia

Permanent middle cerebral artery (MCA) occlusion in the rat produces an area of decreased blood flow in the MCA territory[55] that eventually creates an area of pan-necrosis or territorial infarct 72–96 hours after the arterial occlusion.[56] Lesions of ischemic etiology, restricted to the cerebral WM, have been experimentally induced in cats brains after reperfusing an arterial territory that was made ischemic by clipping the origin of one MCA six hours before removing the clip and restoring anterograde flow.[57] MCA occlusion can be induced in rats by inserting a nylon monofilament in the external carotid artery and advancing it in the internal carotid artery until a point where the origin of the MCA becomes occluded.[58] Using this method to occlude one MCA in rats, Garcia and collaborators have documented structural alterations in the brain affecting different cell types (neurons, glia, and microvessels) at variable intervals after permanently occluding the vessel.[57,59,60] The typical leukoencephalopathy that affects patients with "risk factors" for cerebrovascular diseases and variable degrees of cognitive impairment cannot be attributed to the prolonged occlusion of a large intracranial vessel. Nevertheless we aimed to outline the responses of the WM components to an ischemic insult of predetermined duration utilizing the experimental model of permanent MCA occlusion.

We defined several histological and ultrastructural alterations affecting the subcortical cerebral WM of Wistar rats in experiments electively terminated at periods ranging from 30 minutes to 24 hours after the permanent occlusion of one MCA.[61] The most striking result was the finding of oligodendrocyte's swelling which became detectable as early as 30 minutes after the MCA occlusion.[61] At this early time, the mean diameter of oligodendrocytes nuclei, in the ischemic area, was significantly different from that of oligodendrocytes in the contralateral, nonischemic hemisphere. This difference progressively increased from 30 minutes to 4 hours after the MCA occlusion. Three hours after the arterial occlusion, oligodendrocytes in the WM began displaying changes characteristic of irreversible cell injury, such as nuclear pyknosis and discontinuities in nuclear and plasma membranes. Simultaneously with the appearance of nuclear changes in oligodendrocytes, vacuolation of the WM became apparent. The areas of vacuolation in the WM corresponded to: 1) spaces formed by the separation of the inner myelin sheaths from the axolemma; 2) widened extracellular spaces; and 3) expansion of astrocyte's processes.[61] Each of these changes is remarkable in that it preceded the appearance of irreversible injury to neuronal perikarya (ie, eosinophilia), thus suggesting that under special conditions the early changes induced by ischemia in the WM are independent of injury to the neuronal perikaryon. The selective injury to the WM components was confirmed in a series of subsequent experiments based on transient MCA occlusion of one hour duration followed by up to 21 days reperfusion.[62]

Our own observations have been confirmed by one study that evaluated the response of some components of the myelinated axons (microtubule-associated proteins or MAPs) to ischemia. Using a transcranial approach to permanently occlude the MCA, the authors demonstrated changes in the immunostaining of MAPs 2 hours after the induction of ischemia. While histological evaluation was not performed at earlier times, the changes were accentuated at 6 hours.[63]

Injury to WM components was documented in rat's brains subjected to cerebral thromboembolism.[64] Three days after inducing localized thrombosis of the common carotid artery, by photochemical methods, the authors documented the presence of ipsilateral, small embolic infarcts in the cerebral hemisphere. Interestingly, using β-amyloid precursor protein immunochemistry as a marker of axonal damage,[65] they also described abnormalities of WM bundles distant from the sites of severe gray matter damage.[64] Once more these observations support the concept that under conditions not well characterized as yet, ischemia can cause WM injury independently of damage to neuronal peri-karya.

A recent publication described the selective vulnerability of oligo-dendrocytes in a model of transient global ischemia in rats.[66] The selective damage to the hippocampal neurons produced by the transient occlusion of all 4 major cervical arteries is well known and was detected in these experiments. In addition, one day following the ischemic event, the authors could demonstrate, by the *in situ* end labeling (ISEL) method, DNA fragmentation in oligodendrocytes of the cortex and thalamus, two regions of the brain where neuronal perikaryal injury is, in this type of ischemia, either minimal or totally absent.[66] These experiments reinforce our original observations that suggest high vulnerability of oligodendrocytes to the effects of ischemia.[61]

The above reported experiments are in agreement with data derived from *in vitro* observations that show susceptibility of oligodendrocytes and myelin to hypoxia. The response of the WM to anoxic/hypoxic injuries has been studied *in vitro* in the isolated rat optic nerve. The isolated rat optic nerve can be exposed to periods of anoxia of variable duration; the function of these fibers can be evaluated by measuring the compound action potential either under anoxic conditions or after restoring to the medium the normal concentration of O_2. Immediately after a period of 60 minutes anoxia, the optic nerve shows numerous large, apparently empty vacuoles within myelin sheaths at a site adjacent to the axon.[67] This alteration closely resembles those found in the *in vivo* model of ischemia and described in previous paragraphs. In addition to this vacuolation, Waxman et al. reported mitochondrial swelling, loss of microtubules and neurofilaments, and retraction of the myelin sheaths from the nodes of Ranvier. These alterations partially regressed when the optic nerve was allowed to recover for 60 minutes in normally oxygenated medium.[67] Stys et al. have demonstrated that this anoxic damage to the WM is Ca^{++}- mediated, and consequent to an alteration in the Na^+-Ca^{++} exchanger.[68] That an excess of intracellular influx of Ca^{++} may mediate the injury to the WM is corroborated by the observation that the injection of the Ca^{++} ionophore ionomycin in the dorsal column of the rat spinal cord induces WM alterations characterized by the formation of large intra-myelinic vacuoles, shrinkage of oligodendrocytes, indicative of cellular necrosis, and swelling of astrocytes.[69]

Very recently, some of the possible biochemical mechanisms of Ca^{++}- mediated injury to the WM components have begun to be disclosed. McDonald et al. have shown that oligodendrocytes are extremely vulnerable to excitoxicity mediated by AMPA/kainate receptor both *in vitro* and *in vivo*.[70] Such a mechanism of damage had been previously demonstrated only in neurons. Futhermore, treatment with

NBQX, an antagonist of the AMPA/kainate receptor, blocked this toxicity further supporting the hypothesis that Ca^{++} entry may play an important role in the lethal injury to oligodendrocytes.[70]

Experiments demonstrating the vulnerability of the WM to hypoxic and ischemic insults support the hypothesis of an ischemic origin for the WM changes that are found, by neuroimaging methods in aged, frequently hypertensive patients. We suggest that repetitive but brief ischemic insults to the WM may lead to selective damage involving a restricted number of oligodendrocytes. Since each oligodendrocyte provides the myelin sheath for many widespread axons (up to 50), selective damage to a relatively small number of these cells could result in alterations involving comparatively large regions of the WM. This premise must be examined in appropriate experimental protocols.

Acknowledgment   The authors are grateful to Lorraine Mayberry for expert secretarial support.

References

1. Chauqui R, Tapia J. Histologic assessment of the age of recent brain infarcts in man. *J Neuropathol Exp Neurol* 1993;52:481-489.
2. Auer RN. Histopathology of cerebral ischemia. In Ginsberg MD, Bogouslavsky J (eds): *Cerebrovascular Disease: Pathophysiology, Diagnosis, and Management.* Oxford: Blackwell Science;1998:90-101.
3. Schwedenberg TH. Leukoencephalopathy following carbon monoxide asphyxia. *J Neuropathol Exper Neurol* 1959;18:597-608.
4. Hirano A, Levine S, Zimmerman HM. Experimental cyanide encephalopathy. Electron microscopic observations of early lesions in white matter. *J Neuropathol Exp Neurol* 1967;26:200-213.
5. Dooling EC, Richardson EP Jr. Delayed encephalopathy after strangling. *Arch Neurol* 1976;33:196-199.
6. Sarnat HB. Perinatal hypoxic/ischemic encephalopathy: Neuropathological features. In: *Neuropathology: The Diagnostic Approach.* JH Garcia, et al. (eds): St. Louis, Mosby-Year Book Inc., 1997;541-580.
7. Hommel M, Besson G. Clinical features of lacunar and small deep infarcts at specific anatomical sites. *Adv Neurol* 1993;62:161-179
8. Alex M, Baron EK, Goldenberg S, et al. An autopsy study of cerebrovascular accident in diabetes mellitus. *Circulation* 1962;25:663-673.
9. Furuta A, Ishii N, Nishihara Y, et al. Medullary arteries in aging and dementia. *Stroke* 1991;22:442-446.
10. Ostrow PT, Miller LL. Pathology of small artery disease. *Adv Neurol* 1993;62:93-123.
11. Lammie GA, Brannan F, Slattery J, et al. Nonhypertensive cerebral small-vessel disease. An autopsy study. *Stroke* 1997;28:2222-2229.
12. Millikan C, Futrell N. The fallacy of the lacune hypothesis. *Stroke* 1990;21:1251-1257.

13. Caplan LR. Intracranial branch atheromatous disease: A neglected, understudied, and underused concept. *Neurology* 1989;39:1246-1250.

14. Ferrer I, Bella R, Serrano MT, et al. Arteriolosclerotic leucoencephalopathy in the elderly and its relation to white matter lesions in Binswanger's disease, multi-infarct encephalopathy and Alzheimer's disease. *J Neurol Sci* 1990;98:37-50.

15. Brun A, Englund E. A white matter disorder in dementia of the Alzheimer type: A pathoanatomical study. *Ann Neurol* 1986;19:253-262.

16. Pantoni L, Garcia JH. The significance of cerebral white matter abnormalities 100 years after Binswanger's report. A review. *Stroke* 1995;26:1293-1301.

17. Pantoni L, Garcia JH, Brown GG. Vascular pathology in three cases of progressive cognitive deterioration. *J Neurol Sci* 1996;135:131-139.

18. Pantoni L, Garcia JH. Pathogenesis of Leukoaraiosis: A review. *Stroke* 1997;28:652-659.

19. Hachinski VC, Potter P, Merskey H. Leuko-araiosis. *Arch Neurol* 1987;44:21-23

20. Chimowitz MI, Estes ML, Furlan AJ, et al. Further observations on the pathology of subcortical lesions identified on magnetic resonance imaging. *Arch Neurol* 1992;49:747-752.

21. Fazekas F, Kleinert R, Offenbacher H, et al. The morphologic correlate of incidental punctate white matter hyperintensities on MR images. *AJNR* 1991;12:915-921.

22. Grafton ST, Sumi SM, Stimac GK, et al. Comparison of postmortem magnetic resonance imaging and neuropathologic findings in the cerebral white matter. *Arch Neurol* 1991;48:293-298.

23. Leifer D, Buonanno FS, Richardson EP Jr. Clinicopathologic correlations of cranial magnetic resonance imaging of periventricular white matter. *Neurology* 1990;40:911-918.

24. Moody DM, Brown WR, Challa VR, et al. Periventricular venous collagenosis: Association with leukoaraiosis. *Radiology* 1995;194:469-476.

25. Scarpelli M, Salvolini U, Diamanti L, et al. MRI and pathological examination of post-mortem brains: The problem of white matter high signal areas. *Neuroradiology* 1994;36:393-398.

26. Sze G, De Armond SJ, Brant-Zawadzki M, et al. Foci of MRI signal (pseudolesions) anterior to the frontal horns: Histologic correlations of a normal finding. *AJNR* 1986;7:381-387.

27. van Swieten JC, van Den Hout JHW, van Ketel BA, et al. Periventricular lesions in the white matter on magnetic resonance imaging in the elderly. A morphometric correlation with arteriolosclerosis and dilated perivascular spaces. *Brain* 1991;114:761-774.

28. Jungreis CA, Kanal E, Hirsch WL, et al. Normal perivascular spaces mimicking lacunar infarction: MR imaging. *Radiology* 1988;169:101-104.

29. Braffman BH, Zimmerman RA, Trojanowski JQ, et al. Brain MR. Pathologic correlation with gross and histopathology. 1. Lacunar infarction and Virchow-Robin spaces. *AJNR* 1988;9:621-628.

30. Marshall VG, Bradley WG Jr, Marshall CE, et al. Deep white matter infarction: Correlation of MR imaging and histopathologic findings. *Radiology* 1988;167:517-522.

31. Muñoz DG, Hastak SM, Harper B, et al. Pathologic correlates of increased signals of the centrum ovale on magnetic resonance imaging. *Arch Neurol* 1993;50:492-497.

32. Braffman BH, Zimmerman RA, Trojanowski J, et al. Brain MR. Pathologic correlation with gross and histopathology. 2. Hyperintense white-matter foci in the elderly. *AJNR* 1988;9:629-636.

33. Fazekas F, Kleinert R, Offenbacher H, et al. Pathologic correlates of incidental MRI white matter signal hyperintensities. *Neurology* 1993;43:1683-1689.

34. Révész T, Hawkins CP, du Boulay EPGH, et al. Pathological findings correlated with magnetic resonance imaging in subcortical arteriosclerotic encephalopathy (Binswanger's disease). *J Neurol Neurosurg Psychiatry* 1989;52:1337-1344.

35. Awad IA, Johnson PC, Spetzler RF, et al. Incidental subcortical lesions identified on magnetic resonance imaging in the elderly. II. Postmortem pathological correlations. *Stroke* 1986;17:1090-1097.

36. Janota J, Mirsen TR, Hachinski VC, et al. Neuropathological correlates of leuko-araiosis. *Arch Neurol* 1989;46:1124-1128.

37. Lotz PR, Ballinger WE Jr, Quisling RG. Subcortical arteriosclerotic encephalopathy: CT spectrum and pathologic correlation. *AJNR* 1986;7:817-822.

38. Ho K-L, Garcia JH. Neuropathology of small blood vessels in selected diseases of the cerebral white matter. In: The Matter of White Matter. Pantoni L, Inzitari D, Wallin A (eds): The Netherlands, ICG Publications, 1998.

39. Pantoni L, Garcia JH. Cerebral ischemic and cognitive impairment in the elderly. *Facts Res Gerontol* 1996; (Supplement:Stroke):171-182.

40. Garcia JH, Lassen NA, Weiler C, et al. Ischemic stroke and incomplete infarction. *Stroke* 1996;27:161-165.

41. Shimada K, Kawamoto A, Matsubayashi K, et al. Diurnal blood pressure variations and silent cerebrovascular damage in elderly patients with hypertension. *J Hypertens* 1992;10:875-878.

42. Tohgi H, Chiba K, Kimura M. Twenty-four-hour variation of blood pressure in vascular dementia of the Binswanger type. *Stroke* 1991;22:603-608.

43. McQuinn BA, O'Leary DH. White matter lucencies on computed tomography, subacute arteriosclerotic encephalopathy (Binswanger's disease), and blood pressure. *Stroke* 1987;18:900-905.

44. Harrison MJG, Marshall J. Hypoperfusion in the aetiology of subcortical arteriosclerotic encephalopathy (Binswanger type). *J Neurol Neurosurg Psychiatry* 1984;47:754.

45. Matsushita K, Kuriyama Y, Nagatsuka K, et al. Periventricular white matter lucency and cerebral blood flow autoregulation in hypertensive patients. *Hypertension* 1994;23:565-568.

46. Strandgaard S. Autoregulation of cerebral blood flow in hypertensive patients: The modifying influence of prolonged antihypertensive treatment on the tolerance to acute, drug-induced hypotension. *Circulation* 1976;53:720-727.

47. Young RSK, Hernandez MJ, Yagel SK. Selective reduction of blood flow to white matter during hypotension in newborn dogs: A possible mechanism of periventricular leukomalacia. *Ann Neurol* 1982;12:445-448.

48. Hattori H, Takeda M, Kudo T, et al. Cumulative white matter changes in the gerbil under chronic cerebral hypoperfusion. *Acta Neuropathol* (Berl) 1992;84:437-442.

49. Kudo T, Takeda M, Tanimukai S, et al. Neuropathologic changes in the gerbil brain after chronic hypoperfusion. *Stroke* 1993;24:259-265.

50. Ni J-W, Matsumoto K, Li H-B, et al. Neuronal damage and decrease of central acetylcholine level following permanent occlusion of bilateral common carotid arteries in rat. *Brain Res* 1995;673:290-296.

51. Mickel HS, Kempski O, Feuerstein G, et al. Prominent white matter lesions develop in Mongolian gerbils treated with 100% normobaric oxygen after global brain ischemia. *Acta Neuropathol (Berl)* 1990;79:465-472.

52. Yusa T. Hydrogen peroxide generation in rat brain in-vivo correlates with oxygen pressure. *Jpn J Anesthesiol* 1986;35:1077-1082.

53. Wakita H, Tomimoto H, Akiguchi I, et al. Glial activation and white matter changes in the rat brain induced by chronic cerebral hypoperfusion: An immunohistochemical study. *Acta Neuropathol (Berl)* 1994;87:484-492.

54. Wakita H, Tomimoto H, Akiguchi I, et al. Protective effect of cyclosporin A on white matter changes in the rat brain after chronic cerebral hypoperfusion. *Stroke* 1995;26:1415-1422.

55. Nagasawa H, Kogure K. Correlation between cerebral blood flow and histologic changes in a new rat model of middle cerebral artery occlusion. *Stroke* 1989;20:1037-1043.

56. Garcia JH, Yoshida Y, Chen H, et al. Progression from ischemic injury to infarct following middle cerebral artery occlusion in the rat. *Am J Pathol* 1993;142:623-635.

57. Garcia JH, Kamijyo Y, Cooper J. Temporary middle cerebral artery occlusion: A model of hemorrhagic and subcortical infarction. *J Neuropathol Exper Neurol* 1977;36:338-350.

58. Zea Longa E, Weinstein PR, Carlson S, et al. Reversible middle cerebral artery occlusion without craniectomy in rats. *Stroke* 1989;20:84-91.

59. Garcia JH, Liu K-F, Yoshida Y, et al. Brain microvessels: Factors altering their patency after the occlusion of a middle cerebral artery (Wistar rat). *Am J Pathol* 1994;145:728-740.

60. Garcia JH, Liu K-F, Yoshida Y, et al. Influx of leukocytes and platelets in an evolving brain infarct (Wistar rat). *Am J Pathol* 1994;144:188-199.

61. Pantoni L, Garcia JH, Gutierrez JA. Cerebral white matter is highly vulnerable to ischemia. *Stroke* 1996;27:1641-1647.

62. Gutierrez JA, Ye Z-R, Liu K-F, et al. Moderate focal ischemia selectively injures cerebral white matter in the rat. *J Neuropathol Exp Neurol* [Abstract] 1997;56:573.

63. Dewar D, Dawson DA. Changes of cytoskeletal protein immunostaining in myelinated fibre tracts after focal cerebral ischaemia in the rat. *Acta Neuropathol (Berl)* 1997;93:71-77.

64. Dietrich WD, Kraydieh S, Prado R, et al. White matter alterations following thromboembolic stroke: A β-amyloid precursor protein immunocytochemical study in rats. *Acta Neuropathol* 1998;95:524-531.

65. Yam PS, Takasago T, Dewar D, et al. Amyloid precursor protein accumulates in white matter at the margin of a focal ischaemic lesion. *Brain Res* 1997;760:150-157.

66. Petito CK, Olarte J-P, Roberts B, et al. Selective glial vulnerability following transient global ischemia in rat brain. *J Neuropath Exp Neurol* 1998;57: 231-238.

67. Waxman SG, Black JA, Stys PK, et al. Ultrastructural concomitants of anoxic injury and early post-anoxic recovery in rat optic nerve. *Brain Res* 1992;574:105-119.

68. Stys PK, Waxman SG, Ransom BR. Na^+- Ca^{++} exchanger mediates Ca^{++} influx during anoxia in mammalian central nervous system white matter. *Ann Neurol* 1991;30:375-380.

69. Smith KJ, Hall SM. Central demyelination induced *in vivo* by the calcium ionophore ionomycin. *Brain* 1994;117:1351-1356.

70. McDonald JW, Althomsons SP, Hyrc KL, et al. Oligodendrocytes from forebrain are highly vulnerable to AMPA/kainate receptor-mediated excitotoxocity. *Nat Med* 1998;4:291-297.

Chapter 10

Approaches to the Study of the Cellular and Molecular Pathogenesis of Perinatal White Matter Injury

Stephen A. Back, MD, PhD

Periventricular leukomalacia (PVL) is a developmental lesion of human cerebral white matter (WM) that has its peak incidence in the premature infant. The impact of PVL is enormous. In the US alone each year, 85% of the more than 55,000 preterm infants born with a birth weight of less than 1500g survive beyond the neonatal period.[1] In 5%–10% of the survivors, the major consequence of PVL is permanent motor impairment (ie, "cerebral palsy") that ranges from mild to profound spastic motor deficits. By school age, an additional 25%–50% manifest a broad spectrum of learning disabilities.[2] The estimated cost to society of cerebral palsy is in excess of five billion dollars annually. An understanding of the cellular and molecular basis of PVL is thus urgently needed to develop effective interventions to prevent these life-long neurological handicaps.

Two widely accepted, and not mutually exclusive, potential etiologies for PVL are ischemia-reperfusion[3] and cytotoxic cytokines released during infection, ischemia, or other insults.[4] In addition, a complex inter-

Support is gratefully acknowledged from the National Institutes of Health (NS01855 and P30HD33703), a Grass Foundation Morison Fellowship, a Hearst Foundation Award and a Doernbecher Junior Executive Board Award. We are grateful for the ongoing support of the NIH Brain and Tissue Bank at the University of Miami under the direction of Dr. Carol Petito (NO1-HD-8-3284) and to Drs. Joseph J. Volpe, Hannah C. Kinney and Paul A. Rosenberg for many helpful discussions.

From: Choi D, Dacey RG, Hsu CY, Powers WJ. *Cerebrovascular Disease: Momentum at the End of the Second Millennium.* Armonk, NY: Futura Publishing Company, Inc., © 2002.

play of vascular factors predisposes the human periventricular WM to injury. These include the presence of vascular end zones as well as a propensity for the sick premature neonate to exhibit a pressure-passive circulation that reflects a disturbance of cerebral autoregulation.[2,5,6]

Although the precise cellular and molecular mechanisms that are triggered by these pathogenetic factors are not yet defined, one hypothesis under study is that PVL arises, in part, from injury to a *developmentally-vulnerable target cell*, oligodendrocyte (OL) precursors, in the periventricular WM. A loss of OL precursors in PVL could account for the disrupted myelination that ensues. Delineation of the specific developmental stage of this vulnerable cell type, until now, has not been possible. Recently, the successive stages of OL development which give rise to the mature OL have been defined.[7,8] It has, thus, become feasible to characterize defined stages in the OL developmental lineage both *in vitro* and *in situ* with regard to the intrinsic and extrinsic cellular processes that may predispose to death of OL precursors.

This chapter will examine recent studies that have identified a number of mechanisms intrinsic and extrinsic to OL precursors that are potentially involved in causing OL death at sites of PVL. In support of an *intrinsic* susceptibility of OL precursors to injury are studies *in vitro* that demonstrated a maturation-dependent oxidative stress pathway in OL precursors that when activated causes apoptosis. Oxidative stress ensues from intracellular depletion of glutathione that results in the generation of intracellular oxygen radical species.[9-12]

Cellular events *extrinsic* to the OL may also contribute to the pathogenesis of PVL. A role for cellular mediators is supported by experimentally-induced WM injury by endotoxins,[13-15] the presence of a marked increase in reactive cell types—initially, macrophages and, later, reactive astrocytes at sites of human WM injury[16-18] and the identification of a number of cytokines with toxic or trophic effects on OL survival in tissue culture.[10,19,20] Injury to other cell types present in the cerebral WM that may support the survival and differentiation of OLs may also have deleterious effects on OL viability through mechanisms that include a loss of trophic factors essential for OL survival and differentiation.[21,22]

Pathogenesis Of PVL

Pathological Features of PVL

Current understanding of the pathogenesis of PVL derives from neuropathological and neuroimaging studies.[3,16,18,23,24] The pathological lesions characteristic of PVL may be classified as focal or diffuse. Focal lesions appear to arise from infarction of the WM in the distribution of vascular end zones. Acutely, at the core of the infarct there is a generalized loss of all cellular elements—including OLs, other neuroglia and axonal elements. A key feature is the presence of axonal spheroids that arise from the focal disruption of axons in the territory of the infarct. Subacutely, within 3–10 days after injury, the infarct is infiltrated first by macrophages and microglia and later by reactive hypertrophic astrocytes. Over several weeks this histological lesion may evolve to one of two macroscopic pictures: a cystic lesion, so called cystic PVL, or a region of gliosis. The cystic changes may become quite extensive when adjacent focal lesions become confluent. Subsequently, smaller cystic lesions may be replaced by gliotic scars with no discernible macroscopic cavity. The regions of PVL are later characterized histologically by myelin pallor, based on staining with Luxol-Fast Blue. A second form of cerebral WM injury is characterized by diffuse gliosis and an apparent paucity of OLs (see below). A central question, therefore, is whether diffuse PVL represents the oligodendroglial-specific form of PVL. The more diffuse lesion may coexist with the focal lesions of PVL, but extends widely beyond the territory of focal infarction. Diffuse gliosis is characterized by a generalized increase in hypertrophic reactive astrocytes; the etiology of which remains poorly defined. Diffuse gliosis may be a normal finding related to astrocyte development or a pathological response to WM injury. Further studies are needed to clarify the relationship between diffuse gliosis, OL loss and impaired myelination.

A Developmental Vulnerability Hypothesis of PVL

The pathogenesis of PVL appears to involve a number of interrelated developmental factors that influence the relative vulnerability of the cerebral WM to injury during the course of its maturation. The incidence of PVL increases markedly with decreasing gestational age. PVL was detected by ultrasonography in 5% of premature infants between 26–27 weeks and in 25% at 24 weeks gestational age.[25] Earlier studies had reported a peak incidence around 28–32 weeks gestational age reflecting the bias toward survival at later ages.[26]

Hence, PVL is largely a disorder of prematurity and occurs prior to the onset of active myelination. The appearance of microscopic myelin does not occur until at least after the first postnatal month and myelin tubes are not detected until 11–13 postconceptional months.[27,28] Interestingly, studies with diffusion tensor magnetic resonance imaging identified nonmyelinated fibers in the human corpus callosum as early as 28 weeks gestation, whereas late myelinating regions such as the central cerebral WM were detectable later at term.[29] The significance of these findings must await correlation with the timing of progression of the human OL lineage (see below).

In preterm infants, active myelination is preceded by the appearance of numerous large cells, readily mistaken for reactive astrocytes, which were called "myelination glia."[30] Myelination glia have only been characterized morphologically and are hypothesized to be OL precursors. Rorke reported myelination glia to be conspicuously reduced in number in the brains of preterm infants with evidence of both the least severe form of WM injury (ie, gliosis) as well as PVL.[31] Several studies of long-term survivors with documented PVL have also been observed at autopsy to have histological evidence of delayed myelination.[31-35] Hence, pathological studies of PVL support a developmental vulnerability of the WM to injury that may arise due to loss of OL precursors whose differentiation is critical for myelination.

Definition of the specific stage of development in the OL lineage, when the vulnerability to injury is greatest, would be a critical advance in the understanding of this disorder. This accomplishment may now be feasible with the application of stage-specific antibodies that have been developed against an array of sequentially expressed OL cell-surface and myelin-specific glycolipids and glycoproteins.[7] These antibodies have been used *in vitro* and *in situ* to define the OL developmental lineage. These studies have led to the identification of sequential stages of OL differentiation, each with a distinct phenotype in terms of its morphological, migratory and proliferative features. Isolation of OLs at specific stages in the lineage has been achieved by using OL-selective antibodies in tissue culture protocols based on immunopanning. This technique permits the isolation of nearly pure populations of OLs with elimination of other glial and neural cell types.[36,37] As discussed below, such *in vitro* model systems provide a means to characterize intrinsic differences in the OL lineage relevant to the study of OL loss in PVL.

The OL Developmental Lineage

The OL precursors which give rise to fully mature OLs are, in order of their successive stages, characterized as: the OL progenitor, preoligodendrocyte, immature OL and mature OL. Figure 1 summarizes the salient features of this developmental lineage which are pertinent to a consideration of human OL development. It should be remembered that this scheme is largely a synthesis of animal studies and *in vitro* studies with rodent OLs, and that validation of some of these findings in developing human brain is still required (see next section). *In vitro* studies first identified that, under the influence of a number of molecular

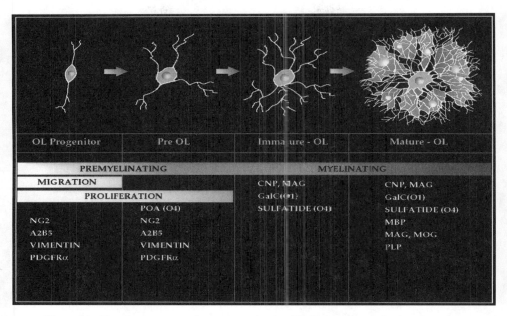

OL Progenitor	Pre OL	Immature - OL	Mature - OL

PREMYELINATING		MYELINATING	
MIGRATION		CNP, MAG	CNP, MAG
PROLIFERATION		GalC(O1)	GalC(O1)
	POA (O4)	SULFATIDE (O4)	SULFATIDE (O4)
NG2	NG2		MBP
A2B5	A2B5		MAG, MOG
VIMENTIN	VIMENTIN		PLP
PDGFRα	PDGFRα		

Figure 1. The four successive stages in the OL lineage are depicted at the top together with the corresponding biological features that distinguish each stage (middle). Also shown at the bottom are the most widely used markers applied to define each stage.

cues, a population of self-renewing, motile glial O2A progenitor cells could be selected to differentiate along either an astrocytic or oligodendroglial lineage.[38-42] Although bipotential progenitors have also been cultured from human fetal[43] and adult[44] brain, *in vivo* evidence has questioned the existence of bipotential glial progenitors.[45] *In vitro* studies indicate that these early progenitors are bipolar, proliferative and migratory. This population is generated over a short period during late gestation and early postnatal development and can be identified *in vitro* by immunoreactivity against the monoclonal antibody (mAb) A2B5, the ganglioside antigen G_{D3}, and vimentin.[39,46,47] These three markers are not specific for OLs but are useful in combination to define *in vitro* a given stage of OL development. A2B5 visualizes both OLs and neurons, and G_{D3} visualizes both OLs and microglia. Vimentin is a marker for proliferating glia, including OLs and astrocytes. The chondroitin sulfate proteoglycan NG2 appears to be an OL-specific marker that is expressed both on OL progenitors and preOLs,[48-51] and co-localizes with the platelet derived growth factor-α receptor (PDGF-αR),[52] which is also expressed on OL progenitors and preOLs.[53]

Next in progression is the preoligodendrocyte (preOL), a multipolar mitotically active late OL progenitor defined by expression of specific cell surface glycolipids, including POA (prooligodendroblast antigen),[54] and identified by reactivity to the O4 mAb but not the O1 mAb. A population of preOLs committed to the OL lineage has been identified to originate in the subventricular zone of the lateral ventricles.[55] It is noteworthy that restricted foci of late OL progenitors that bind the O4 antibody were detected in the ventral ventricular zone of the human spinal cord as early as 6 weeks gestation.[56] Immunoreactivity to the O4 mAb persists in subsequent stages.[57-61]

The preOL gives rise to immature OLs that are postmitotic, have more extensively branched processes and constitute a stage committed to terminal progression into a mature OL. Labeling of immature OLs with O1 is correlated with cell surface expression of several antigens, including galactocerebroside, 3'-sulfate galactocerebroside (sulfatide) and seminolipid.[54,59] The mature OL is characterized by expression of proteolipid protein (PLP)[62,63] and myelin basic protein (MBP).[64-67] The developmental expression of MBP in cells presumed to be OLs by morphological criteria has been defined in human deep, intermediate and superficial WM.[68]

Definition of the Human OL Developmental Lineage

Test of the hypothesis that the pathogenesis of PVL involves death of OL precursors has been hampered by limited information about the progression of the human OL lineage during fetal brain development. Such studies require suitable means to visualize OL precursors in human postmortem tissue. However, OL-specific antibodies are not amenable to localization via conventionally used neuropathological methods for handling and processing of human brain tissue. We have developed several approaches that optimized the visualization of OL-specific antibodies in human postmortem tissues. We examined in 25 autopsy human brains whether anti-NG2, O4, O1 and anti-MBP antibodies could visualize OLs in a standardized region of human parietal cerebral WM that has a high predilection for PVL.[69,70] These studies addressed the morphological features and timing of OL lineage progression between 18 to 40 weeks gestation.

As summarized in Figure 2, between 18–28 weeks postconceptional age, the WM is populated almost exclusively by NG2+O4+O1- preOLs. Although a small number of O1+ immature OLs are present during this period in brain development, they do not show evidence of active myelination. A commitment to myelination, occurs around 30 weeks, at which time ensheathment of axons by early myelin can be detected in the deep WM adjacent to the germinal matrix. Hence, the WM, at this time is populated mostly by OL precursors and a restricted population of myelin-producing cells. Interestingly, we detected many MBP-negative premyelin sheaths which further supports a relative

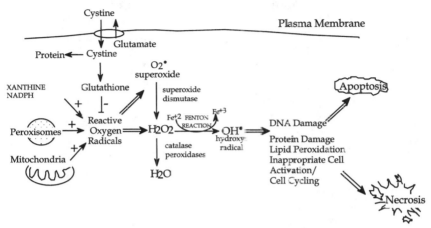

Hypothetical pathway for reactive oxygen radical mediated oligodendrocyte death.

Figure 2. This model depicts an oxidative stress pathway in which the depletion of intracellular glutathione mediates the death of OL precursors via the accumulation of toxic reactive oxygen radicals. Intracellular glutathione is depleted via a glutamate receptor-independent mechanism that involves a plasma membrane-associated glutamate-cystine antiporter.

immaturity of the OLs that populate the WM when the incidence of PVL is high. By contrast, progressively more MBP-positive myelin sheaths are detected in the WM closer to term gestation when the incidence of PVL falls off markedly.

In summary, the peak incidence of PVL corresponds to a period in WM development before the onset of active myelination. The impaired myelination that occurs in PVL may arise from death of OL precursors whose differentiation into mature OLs is critical for active myelination. Further studies are needed to evaluate whether the immaturity of OL precursors and the limited myelination of the WM contribute to the susceptibility of the cerebral WM to injury. This maturational vulnerability hypothesis is the focus of much current basic research on PVL, as discussed below.

Mechanisms of
Death of Oligodendrocyte Precursors

Much of the study of OL death has focused on the mature OL with the aim of characterizing the mechanisms underlying adult demyelinating disorders, including multiple sclerosis.[71] A variety of studies now indicate that the biology of OL precursors differs from that of the mature OL.[7] Hence, it remains to be determined whether the mechanisms that mediate death of developing OLs differ from those that act in mature OLs. Studies of OL death have centered around three main areas to be reviewed below: 1) the role of glutamate on the survival and differentiation of OL precursors; 2) the vulnerability of OL precursors to free radical-mediated toxicity triggered by intracellular depletion of glutathione; and 3) the toxicity to OLs of cellular mediators, including cytokines and growth factors.

Role of Glutamate Receptors in OL Differentiation and Death

The actions of glutamate on OL survival and differentiation appear to be developmentally regulated and to be mediated through both receptor and non-receptor-mediated mechanisms. Several recent *in vitro* studies have begun to clarify the role of receptor-mediated actions of glutamate on the differentiation and survival of OL progenitors.[72] OL progenitors prinicipally express the AMPA/kainate classes of glutamate receptors.[73] There is no compelling evidence for functionally active N-methyl-D-aspartate (NMDA) receptor expression at any OL stage. Glutamate has been proposed to block the differentiation of early OL progenitors through an AMPA receptor-mediated mechanism involving potassium influx via a delayed-rectifier potassium channel.[74-77] These cells were relatively resistant to a 24 hour exposure to 1 mM kainate, which caused less than a 20% appearance of apoptotic cells. Similarly, mixed populations of OL progenitors and GC-positive cells were only partially killed by a 24-hour exposure to 1mM kainate.[78] Maturation of OLs is associated with increased vulnerability to AMPA-kainate receptor agonists or oxygen-glucose deprivation via a mechanism of receptor-mediated excitotoxicity blocked by a selective AMPA receptor antagonist, but not by growth factors or antioxidants.[79-81] Future studies are needed to clarify the role of maturation-related factors in determining the sensitivity of OLs to glutamate-mediated toxicity. Changing patterns of glutamate receptor and ion channel expression may significantly alter the responsiveness of OLs to the effects of glutamate as a survival and differentiation factor.

Mechanisms of Oxidative Stress-Mediated Death of OL Precursors

Role of Glutamate Uptake Mechanisms in OL Differentiation and Death

Precedent for nonreceptor-mediated glutamate cytotoxicity was first reported in immature cortical neurons that were shown to be killed *in vitro* via a glutamate uptake-mediated mechanism.[82,83] Immature cortical neurons are vulnerable to an apoptotic form of death that is triggered by uptake of glutamate or homocysteate, a glutamate analog that blocks cystine uptake via a glutamate-cystine antiporter.[84,85] Glutamate uptake causes a depletion of intracellular cysteine, a precursor for glutathione. Glutamate toxicity is accompanied by a depletion of intracellular glutathione. Buthionine sulfoximine, an inhibitor of glutathione synthesis, is also neurotoxic.

We have identified a developmentally-regulated oxidative stress pathway in OL precursors that when activated causes apoptosis. Initial studies on OL susceptibility to glutamate exposure *in vitro* found a delayed form of death to immature OLs that occurred over hours with an EC_{50} of 200 μM glutamate.[9] Cell killing involved a nonreceptor-mediated mechanism. Neither the NMDA receptor antagonist, MK-801, nor CNQX, a competetive antagonist of nonNMDA receptors, protected OLs from glutamate toxicity. Rather, the toxicity of glutamate occurred via an apparently novel sodium-dependent transport system and was completely prevented by inhibition of glutamate uptake by D,L-threo-β-hydroxybutyrate. The novel nature of this form of glutamate-triggered OL death was supported by the observation that death was preceded by intracellular depletion of glutathione, a key scavenger of oxygen free radicals.[9] A role for free radical toxicity in triggering the death of OL precursors was supported by the prevention of cell death by a number of structurally distinct free radical scavengers, including ascorbate, α-tocopherol and idebenone.[9] Further insight into the mechanism of glutamate-mediated OL toxicity came from the observation that the toxicity could be enhanced by exposing OLs to glutamate under cystine-free conditions.[9,11] Cystine is the oxidized form of the amino acid cysteine and the principal *in vitro* form of this crucial amino acid. In addition, cystine was found to protect against glutamate-toxicity in a dose-dependent manner with an EC_{50} of 200 μM and exposure to cystine-depleted conditions alone (ie, cystine deprivation) induced a form of death indistinguishable from glutamate exposure. These studies supported that glutamate toxicity occurred by inducing intracellular cystine deficiency via the action of a glutamate-cystine exchanger, with uptake of glutamate accompanied by cystine efflux. Studies of OLs preloaded with radiolabeled cystine, in fact, showed an increased efflux of the radiolabel from OLs exposed to glutamate, supporting the presence of a glutamate-cystine exchanger in OL precursors. This putative X_c exchanger is operative in both central nervous system (CNS) and non-CNS cell types[85] and has been recently cloned.[87]

The basis for the critical dependence of OL precursors for cystine appears to derive from the fact that cystine is not only required for protein synthesis but is also a precursor for the tripeptide, glutathione, a key scavenger of intracellular free radicals. When OLs were deprived of cystine, death was preceded by a steady decline in intracellular glutathione.[11] In addition, the free radical scavenger, N-acetylcysteine, also protected OLs from glutamate toxicity by supplying a precursor for glutathione synthesis.[10]

Maturation-Dependent Vulnerability of OLs to Glutathione Depletion.

If death of OL precursors is important to the pathogenesis of PVL, then one might predict that the mechanism of OL death should be developmentally regulated. Since preOLs predominate in the human cerebral WM when the peak incidence of PVL occurs,[69] we examined whether preOLs were more susceptible to oxidative stress induced by glutathione depletion than were mature OLs. Using immunopanning to isolate rat preOLs, we generated highly enriched populations of preOLs and mature OLs under chemically defined conditions. When these two populations of OLs were subjected to the toxicity of various means of glutathione depletion, we found that preOLs were markedly more vulnerable. Hence, OL maturation was associated with increased resistance to cell death induced by glutathione depletion.[12] Moreover, glutathione depletion caused a variety of ultrastructural changes that were consistent with a mechanism of preOL death induced by apoptosis.

Further support for maturation-dependent susceptibility of preOLs to oxidative stress came from studies that demonstrated that the same degree of glutathione depletion markedly increased free radical production in preOLs but not in mature OLs. Moreover, when free radical production in preOLs was suppressed by the free radical scavengers α-tocopherol or idebenone or by intracellular glutathione replenishment with glutathione monoethylester, preOL death was prevented. These studies thus indicated that the death of preOLs was linked to a mechanism that was not uniquely triggered by glutamate or cystine deprivation. Rather, death might be induced by a variety of conditions that caused a depletion of intracellular glutathione, thereby rendering cells susceptible to injury from a form of oxidative stress.

The enhanced susceptibility of OL precursors to oxidative stress has been confirmed in a number of studies. We found that preOLs were also more vulnerable than mature OLs to exogenous free radical toxicity derived from xanthine-xanthine oxidase exposure.[12] C2-ceramide was also more toxic to O2A progenitors or CG-4 cells than to mature OLs,[88,89] and the mechanism of ceramide-induced apoptosis appeared to involve an early rise in mitochondrial reactive oxygen species (ROS) generation.[90] OL precursors also generated higher levels of ROS than astrocytes when made hypoxic or upon exposure to photochemically generated intracellular reactive oxygen species, but mature OLs were not examined.[91,92] OL precursors in the 1-week-old rat pup showed degenerative changes after a brief period of hypoxia-ischemia, but mature OLs were not examined.[93] The response of OLs to nitric oxide is complex. Nitric oxide can trigger necrotic OL death.[94] In immortalized OLs, nitric oxide had minimal toxicity to the least and most mature cell lines.[95] Although several nitric oxide donors were similarly toxic to OL precursors and mature OLs, a protective role for nitric oxide was demonstrated when the redox state of the cell was altered by depletion of intracellular thiols.[96] Hence, OL precursors may utilize nitric oxide as one defense mechanism against oxidative stress in the developing WM. Since mature OLs are not completely resistant to some forms of free radical toxicity (Griot et al., 1990; Kim and Kim 1991), the mechanisms that may determine the maturational susceptibility of OLs to oxidative stress is examined below.

A Role for Iron in Free-radical-Mediated Death of OL Precursors?

What may be the basis for the increased susceptibility of preOLs to oxidative stress? Several in vitro studies are consistent with a role for iron in triggering free-radical mediated OL injury. We reported that cystine deprivation-induced death of OL precursors was prevented by pretreatment with the iron chelator desferrioxamine.[11] A photochemically-induced rise in ROS was also blocked in OLs by desferrioxamine.[92] In a pertinent recent study in embryonic cortical neurons, a broader role for iron chelators was proposed based upon the finding that the protection rendered by such compounds against oxidative-stress induced apoptosis involves the activation of a collection of hypoxia-responsive genes.[97]

Although a variety of intracellular trace metals might be a potential source of oxygen radicals, multiple studies indicate that OLs play a central role in CNS iron metabolism and, thus, may be at risk for iron-mediated oxygen radical toxicity. Within the adult rodent and human CNS, including the WM, ferric iron, ferritin, and transferrin localize primarily to OLs, as well as to some restricted populations of neurons, microglia and astrocytes.[98-103] Myelin deficient rats, in which OLs fail to mature, show significant reductions in the distribution of iron, transferrin, and the transferrin receptor in the CNS.[104-106]

The timing of the developmental expression of iron and iron-binding proteins is highly regulated within the rodent[107] and human[68,102,108] brain. Systems for iron storage and metabolism appear to be established relatively early during human brain development. Iron storage by ferritin is observed in WM as early as 19 weeks gestation in human fetal brainstem.[102,109] Ferritin-positive OLs, identified by morphological criteria, increase markedly in cerebral WM, from deep to superficial regions, from approxiately 30 weeks of gestation.[68] The peak utilization of iron appears to occur in the early perinatal period with the onset of myelinogenesis. In the neonatal rat, rapid brain growth in the first 2 weeks of life is accompanied by a commensurate increase in the rate of iron uptake that peaks by day 15 of life.[110] Iron-positive cells are localized predominantly in the subcortical WM as early as postnatal day 3 in the rat, and between 14 and 28 days of age reach an adult pattern in which clusters of iron-positive cells localize near blood vessels.[111] Moreover, OLs are enriched in heavy-chain (H) ferritin early in development; H-ferritin is associated with high iron utilization and low iron storage.[103]

Prior to birth in the rodent the distribution of transferrin is most prominent in the choroid plexus, probably reflecting a role for transferrin in the CSF uptake and transport of iron into the CNS via receptor-mediated transport of iron across cell membranes.[112,113] In contrast to ferritin, there is limited transferrin expression in WM until near term, after which transferrin most heavily localizes to WM tracts which are beginning to myelinate.[99,101,107,109] Studies in developing rat optic nerve found that expression of the transferrin receptor preceded the appearance of staining for transferrin, myelin-basic protein and galactocerebroside.[114]

Taken together, these observations support an important role for iron and transferrin during active myelination of WM, and suggest that a variety of ROS may be normally produced as a byproduct of iron-requiring metabolic processes that are activated near the onset of myelination. Under physiological conditions, for example, ferritin can function as an iron donor for microsomal lipid peroxidation.[115] Moreover, the timing of expression of iron regulatory proteins may crucially influence the developmental vulnerability of human cerebral WM to injury. Several intriguing studies have begun to elucidate the functional importance of these proteins under physiological and pathophysiological conditions. Ferritin can function as an antioxidant that sequesters intracellular iron stores to prevent iron-induced toxicity.[116] Furthermore, under hypoxic or acidotic conditions, OLs in culture show both a reversible inhibition of myelin basic protein synthesis and a marked induction in the ferritin H chain.[117,118] Ferritin induction appears to occur in response to increased free intracellular iron or iron-mediated ROS generation under acidotic conditions.[119,120] It, thus, appears that iron stores are tightly regulated under both normal and hypoxic conditions, probably reflecting the essential but potentially deleterious effects of this ion on OL survival. It is an intriguing possibility that, in the setting of WM injury, regulation of iron might fail, if the death of ferritin-rich OLs were to release excessive iron into the surrounding

WM, thus, potentially leading to a self-perpetuation of free-radical mediated cell death.

What Role Do Antioxidant Enzymes Play in OL Susceptibility to Oxidative Stress?

An elevation in a variety of ROS is a well established sequela of ischemia.[121,122] It remains to be determined whether a rise in ROS could result in cell death by exceeding the capacity of antioxidant enzymes in the OL precursor to handle ROS. The vulnerability of immature OLs to oxidative stress may in part be due to a lack or imbalance in expression of antioxidant enzymes early in development. Little is known *in vitro* about the developmental expression in OLs of the antioxidant enzymes catalase, superoxide dismutase (SOD) and glutathione peroxidase, which are the primary enzymes required by most cell types to inactivate ROS. Exogenous catalase will protect against OL death induced *in vitro* by oxygen radicals.[123,124] Recent studies suggest that OLs at several stages have lower levels of some antioxidant enzymes than do other types of glia. Manganese superoxide dismutase was not immunocytochemically detected in either apparent OL progenitors or mature OLs, but was strongly visualized in both astrocytes and microglia.[125] Glutathione peroxidase levels were reported to be lower in OLs at several stages compared to astrocytes.[126]

In human brain, limited data suggest a progressive maturation of antioxidant systems near the time of birth as myelination begins. A temporal gradient is observed for catalase immunoreactive glial cells, which are first visualized in deep cerebral WM by 32 post conceptional weeks.[127] At term, all layers of the cerebral WM contain glia which stain for catalase. It may also be significant that whereas SOD demonstrates a steady increase in activity in the early postnatal rat brain, catalase levels show more fluctuation.[128] At birth, catalase levels are markedly higher than adult levels but steadily decline until 11 weeks of age, after which catalase gradually increases to adult levels by 40 weeks. A particular vulnerability of immature brain to hydrogen peroxide and hydroxyl radical production was suggested by the demonstration of accentuated brain injury after hypoxia-ischemia in copper/zinc SOD transgenic mice in the perinatal period but not in the adult.[129] This study did not specifically examine WM injury in these animals, however.

Summary: Mechanisms of Oxidative Stress-Mediated Death of OL Precursors

The pathogenesis of PVL relates to a developmental predilection of the WM to injury from cerebral ischemia induced by a pressure passive circulation or possibly vasoactive cytokines (see below). Since ischemia is well established to result in oxidative stress via the production of injurious free radicals,[130,131] recent studies have sought a cellular explanation that links oxidative stress to the disrupted myelination that characterizes chronic PVL. Since we identified that preOLs predominate in the cerebral WM when the risk of PVL is high (Figure 2), we examined whether preOLs might display increased susceptibility to oxidative stress. We identified an oxidative stress pathway in preOLS that is active when preOLs undergo glutathione depletion (Figure 3). The resistance of mature OLs to death via this oxidative stress pathway supports a cellular explanation for the developmental specificity of PVL. In this pathway, glutathione depletion is triggered by excess extracellular glutamate or a depletion of intracellular cystine acting at the site of a glutamate-cystine exchanger. Pharmacologic agents that deplete glutathione distal to the exchanger are also toxic to OL precursors. The net result of a decline in glutathione is a rise in intracellular ROS levels. ROS toxicity directly or indirectly mediates the death of OL precursors via apoptosis. Cell death is prevented by several structurally distinct free radical scavengers (ie, α-tocopherol, ascorbate or idebenone) or by supplying glutathione to the cell.

Future studies are required to clarify whether the selective vulnerability of OL precursors to oxidative stress relates to a delay in the expression of antioxidant enzymes, which may be upregulated later in WM development to inactivate ROS generated from myelinogensis. It is unknown which free radicals may be toxic to OLs, but the fact that the OL is the major CNS cell type that utilizes iron, transferrin, and ferritin suggests that iron catalyzed intracellular ROS generation may contribute to the downstream mechanisms leading to death of OL precursors. It should be recognized that the active production of extracellular ROS in the cerebral WM may be accentuated in the premature infant by hypoxia, ischemia-reperfusion, actions of cytokines, inflammatory cells and phagocytes. The importance of ROS-mediated toxicity in the genesis of disorders such as bronchopulmonary dysplasia and retinopathy of prematurity is supported by clinical and experimental data.[132-135]

Regulation of OL Survival by Cellular Mediators

Cytotoxic Cytokines

As discussed below, a role for cellular mediators in the pathogenesis of PVL is suggested by cerebral WM injury after exposure to endotoxin, a marked increase in reactive cell types—initially, macrophages and, later, reactive astrocytes at sites of PVL, and the identification of cytokines with toxic or protective effects on survival of OLs in tissue culture.

Gilles and colleagues first studied the potential link between cellular mediators released as a result of neonatal gram negative sepsis and PVL in a feline model of *E. coli* endotoxin-induced cerebral WM injury.[136] In this model, 1-2 weeks of daily intraperitoneal injections of endotoxin were found to produce injury largely restricted to the telencephalic WM in the kitten but not in the adult cat. Subsequently, a single intraperitoneal injection of bacterial endotoxin was also shown to produce cystic periventricular WM necrosis in both the neonatal kitten and monkey, but the effects were more variable in the rabbit and rat.[13] A shortcoming of these studies was a lack of monitoring for adverse systemic reactions to endotoxin, including hypoglycemia, acidosis, hypotension and a failure of cerebral autoregulation. Subsequent studies in 2-week-old rabbit pups[15] and in neonatal dogs[14] demonstrated that cerebral WM lesions occurred within 1–3 days of endotoxin exposure in the setting of transient acute arterial hypotension. Hence, the diverse forms of WM pathology induced by endotoxin in the five species studied to date might be due, at least in part, to systemic-vascular effects.

A role for direct OL injury by cellular mediators in the pathogenesis of PVL remains unresolved. Endotoxin does not cross the blood brain barrier,[137] but does produce disruption of the blood-brain barrier[138] and an inflammatory response of both the vascular endothelium and brain parenchyma in experimental animals.[14] The occurrence of such an inflammatory response *in vivo* in the human infant brain has not been demonstrated. Nevertheless, the release of cytokines as part of an acute inflammatory process represents a potential sequela of endotoxemia that could contribute to cerebral WM injury. A role for cellular mediators is suggested by recent epidemiological studies seeking an etiology for PVL in cases for which no apparent hypoxic-ischemic or hypotensive event could be identified. For example, an increased incidence of PVL has been reported in preterm infants born to mothers with chorioamnionitis or premature rupture of membranes.[139] Moreover, elevation of interleukin-6 (IL-6), but not TNFα, in umbilical cord blood has also been associated with increased risk of PVL.[140] Interestingly, as noted below, however, IL-6 enhances the *in vitro* survival of OLs.[20,36,141] Finally, it is noteworthy that IL-6, but not TNF, was elevated in critically ill neonates with bacterial sepsis and necrotizing enterocolitis.[142] These studies do not exclude potential *in vivo* toxicity to OLs from TNF, as TNF levels have been reported to peak within 90 minutes in a baboon model of *E. coli* sepsis and fall rapidly to baseline.[143] In summary, it remains unclear whether such cellular mediators might act directly or indirectly to cause WM injury or whether they are epiphenomena or markers of another primary insult.

Could cytokines produced by reactive astrocytes or microglia be a potential source of inflammation-mediated injury to OLs at sites of PVL? Acute PVL is characterized histologically by an initial tissue reaction in which infiltrates of macrophages/microglia predominate.[18,23] During the subacute phase of PVL, hypertrophic astrocytes increase in number in and around the injury site. Among the cell mediators which produce reactive astrocytosis are a number of cytokines and growth factors which have trophic or toxic effects upon OLs *in vitro*. Microglia induce reactive astrocytosis via release of TNF, IL-1, IL-6 and interferon-γ (INF-γ).[144] *In vitro* studies, limited to mature OLs, have shown that TNF/lymphotoxin or INF-γ have toxic effects upon OLs in culture.[10,19,20,145-148] TNF mediates a slow form of OL injury occuring over 48–96 hours, consistent with apoptosis. Toxic effects of lymphotoxin occur more rapidly and at lower doses than TNF.[19] By contrast, three members of the interleukin-6 family of cytokines, IL-6, LIF and CNTF, enhance the *in vitro* survival of OLs.[20,36,141] A number of other blood-borne mediators of astrogliosis, including PDGF, steroids, and insulin-like growth factor (IGF), also promote the survival of OLs (see below). Future study is required to determine the conditions that might promote cytokine-mediated tissue injury in PVL. The variable degree of toxicity to OL precursors observed *in vitro* with some cytokines, including TNF and INF-γ, may reflect a requirement for cooperation among multiple cell types to initiate the actions of a given cytokine. Under some conditions, the activation of microglia requires the subsequent expression of astrocytic cytokines.[149,150] Microglia, but not astrocytes, for example, are potently stimulated by bacterial endotoxin to produce IL-1β which secondarily stimulates astrocytic expression of both TNF-α and IL-6.[151] Finally, cytokines may be necessary but not sufficient to produce OL death *in vivo*; eg, a speculative possibility is that cytokines may mediate injury in combination with processes that impair local cerebral perfusion.

Growth Factors and Regulation of Oligodendrocyte Survival

Two pathological processes, which occur in the setting of PVL, may impair the normal release of growth factors that promote the survival, proliferation or differentiation of OL precursors: acute axonal injury and subacute reactive astrocytosis. Both neurons and astrocytes produce growth factors which affect the survival of OLs.[152] The identification of these growth factors represents an emerging field of great potential importance to understanding the pathogenesis of PVL.

The fate of each stage in the OL developmental lineage is regulated by a competition for selected growth factors, such that the mechanisms that promote OL survival are closely linked to those that promote OL death via apoptosis.[153] Hence, the timing of PVL might affect one or more populations of OL precursors, depending upon the OL stages that predominate and the required growth factors that may be disrupted.

Among the growth factors that regulate the survival of OL precursors are basic fibroblast growth factor (bFGF), neurotrophin-3 (NT-3), PDGF, and IGF-1. Basic FGF inhibits the differentiation and promotes the proliferation of OL precursor cells *in vitro*.[154-157] Neurotrophin-3 derives from both astroyctes and neurons and promotes the survival and proliferation of OL precursors *in vitro*.[36,158] *In vivo* studies, in which anti-NT-3 monoclonal antibodies were delivered by hybridoma cells implanted in the vicinity of the optic nerve, also supported a role for NT-3 in stimulating the proliferation of OL precursors.[158]

The insulin-like growth factors derive from astrocytes[159,160] and their primary action on OL precursors may be to promote their short-term survival.[21] Insulin and IGF-1 receptors localize to OL precursors *in vitro* or *in vivo*.[159,161] IGF-1 mRNA localizes to the subventricular zone at the time of appearance of OL progenitors[162] and autocrine expression of IGF-1 by OL precursors is suggested by detection of IGF-1 mRNA in OL precursors *in vitro*.[163] An increase in astrocytic IGF-1 gene expression has been observed in models of experimentally-induced myelin regeneration in adult rats in association with transient OL expression of IGF receptors[159] or expression of myelin basic protein mRNA.[160] It remains to be determined whether release of IGF-1 from reactive astrocytes at sites of PVL may represent a potential mechanism to promote survival of OL precursors.

Platelet-derived growth factor derives largely from neurons,[164,165] is a potent mitogenic,[166] chemotactic,[41] and survival factor[21] for OL precursors and blocks their differentiation toward immature OLs.[166-168] *In vitro*, PDGF potentiates the migratory and proliferative effects of bFGF on OL progenitor cells.[156] In combination with FDGF, NT-3 promotes the proliferation of OL precursors *in vitro*.[36] *In vivo*, PDGF functions largely as a survival factor. Implants of the COS-7 cell line, which were transfected with a PDGF plasmid expression vector, released exogenous PDGF into the vicinity of the optic nerve and caused a two-fold increase in the number of immature OLs.[21] The increase was consistent with enhanced OL survival but not an increase in cell proliferation, since the number of mitotic figures did not change. In the developing rat forebrain, Ellison and de Vellis localized the PDGFα receptor exclusively to OL precursors of two distinct lineage stages— the OL progenitor and preOL and failed to find receptor expression on immature OLs or other CNS cell types.[53] Taken together, these *in vivo* studies support a key role for PDGF in promoting the survival of proliferative OL precursor populations. It remains to be determined *in vivo* whether focal axonal injury, as occurs in acute PVL, might affect the survival of proliferative OL precursors by disrupting the actions of PDGF, NT-3 or other factors.

In addition to OL precursors, post-mitotic immature and mature OLs populate the cerebral WM in increasing numbers as term gestation approaches. *In vitro* studies have shown that the survival of these later OL stages is promoted by at least three classes of trophic factors: insulin and insulin-like growth factors;[36,169] neurotrophins, principally NT-3;[36] and members of the interleukin-6 family, IL-6, CNTF, and leukemia inhibitory factor (LIF).[20,36,141] Exogenous sources of NT-3[158] and CNTF[36] each promote the *in vivo* survival of GC-positive OLs in developing optic nerve. In addition to a role in OL survival, IGF-1 is an important inducer of CNS myelination *in vivo*. An IGF-1 knock-out mouse displayed a reduction in the size of WM tracts that was associated with decreased numbers of OLs and myelinated axons.[170] Similarly, transgenic mice that ectopically express IGF binding protein, which inhibits the action of IGF-1, show a decrease in the number of myelinated axons and of callosal and cortical OLs.[171] Transgenic mice that overexpress IGF-1 show an increase in OL number, myelin content and expression of myelin protein genes.[171,172]

In summary, a number of trophic factors, that include PDGF, NT-3, IGF-1 and CNTF, have been identified through *in vitro* and animal studies to play a role in OL precursor survival. Withdrawal of these factors can result in OL death via apoptosis. At present, little is known about the actions of these factors during human cerebral WM development. It is possible that focal axonal injury or diffuse gliosis may contribute to the pathogenesis of PVL by disrupting the release or altering the balance of trophic factors required for OL survival and maturation in cerebral WM. Future studies are needed to determine what role these and other trophic factors may play acutely and chronically to mitigate or promote OL death or disrupt myelination following cerebral WM injury.

Conclusions and Future Directions

PVL is the major type of brain injury in the premature infant and results in enormous long-term neurological disability in the survivors of the intensive care nursery. The hallmark of PVL is focal or diffuse cerebral WM injury with subsequent impairment of myelination. A specific window of vulnerability exists during human cerebral WM development when the risk for PVL is increased. Although the molecular basis for this vulnerability is unknown, the WM is populated by OL precursors, a hypothetical target cell in this disorder, when the risk for PVL is high. Two widely accepted potential etiologies for the pathogenesis of PVL are hypoxia-ischemia and cytotoxic cytokines, both of which may triggers death of OL precursors via oxidative stress. Our studies indicate that death of OL precursors is triggered by an oxidative stress pathway in which depletion of intracellular glutathione is accompanied by a rise in intracellular reactive oxygen species and subsequent death via apoptosis. The increased susceptibility of OL precursors to oxidative stress suggests an explanation for the developmental specificity of PVL

There are several avenues of future investigation into potential interventions to prevent PVL. More work is needed to understand the intrinsic molecular differences that render OL precursors more vulnerable to cell death than mature OLs. It remains to be determined whether free radicals are generated in PVL as a result of ischemia-reperfusion or the action of inflammatory mediators. The OL precursor is particularly vulnerable *in vitro* to free-radical mediated injury. This raises the possibility that free radical scavengers may be one potential intervention to disrupt the cascade of events which triggers OL death. Several triggers for death of OL precursors via apoptosis have been identified. Future advances in the elucidation of the mechanisms that promote apoptosis may thus provide selective means to pharmacologically block OL death arising from acute WM insults. Alternatively, death of OL precursors may be circumvented by strategies to replete damaged OLs by implantation of OL progenitors. Notably, such progenitors can be isolated in large number from adult rodent optic nerve[173] and adult human subcortical WM[174] and were capable of remyelination in the adult rat spinal cord.[175] Strategies are also under investigation to generate OL progenitors with myelinogenetic potential from totipotent embryonic stem cells.[176] Transplantation of such cells into a myelin-deficient fetal rat model resulted in myelin formation at multiple levels in the neuraxis.[177]

It remains to be determined whether subacute responses to injury may further contribute to the pathogenesis of PVL. Cytotoxic cell mediators, including cytokines, may be released from microglia or reactive astrocytes acting in response to acute WM injury. In addition, these reactive cell types, as well as axonal injury, may disrupt mechanisms that mediate the actions of OL trophic factors. One result might be a failure of OL maturation at sites of axonal injury[178] or decreased OL survival. The selective delivery of OL growth and differentiation factors represents a potential intervention to sustain populations of OL precursors that might promote myelination and axon development.[8]

Further insight is also needed into the effects of PVL on axonal integrity. Pertinent to this question is a need for greater insight into the excitoxic mechanisms that may result in axonal injury in the developing WM. Moreover, the importance of the OL to direct neuronal maturation is indicated by recent studies that demonstrated that some aspects of axonal maturation are mediated by OLs independent of myelination status,[179] whereas others require compact myelin formation.[180] Interestingly, a recent clinical study demonstrated a reduction in cerebral cortical gray matter volume in premature infants with PVL.[181] Future studies are thus needed to determine what role OL precursors might play in sustaining axonal function. Clearly, the ultimate success of interventions to circumvent the clinical sequelae of PVL will depend upon sustaining the functional integrity of axonal-oligodendroglial interactions.

References

1. Hack M, Friedman H, Avroy A, et al. Outcomes of extremely low birth weight infants. *Pediatrics* 1996;98:931-937.

2. Volpe J. Brain injury in the premature infant: Overview of clinical aspects, neuropathology, and pathogenesis. *Seminars in Pediatric Neurology* 1998; 5:135-151.

3. Volpe JJ. Neurology of the Newborn. Philadelphia: W.B. Saunders; 1995.

4. Dammann O, Levition A. Infection remote from the brain, neonatal white matter damage, and cerebral palsy in the preterm infant. *Seminars in Pediatric Neurology* 1998;5:190-201.

5. Pyrds O. Control of cerebral circulation in the high-risk neonate. *Ann Neurol* 1991;30:321-329.

6. Nakamura Y, Okudera T, Hashimoto T. Vascular architechture in white matter of neonates: its relationship to periventricular leukomalacia. *J Neuropath Exp Neurol* 1994;53:582-589.

7. Pfeiffer SE, Warrington AE, Bansal R. The oligodendrocyte and its many cellular processes. *Trends Cell Biol* 1993;3:191-197.

8. McMorris FA, McKinnon RD. Regulation of oligodendrocyte development and CNS myelination by growth factors: Prospects for therapy of demyelinating disease. *Brain Pathol* 1996;6:313-329.

9. Oka A, Belliveau MJ, Rosenberg PA, et al. Vulnerability of oligodendroglia to glutamate: Pharmacology, mechanisms, and prevention. *J Neurosci* 1993;13(4):1441-1453.

10. Mayer M, Noble M. N-acetyl-L-cysteine is a pluripotent protector against cell death and enhancer of trophic factor-mediated cell survival in vitro. *Proc Natl Acad Sci USA* 1994;91:7496-7500.

11. Yonezawa M, Back SA, Gan X, et al. Cystine deprivation induces oligodendroglial death: Rescue by free radical scavengers and by a diffusible glial factor. *J Neurochem* 1996;67:566-573.

12. Back S, Gan X-D, Li Y, et al. Maturation-dependent vulnerability of oligodendrocytes to oxidative stress-induced death caused by glutathione depletion. *J Neurosci* 1998;18:6241-6253.

13. Gilles FH, Averill DR, Kerr CS. Neonatal endotoxin encephalopathy. *Ann Neurol* 1977;2:49-56.

14. Young RSK, Yagel SK, Towfighi J. Systemic and neuropathologic effects of *E. coli* endotoxin in neonatal dogs. *Pediatr Res* 1983;17:349-353.

15. Ando M, Takashima S, Mito T. Endotoxin, cerebral blood flow, amino acids and brain damage in young rabbits. *Brain Devel* 1988;10:365-370.

16. Banker B, Larroche J. Periventricular leukomalacia of infancy. A form of neonatal anoxic encephalopathy. *Arch Neurol* 1962;7:386-410.

17. Rorke LB. Perinatal brain damage. 5th ed. London: Edward Arnold; 1992.

18. Leviton A, Gilles F. Acquired perinatal leukoencephalopathy. *Ann Neurol* 1984;16:1-10.

19. Selmaj K, Raine CS, Farooq M, et al. Cytokine cytotoxicity against oligodendrocytes: Apoptosis induced by lymphotoxin. *J Immunol* 1991;147:1522-1529.

20. Louis J-C, Magal E, Takayama S, et al. CNTF protection of oligodendrocytes against natural and tumor necrosis factor-induced death. *Science* 1993;259:689-692.

21. Barres BA, Hart IK, Coles HSR, et al. Cell death and control of cell survival in the oligodendrocyte lineage. *Cell* 1992;70:31-46.

22. Raff M, Barres B, Burne J, et al. Programmed cell death and the control of cell survival: Lessons from the nervous system. *Science* 1993;262:695-700.

23. Rorke LB. Anatomical features of the developing brain implicated in pathogenesis of hypoxic-ischemic injury. *Brain Pathol* 1992;2:211-221.

24. Kinney H, Back S. Human oligodendroglial development: Relationship to periventricular leukomalacia. *Seminars in Pediatric Neurology* 1998;5:180-189.

25. Claris O, Besnier S, Lapillonne A, et al. Incidence of ischemic-hemorrhagic cerebral lesions in premature infants of gestational age ≤ 28 weeks: A prospective ultrasound study. *Biol Neonate* 1996;70:29-34.

26. Leviton A, Paneth N. White matter damage in preterm newborns—an epidemiologic perspective. *Early Hum Dev* 1990;24:1-22.

27. Brody BA, Kinney HC, Kloman AS, et al. Sequence of central nervous system myelination in human infancy. I. An autopsy study of myelination. *J Neuropath Exp Neurol* 1987;46:283-301.

28. Kinney HC, Brody BA, Kloman AS, et al. Sequence of central nervous system myelination in human infancy. II. Patterns of myelination in autopsied infants. *J Neuropathol Exp Neurol* 1989;47:217-234.

29. Huppi P, Maier S, Peled S, et al. Microstructural development of human newborn cerebral white matter assessed *in vivo* by diffusion tensor magnetic resonance imaging. *Pediatr Res* 1998;44:584-590.

30. Friede RL. Developmental Neuropathology. 2nd ed. Berlin: Springer-Verlag; 1989.

31. Rorke LB. Pathology of Perinatal Brain Injury. New York: Raven Press; 1982.

32. De Vries L, Wigglesworth J, Regev R, et al. Evolution of periventricular leukomalacia during the neonatal period and infancy: Correlation of imaging and postmortem findings. *Early Human Development* 1988;17:205-219.

33. Dambska M, Laure-Kamionowska M, Schmit-Sidor B. Early and late neuro-pathological changes in perinatal white matter damage. *J Child Neurol* 1989;4:291-298.

34. Paneth N, Rudelli R, Monte W, et al. White matter necrosis in very low birth weight infants: Neuropathologic and ultrasonographic findings in infants surviving six days or longer. *J Pediatr* 1990;116:975-984.

35. Golden J, Gilles F, Rudewill R. Frequency of neuropathological abnormalities in very low birth weight infants. *J Neuropathol Exper Neurol* 1997;56:472-478.

36. Barres B, Schmid R, Sendnte M, et al. Multiple extracellular signals are required for long-term oligodendrocyte survival. *Development* 1993;118:283-295.

37. Gard AL, Pfeiffer SE, Williams WC III. Immunopanning and developmental stage-specific primary culture of oligodendrocyte progenitors (O4+GalC−) directly from postnatal rodent cerebrum. *Neuroprotocols* 1993;2:209-218.

38. Noble M, Murray K. Purified astrocytes promote the in vitro division of a bipotential glial progenitor cell. *EMBO J* 1984;3:2243-7.

39. Raff MC, Williams BP, Miller RH. The in vitro differentiation of a bipotential glial progenitor cell. *EMBO J* 1984;3:1857-1864.

40. Aloisi F, Agresti C, D'Urso D, et al. Differentiation of bipotential glial precursors into oligodendrocytes is promoted by interaction with type-1 astrocytes in cerebellar cultures. *Proc Natl Acad Sci USA* 1988;85:6167-6171.

41. Armstrong RC, Harvath L, Dubois-Dalcq ME. Type 1 astrocytes and oligo-dendrocyte-type 2 astrocyte glial progenitors migrate toward distinct molecules. *J Neurosci Res* 1990;27:400-407.

42. Wren D, Wolswijk G, Noble M. In vitro analysis of the origin and mainte-nance of 0-2Adult progenitor cells. *The J Cell Biol* 1992;116:167-176.

43. Rivkin MJ, Flax J, Mozell R, et al. Oligodendroglial development in human fetal cerebrum. *Ann Neurol* 1995;38:92-101.

44. Scolding N, Rayner P, Sussman J, et al. A proliferative adult human oligode-ndrocyte progenitor. *Neuroreport* 1995;6:441-445.

45. Espinosa de los Monteros A, S ZM, De Vellis J. O2A progenitor cells transplanted into the neonatal rat brain develop into oligodendrocytes but not astrocytes. *Proc Natl Acad Sci USA* 1993;90:50-54.

46. Fredman P, Magnani JL, Nirenberg M, et al. Monoclonal antibody A2B5 reacts with many gangliosides in neuronal tissue. *Arch Biochem Biophys* 1984;33:661-666.

47. Dubois C, Manuguerra J-C, Hauttecoeur B, et al. Monoclonal antibody A2B5, which detects cell surface antigens, binds to ganglioside GT3 (II3(-NeuAc)3LacCer) and to its 9-O-acetylated derivative. *J Biol Chem* 1990;265:2797-2803.

48. Levine J, Stallcup W. Plasticity of developing cerebellar cells in vitro studied with antibodies against the NG2 antigen. *J Neurosci* 1987;7:2721-2731.

49. Reynolds R, Hardy R. Oligodendroglial progenitors labeled with the O4 antibody persist in the adult rat cerebral cortex in vivo. *J Neurosci Res* 1997;47:455-470.

50. Trapp B, Nishiyama A, Cheng D, et al. Differentiation and death of premy-elinating oligodendrocytes in developing rodent brain. *J Cell Biol* 1997;137:459-468.

51. Keirstead H, Levine J, Blakemore W. Response of the oligodendrocyte progenitor cell population (defined by NG2 labelling) to demyelination of the adult spinal cord. *Glia* 1998;22:161-170.

52. Nishiyama A, Lin X-H, Giese N, et al. Co-localization of NG2 proteoglycan and PDGF α receptor on O2A progenitor cells in the developing rat brain. *J Neurosci Res* 1996;42:299-314.

53. Ellison JA, de Vellis J. Platelet-derived growth factor receptor is expressed by cells in the early oligodendrocyte lineage. *J Neurosci Res* 1994;37:116-128.

54. Bansal R, Stefansson K, Pfeiffer SE. Proo igodendroblast antigen (POA), a developmental antigen expressed by AO07/04-positive oligodendrocyte progenitors prior to the appearance of sulfatide and galactocerebroside. *J Neurochem* 1992;58:2221-2229.

55. Hardy R. Dorsoventral patterning and oligodendroglial specification in the developing central nervous system. *J Neurosci Res* 1997;50:139-145.

56. Hajihosseini M, Tham T, Dubois-Dalcq M. Origin of oligodendrocytes within the human spinal cord. *J Neurosc* 1996;16:7981-7984.

57. Sommer I, Schachner M. Cells that are O4-antigen positive and O1-negative differentiate into O1 antigen-positive oligodendrocytes. *Neurosci Lett* 1982;29:183-188.

58. Schachner M, Kim SK, Zehnle R. Developmental expression in central and peripheral nervous system of oligodendrocyte cell surface antigens (O antigens) recognized by monoclonal antibodies. *Dev Biol* 1981;83:328-338.

59. Bansal R, Warrington A, Gard A, et al. Multiple and novel specificities of monoclonal antibodies O1, O4, and R-mAb used in the analysis of oligodendrocyte development. *J Neurosci Res* 1989;24:548-557.

60. Gard AL, Pfeiffer SE. Two proliferative stages of the oligodendrocyte lineage (A2B5+O4- and O4+GalC-) under different mitogenic control. *Neuron* 1990;5:615-625.

61. Armstrong RC, Dorn HJ, Kufta CV, et al. Pre-oligodendrocytes from adult human CNS. *J Neurosci* 1992;12:1538-1547.

62. Dubois-Dalcq M, Behar T, Hudson L, et al. Emergence of three myelin proteins in oligodendrocyte cultures without neurons. *J Cell Biol* 1986;102:384-392.

63. Macklin W, Weil CL, Deininger PL. Expression of myelin proteolipid and basic protein mRNA's in cultured cells. *J Neurosci Res* 1986;16:203-217.

64. Mirsky R, Winter J, Abney ER, et al. Myelin-specific proteins and galactolipids in rat Schwann cells and oligodendrocytes in culture. *J Cell Biol* 1980;84:483-494.

65. Zeller NK, Behar TN, Dubois-Dalcq M, et al. The timely expression of myelin basic protein gene in cultured rat brain oligodendrocytes is independent of continuous neuronal influences. *J Neurosci* 1985;5:2955-2962.

66. Barbarese E, Pfeiffer SE. Developmental regulation of myelin basic protein in dispersed cultures. *Proc Natl Acad Sci USA* 1981;74:3360-3364.

67. Gard AL, Pfeiffer SE. Oligodendrocyte progenitors isolated directly from developing telencephalon at a specific phenotypic stage: Myelinogenic potential in a defined environment. *Development* 1989;106:119-132.

68. Iida K, Takashima S, Ueda K. Immunohistochemical study of myelination and oligodendrocyte in infants with periventricular leukomalacia. *Pediatr Neurol* 1995;13:296-304.

69. Back SA, Volpe JJ, Kinney HH. Immunocytochemical characterization of oligodendrocyte development in human cerebral white matter. *Soc Neurosci Abstr* 1996;20:1722.

70. Back S, Borenstein N, Volpe J, et al. Immunocytochemical delineation of oligodendrocyte lineage progression in human cerebral white matter. *Soc Neurosci Abstr* 1999.

71. Back S, Volpe J. Approaches to the study of diseases involving oligodendroglial death. In: Koliatsos V, et al. (eds): Cell death and diseases of the nervous system. Totowa, New Jersey: Humana Press; 1999:401-428.

72. Gallo V, Russell JT. Excitatory amino acid receptors in glia: Different subtypes for distinct function? *J Neurosci Res* 1995;42:1-8.

73. Borges K, Wolswijk G, Ohlemeyer C, et al. Adult rat optic nerve oligodendroctye progenitor cells express a distinct repertoire of voltage and ligand-gated ion channels. *J Neurosci Res* 1995;40:591-605.

74. Borges K, Ohlemeyer C, Trotter J, et al. AMPA/Kainate receptor activation in murine oligodendrocyte precursor cells leads to activation of a cation conductance, calcium influx and blockade of delayed rectifying K+ channels. *Neuroscience* 1994;63:135-149.

75. Gallo V, Zhou JM, McBain CJ, et al. Oligodendrocyte progenitor cell proliferation and lineage progression are regulated by glutamate receptor-mediated K+ channel block. *J Neurosci* 1996;16:2659-2670.

76. Yuan X, Eisen A, McBain C, et al. A role for glutamate and its receptors in the regulation of oligodendrocyte development in cerebellar tissue slices. *Development* 1998;125:2901-2914.

77. Ghiani C, Yuan X, Eisen A, et al. Voltage-activated K+ channels and membrane depolarization regulate accumulation of the cyclin-dependent kinase inhibitors P27 Kip1 and p21CIP1 in glial progenitor cells. *J Neurosci* 1999;19:5380-5392.

78. Yoshioka A, Hardy M, Younkin DP, et al. α-Amino-3-hydroxy-5-methyl-4-isoxazolepropionate (AMPA) receptors mediate excitotoxicity in the oligodendroglial lineage. *J Neurochem* 1995;64:2442-2448.

79. McDonald JW, Althomsons S, Hyrc K, et al. Oligodendrocytes from forebrain are highly vulnerable to AMPA/kainate receptor-mediated excitotoxicity. *Nature Medicine* 1998;4:291-297.

80. Lyons S, Kettenmann H. Oligodendrocytes and microglia are selectively vulnerable to combined hypoxia and hypoglycemia injury *in vitro. J Cereb Blood Flow Metab* 1998;18:521-530.

81. McCarthy KD, de Vellis J. Preparation of separate astroglial and oligodendroglial cell cultures from rat cerebral tissue. *J Cell Biol* 1980;85:890-902.

82. Murphy T, Miyamoto M, Sastre A, et al. Glutamate toxicity in a neuronal cell line involves inhibition of cystine transport leading to oxidative stress. *Neuron* 1989;2:1547-1558.

83. Murphy T, Schnaar R, Coyle J. Immature cortical neurons are uniquely sensitive to glutamate toxicity by inhibition of cystine uptake. *FASEB J* 1990;4:1624-1633.

84. Ratan RR, Murphy TH, Baraban JM. Macromolecular synthesis inhibitors prevent oxidative stress-induced apoptosis in embryonic cortical neurons by shunting cysteine from protein synthesis to glutathione. *J Neurosci* 1994;14:4385-4392.

85. Ratan RR, Murphy TH, Baraban JM. Oxidative stress induces apoptosis in embryonic cortical neurons. *J Neurochem* 1994;62:376-379.
86. Bannai S, Kitamura E. Transport interaction of L-cystine and L-glutamate in human diploid fibroblasts in culture. *J Biol Chem* 1980;255:2372-2376.
87. Sato H, Tamba M, Ishii T, et al. Cloning and expression of a plasma membrane cystine/glutamate exchange transporter composed of two distinct proteins. *J Biol Chem* 1999;274:11455-11458.
88. Cassaccia-Bonnefil P, Aibel L, Chao M. Central glial and neuronal populations display differential sensitivity to ceramide-dependent cell death. *J Neurosci Res* 1996;43:382-389.
89. Brogi A, Strazza M, Melli M, et al. Induction of intracellular ceramide by interleukin-1β in oligodendrocytes. *J Cell Biochem* 1997;66:532-541.
90. Quillet-Mary A, Jaffrezou J-P, Mansat V, et al. Implication of mitochondrial hydrogen peroxide generation in ceramide-induced apoptosis. *J Biol Chem* 1997;272:21388-21395.
91. Husain J, Juurlink BHJ. Oligodendroglial precursor cell susceptibility to hypoxia is related to poor ability to cope with reactive oxygen species. *Brain Res* 1995;698:86-94.
92. Thorburne SK, Juurlink BHJ. Low glutathione and high iron govern the susceptibility of oligodendroglial precursors to oxidative stress. *J Neurochem* 1996; 67:1014-1022.
93. Jelinski S, Yager J, Juurlink B. Preferential injury of oligodendroblasts by a short hypoxic-ischemic insult. *Brain Res* 1999;815:150-153.
94. Mitrovic B, Ignarro LJ, Vinters HV, et al. Nitric oxide induces necrotic but not apoptotic death in oligodendrocytes. *Neuroscience* 1995;65:531-539.
95. Mackenzie-Graham A, Mitrovic B, Smoll A, et al. Differential sensitivity to nitric oxide in immortalized, cloned murine oligodendrocyte cell lines. *Dev Neurosci* 1994;16:162-171.
96. Rosenberg P, Ya L, Ali S, et al. Intracellular redox state determines whether nitric oxide is toxic or protective to rat oligodendrocytes in culture. *J Neurochem* 1999;73:476-484.
97. Zaman K, Ryu H, Hall D, et al. Protection from oxidative stress-induced apoptosis in cortical neuronal cultures by iron chelators is associated with enhanced DNA binding of hypoxia-inducible factor-1 and ATF-1/CREB and increased expression of glycolytic enxymes, p21 waf1/cip1, and erythropoietin. *J Neurosci* 1999;19:9821-9830.
98. Hill JM, Switzer RC. The regional distribution and cellular localization of iron in the rat brain. *Neuroscience* 1984;11:595-603.
99. Dwork AJ, Schon EA, Herbert J. Nonidentical distribution of transferrin and ferric iron in human brain. *Neuroscience* 1988;27:333-345.
100. Gerber MR, Connor JR. Do oligodendrocytes mediate iron regulation in the human brain? *Ann Neurol* 1989;26:95-98.
101. Connor JR, Menzies SL, St. Martin SM, et al. Cellular distribution of transferrin, ferritin, and iron in normal and aged human brains. *J Neurosci Res* 1990;27:595-611.
102. Ozawa H, Nishida A, Mito T, et al. Development of ferritin-containing cells in the pons and cerebellum of the human brain. *Brain Devel* 1994;16:92-95.
103. Connor JR, Menzies SL. Relationship of iron to oligodendrocytes and myelination. *Glia* 1996;17:83-93.

104. Connor JR, Phillips TM, Lakshman MR, et al. Regional variations in the levels of transferrin in the CNS of normal and myelin-deficient rats. *J Neurochem* 1987;49:1523-1529.

105. Connor JR, Menzies SL. Altered distribution of iron in the central nervous system of myelin deficient rats. *Neuroscience* 1990;34:265-261.

106. Roskams AJ, Connor JR. Transferrin receptor expression in myelin deficient (md) rats. *J Neurosci Res* 1992;31:421-427.

107. Connor JR, Fine RE. Development of transferrin-positive oligodendrocytes in the rat central nervous system. *J Neurosci Res* 1987;17:51-59.

108. Jacobsen M, Lassen LC, Mollgard K. Immunohistochemical evidence for intracellular localization of plasma proteins in CNS and some neural crest derivatives in human embryos. *Tumor Biol* 1984;5:53-60.

109. Mollgard K, Stagaard M, Saunders NR. Cellular distribution of transferrin immunoreactivity in the developing rat brain. *Neurosci Lett* 1987;78:35-40.

110. Taylor EM, Morgan EH. Developmental changes in transferrin and iron uptake by brain in the rat. *Brain Res Dev Brain Res* 1990;55:35-42.

111. Connor JR, Pavlick G, Karli D, et al. A histochemical study of iron-positive cells in the developing rat brain. *J Comp Neurol* 1995;355:111-123.

112. Crickton RR, Charloteaux-Wauters M. Iron transport and storage. *Eur J Biochem* 1987;164:485-506.

113. Gocht A, Keith AB, Candy JM, Morris CM. Iron uptake in the brain of the myelin-deficient rat. *Neurosci Lett* 1993;154:187-190.

114. Lin HH, Connnor JR. The development of the transferrin-transferrin receptor system in relation to astroyctes, MBP and galactorcerebroside in normal and myelin-deficient rat optic nerves. *Brain Res* 1989;49:281-293.

115. Koster JF. Ferritin, a physiological iron donor for microsomal lipid peroxidation. *FEBS Lett* 1986;199:85-88.

116. Balla G, Jacob HS, Balla J, et al. Ferritin: A cytoprotective antioxidant strategem of endothelium. *J Biol Chem* 1992;267:18148-18153.

117. Qi Y, Dawson G. Hypoxia induces synthesis of a novel 22-kDa protein in neonatal rat oligodendrocytes. *J Neurochem* 1992;59:1709-1716.

118. Qi Y, Dawson G. Hypoxia specifically and reversibly induces the synthesis of ferritin in oligodendrocytes and human oligodendrogliomas. *J Neurochem* 1994;63:1485-1490.

119. Rehncrona S, Nielsen Hauge H, Siejsö BK. Enhancement of iron-catalyzed free radical formation by acidosis in brain homogenates: Difference in effect by lactic acid and CO_2. *J Cereb Blood Flow Metab* 1989;9:65-70.

120. Qi Y, Jamindar T, Dawson G. Hypoxia alters iron homeostasis and induces ferritin synthesis in oligodendrocytes. *J Neurochem* 1995;64:2458-2464.

121. Kelly FJ. Free radical disorders of preterm infants. *Brit Med Bull* 1993;49:668-678.

122. Chan PH. Role of oxidants in ischemic brain damage. *Stroke* 1996;27:1124-1129.

123. Kim YS, Kim SU. Oligodendroglial cell death induced by oxygen radicals and its protection by catalase. *J Neurosci Res* 1991;29:100-106.

124. Noble PG, Antel JP, Yong VW. Astrocytes and catalase prevent the toxicity of catecholamines to oligodendrocytes. *Brain Res* 1994;663:83-90.

125. Pinteaux E, Perraut M, Tholey G. Distribution of mitochondrial manganese superoxide dismutase among rat glial cells in culture. *Glia* 1998;22:408-414.

126. Juurlink B, Thorburne S, Hertz L. Peroxide-scavenging deficit underlies oligodendrocyte susceptibility to oxidative stress. *GLIA* 1998;22:371-378.

127. Houdou S, Kuruta H, Hasegawa M, et al. Developmental immunohistochemistry of catalase in the human brain. *Brain Res* 1991;556:267-270.

128. Del Maestro R, McDonald W. Distribution of superoxide dismutase, glutathione peroxidase and catalase in developing rat brain. *Mech Ageing Devel* 1987;41:29-38.

129. Ditelberg JS, Sheldon RA, Epstein CJ, et al. Brain injury after perinatal hypoxia-ischemia is exacerbated in copper/zinc superoxide dismutase transgenic mice. *Pediatric Research* 1996;39:204-208.

130. Traystman RJ, Kirsch JR, Koehler RC. Oxygen radical mechanisms of brain injury following ischemia and reperfusion. *Am J Physiol* 1991;71:1185-1195.

131. Perlman J, Vannucci R. Perinatal hypoxic-ischemic encephalopathy. *Pediatrics* 1997;100:1004-1014.

132. Varsila E, Pitkanen O, Hallman M, et al. Immaturity-dependent free radical activity in premature infants. *Pediatr Res* 1994;36:55-59.

133. Sanderud J, Kumlin M, Granstrom E, et al. Effects of oxygen radicals on cysteinyl leukotriene metabolism and pulmonary circulation in young pigs. *Eur Surg Res* 1995;27:117-126.

134. Lackmann G, Hesse L, Tollner U. Reduced iron-associated antioxidants in premature newborns suffering intracerebral hemorrhage. *Free Radical Biol Med* 1996;20:407-409.

135. Lubec G, Widness J, Hayde M. Hydroxyl radical generation in oxygen-treated infants. *Pediatrics* 1997;100:700-704.

136. Gilles FH, Leviton A, Kerr CS. Susceptibility of the neonatal feline telencephalic white matter to a lipopolysaccharide. *J Neurol Sci* 1976;27:183-191.

137. Trippodo NC, Jorgensen JH, Priano LL, et al. Cerebrospinal fluid levels of endotoxin during endotoxemia. *Proc Soc Exp Biol Med* 1973;143:932-937.

138. Clawson CC, Hartman JF, Vernier RL. Electron microscopy of the effect of gram negative endotoxin on the blood brain barrier. *J Comp Neurol* 1966;127:183.

139. Perlman JM, Risser R, Broyles RS. Bilateral cystic periventricular leukomalacia in the premature infant: Associated risk factors. *Pediatrics* 1996;97:822-827.

140. Yoon BH, Romero R, Yang SH, et al. Interleukin-6 concentrations in umbilical cord plasma are elevated in neonates with white matter lesions associated with periventricular leukomalacia. *Am J Obstet Gynecol* 1996;174:1433-1440.

141. Kahn MA, De Vellis J. Regulation of an oligodendrocyte progenitor cell line by the interleukin-6 family of cytokines. *GLIA* 1994;12:87-98.

142. Harris MC, Constantino AT, Sullivan JS, et al. Cytokine elevations in critically ill infants with sepsis and necrotizing enterocolitis. *J Pediatr* 1994;124:105-111.

143. Fong Y, Lowry SF. Tumor necrosis factor in the pathophysiology of infection and sepsis. *Clin Immunol Immunpathol* 1990;55:157-170.

144. Norenberg MD. Astrocyte response to CNS injury. *J Neuropath Exp Neurol* 1994;53:213-220.

145. Robbins DS, Shirazi Y, Drysdale B-E, et al. Production of cytotoxic factor for oligodendrocytes by stimulated astrocytes. *J Immunol* 1987;139:2593-2597.

146. Merrill JE. Effects of interleukin-1 and tumor necrosis factor-α on astrocytes, microglia, oligodendrocytes, and glial precursors in vitro. *Dev Neurosci* 1991;13:130.

147. Prabhakar S, D'Souza S, Antel JP, et al. Phenotypic and cell cycle properties of human oligodendrocytes in vitro. *Brain Res* 1995;672:159-169.

148. Vartanian T, Li Y, Zhao M, et al. Interferon-γ-induced oligodendrocyte cell death: Implications for the pathogenesis of multiple sclerosis. *Mol Med* 1995;1:732-743.

149. Merrill JE, Ignarro LJ, Sherman MP, et al. Microglial cell cytotoxicity of oligodendrocytes is mediated through nitric oxide. *J Immunol* 1993;151:2132-2141.

150. Mitrovic B, Martin FC, Charles AC, et al. Neurotransmitters and cytokines in CNS pathology. *Prog Br Res* 1994;103:319-330.

151. Lee SC, Liu W, Dickson DW, et al. Cytokine production by human fetal microglia and astrocytes: Differential induction by lipopolysaccharide and IL-1β. *J Neurosurg* 1993;150:2659-2667.

152. Collarini EJ, Pringle N, Mudhar H, et al. Growth factors and transcription factors in oligodendrocyte development. *J Cell Sci Supp* 1991;15:117-123.

153. Barres BA, Raff MC. Control of oligodendrocyte number in the developing rat optic nerve. *Neuron* 1994;12:935-942.

154. Bogler O, Wren D, Barnett SC, et al. Cooperation between two growth factors promotes extended self-renewal and inhibits differentiation of oligodendrocyte-type-2 astrocyte(O-2A) progenitor cells. *Proc Natl Acad Sci USA* 1990;87:6368-6372.

155. McKinnon RD, Matsui T, Dubois-Dalcq M, et al. FGF modulates the PDGF-driven pathway of oligodendrocyte development. *Neuron* 1990;5:603-614.

156. Wolswijk G, Noble M. Cooperation between PDGF and FGF converts slowly dividing 0-2Aadult progenitor cells to rapidly dividing cells with characteristics of 0-2A perinatal progenitor cells. *J Cell Biol* 1992;118:889-900.

157. Bansal R, Pfeiffer SE. Inhibition of protein and lipid sulfation in oligodendrocytes blocks biological responses to FGF-2 and retards cytoarchitechtural maturation, but not developmental lineage progression. *Dev Biol* 1994;162:511-524.

158. Barres BA, Raff MC, Gaese F, et al. A crucial role for neurotrophin-3 in oligodendrocyte development. *Nature* 1994;367:371-375.

159. Komoly S, Hudson DL, Dewebster H, et al. Insulin-like growth factor I gene expression is induced in astrocytes during experimental demyelination. *Proc Natl Acad Sci USA* 1992;89:1894-1898.

160. Yao DL, West NR, Bondy CA, et al. Cryogenic spinal cord injury induces astrocytic gene expression of insulin-like growth factor I and insulin-like growth factor binding protein 2 during remyelination. *J Neurosci Res* 1995;40:647-659.

161. Baron-Van Evercooren A, Olichon-Berthe C, Kowalski A, et al. Expression of IGF-1 and insulin receptor genes in the rat central nervous sytem: A developmental, regional and cellular analysis. *J Neurosci Res* 1991;28:244-253.

162. Bartlett WP, Li X-s, Williams M. Expressior. of IGF-1 mRNA in the murine subventricular zone during postnatal development. *Mol Brain Res* 1992;12:285-291.

163. Shinar Y, McMorris FA. Developing oligodendroglia cells express mRNA for insulin-like growth factor-1, a regulator of oligodendrocyte development. *J Neurosci Res* 1995;42:516-527.

164. Yeh H-J, Ruit K, Wang Y-X, et al. PDGF A-chain gene is expressed by mammalian neurons during development and in maturity. *Cell* 1991;64:209-216.

165. Ellison JA, Scully SA, de Vellis J. Evidence for neurcnal regulation of oligodendrocyte development: Cellular localization of platelet-derived growth factor α receptor and A-chain mRNA during cerebral cortex development in the rat. *J Neurosci Res* 1996;45:28-39.

166. Raff MC, Lillien LE, Richardson WD, et al. Platelet-derived growth factor from astrocytes drives the clock that times oligodendrocyte development in culture. *Nature* 1988;333:562-565.

167. Noble M, Murray K, Stroobant P, et al. Platelet-derived growth factor promotes division and motility and inhibits premature differentiation of the oligodendrocyte/type-2 astrocyte progenitor cell. *Nature* 1988;333:560-562.

168. Hart IK, Richardson WD, Bolsover SR, et al. PDGF and intracellular signalling in the timing of oligodendrocyte differentiation. *J Cell Biol* 1989;109:3411-3417.

169. McMorris FA, Mozell RL, Carson MJ, et al. Regulation of oligodendrocyte development and central nervous system myelinatior. by insulin-like growth factors. *Ann N Y Acad Sci* 1993;692:321-324.

170. Beck KD, Powell-Braxton L, Widmer HR, et al. Igf1 gene disruption results in reduced brain size, CNS hypomyelination, and loss of hippocampal granule and striatal parvalbumin-containing neurons. *Neuron* 1995;14:717-730.

171. Carson MJ, Behringer RR, Brinster RL, et al. Insulin-like growth factor I increases brain growth and central nervous system myelination in transgenic mice. *Neuron* 1993;10:729-740.

172. Ye P, Carson J, D'Arcole AJ. In vivo actions of insulin-like growth factor-1 (IGF-1) on brain myelination: Studies of IGF-1 and IGF binding protein-1 (IGFBP-1) transgenic mice. *J Neurosci* 1995;15:7344-7356.

173. Shi J, Marinovich A, Barres B. Purification and characterization of adult oligodendrocyte precursor cells from the rat optic nerve. *J Neurosci* 1998;18:4627-4636.

174. Roy N, Wang S, Harrison-Restelli C, et al. Identification, isolation, and promoter-defined separation of mitotic oligodendroctye progenitor cells from the adult subcortical white matter. *J Neurosci* 1999;19:9986-9995.

175. Keirstead H, Ben-Hur T, Rogister B, et al. Polysialated neural cell adhesion molecule-positive CNS precursors generate both oligodendrocytes and schwann cells to remyelinate the CNS after transplantation. *J Neurosci* 1999;19:7529-7536.

176. Brustle O, Kimberly N, Learish R, et al. Embryonic stem cell-derived glial precursors: A source of myelinating transplants. *Science* 1999;285:754-756.

177. Learish R, Brustle O, Zhang S, et al. Intraventricular transplantation of oligodendrocyte progenitors into a fetal myelin mutant results in widespread formation of myelin. *Ann Neurol* 1999;46:716-722.

178. Butt AM, Colquhoun K. Glial cells in transected optic nerves of immature rats. I. An analysis of individual cells by intracellular dye-injection. *J Neurocytol* 1996; 25:365-380.

179. Sanchez I, Hassinger L, Paskevich P, et al. Oligodendroglia regulate the regional expansion of axon caliber and local accumulation of neurofilaments during development independently of myelin formation. *J Neurosci* 1996;16:5095-5105.

180. Brady S, Witt A, Kirkpatrick L, et al. Formation of compact myelin is required for maturation of the axonal cytoskeleton. *J Neurosci* 1999;19: 7278-7288.

181. Inder T, Huppi P, Warfield S, et al. Periventricular white matter injury in the premature infant is followed by reduced cerebral cortical gray matter volume at term. *Ann Neurol* 1999;46:755-760.

Chapter 11

White Matter Ischemia—Unique Mechanisms of Injury

Peter K. Stys, MD, FRCP(C)

Stroke is a prevalent disorder resulting is serious morbidity and mortality, with an estimated 600,000 new cases every year in the U.S. alone.[1] Functional integrity of the central nervous system depends on a number of interdependent tissues in the brain, including an intact vascular bed for supplying the brain with nutrients and clearing metabolic waste, gray matter consisting largely of neurons, synaptic machinery and supporting glia, and white matter, containing the mostly myelinated axons that support transmission of signals within the nervous system. Gray and white matter elements are uniquely designed to carry out their respective roles, and not surprisingly, display unique cellular and molecular architectures. By extension, one might expect that responses to injurious stimuli and ultimately molecular mechanisms of irreversible damage in gray and white matter may differ significantly, in turn implying that therapy aimed at one area may be ineffective in the other tissue. For these reasons it is important to elucidate the potentially unique mechanisms of injury in white matter, to complement what is known about gray matter injury, so that effective treatments can be proposed to maximize recovery in both tissue types, thus maximizing protection of the central nervous system (CNS) as a whole during stroke.

From: Choi D, Dacey RG, Hsu CY, Powers WJ. *Cerebrovascular Disease: Momentum at the End of the Second Millennium.* Armonk, NY: Futura Publishing Company, Inc., © 2002. The author is supported by a Carrer Investigator Award from the Heart and Stroke Foundation of Ontario. Work in the author's laboratory has been supported by grants from the Medical Research Council of Canada, Heart and Stroke Foundation of Ontario, Ontario Neurotrauma Foundation and the National Institute of Neurological Disorders and Stroke.

White Matter Energy Requirements

Much of what we have learned about the basic mechanisms of white matter anoxic/ischemic injury originated from studies carried out on the *in vitro* rat optic nerve (RON). The RON is a prototypical central white matter tract composed of myelinated axons, myelinating oligodendroglia and supporting astrocytes.[2,3] To date, corroborating experiments appear to support the assumption that the RON is generally representative of CNS white matter with respect to responses to anoxia/ischemia,[4,5] though minor differences between various white matter tracts are likely to emerge as our understanding of precise injury mechanisms in this tissue improves.

Although the rate of energy consumption is less in white matter compared to gray matter,[6] both require a continuous supply of oxygen and glucose to maintain function and integrity. Much of the energy is consumed by the Na^+-K^+-ATPase, fueled largely by ATP derived from oxidative phosphorylation rather than glycolysis.[7] As illustrated in Figure 1, *in vitro* anoxia causes a rapid loss of excitability in the adult RON within minutes. Similar studies in rat spinal cord using isolated dorsal columns also reveal that this white matter tract rapidly becomes inexcitable soon after the onset of anoxia.[4] This loss of electrogenesis is paralleled by a quick and substantial depolarization of the resting membrane potential as measured by the grease gap technique.[7] Interestingly, inhibition of glycolysis using iodoacetic acid, but with oxygen present, first induces a Ca^{2+}-dependent *hyperpolarization* of resting membrane potential, followed by rapid depolarization and loss of excitability, which occurs only ≈ 20 min after application of the inhibitor.[7,8] Why the effects of glycolytic failure are delayed is not known, but may reflect direct utilization by the tricarboxylic acid cycle of alternate substrates such as amino acids;[9] with oxygen available, white matter axons can continue to enjoy the high ATP yield of oxidative metabolism. Also of interest is the difference between aglycemia alone compared to aglycemia with the addition of glycolytic inhibitors such as iodoacetate or 2-deoxyglucose. Omitting glucose without inhibitors causes a far more gradual loss of function,[7,10] which is greatly accelerated by the addition of glycolytic blockers.[7,8,11] The reasons for these differences are not precisely understood. Slow washout of glucose from the extracellular space of the RON is unlikely.[10,11] A more plausible and intriguing explanation may involve the transfer of metabolic substrates from astrocytes. Glia contain most of the brain's stores of glycogen,[12] which can be broken down through glycolysis to supply axons with energy. This process would be impaired in the presence of glycolytic

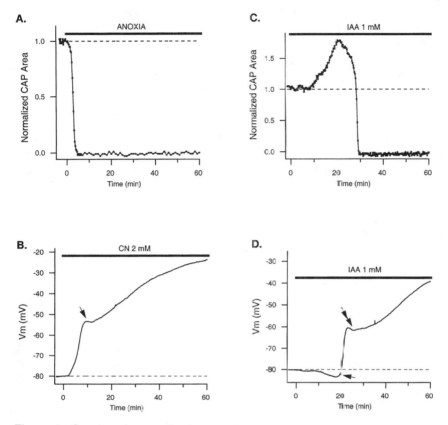

Figure 1. Graphs of normalized rat optic nerve compound action potential (CAP) areas (panels A and C), and compound resting membrane potentials (Vm) (panels B and D), during anoxia or glycolytic block, beginning at time 0 in each graph. **A.** Area under the CAP typically falls to half of control after ~ 5 min of anoxia. **B.** Vm was recorded in a grease gap chamber, with readings normalized to the nominal intra-axonal resting potential of -80 mV.[81] Chemical anoxia using 2 mM cyanide induces a rapid membrane depolarization that coincides with the loss of excitability as shown in panel A. After 10-15 min of anoxia, invariably there is an abrupt change in the *rate* of depolarization (arrow), which is never seen with pure Na⁺-K⁺-ATPase inhibition alone under normoxic conditions (eg, using ouabain, not shown).[82] This may reflect intrinsic mechanisms triggered by energy depletion designed to limit or delay a potentially deleterious membrane depolarization. **C.** In contrast to anoxia, the effects of glycolytic inhibition with 1 mM iodoacetate (IAA) applied at time zero are delayed 10-20 min. There is an initial *rise* in the CAP area likely due to a transient hyperpolarization (see panel D). Excitability then fails abruptly. **D.** Vm during glycolytic inhibition with 1 mM iodoacetate from a different optic nerve illustrates the delayed effects, with the initial change being a transient hyperpolarization (arrow) which closely coincides with the increase in CAP area illustrated in panel C. This is then followed by a rapid and massive depolarization
(continued)

blockers, and in turn would result in a more rapid failure of axonal function, as is observed experimentally.

The susceptibility of optic nerves to anoxic or aglycemic injury greatly depends on the degree of maturity of the tissue. The characteristics described above apply to mature adult RON. Neonatal nerves, on the other hand, are far more resistant. For example, nerves from rats 1 week of age or younger are able to withstand a 60 minute anoxic exposure with no depression of compound action potential amplitude; the nerves remain normally excitable even during the anoxic exposure. While glycolysis can be invoked to explain this resistance to anoxia, even more interesting is an equal resistance of neonatal RON to similar periods of aglycemia; as in anoxia, the response amplitudes are not significantly affected either during or following 60 minutes of aglycemic exposure.[10] Combining anoxia with aglycemia results in more injury than either treatment alone; even neonatal nerves suffer some depression of excitability during the insult, but still manage to recover almost fully with reperfusion/reoxygenation. Generally speaking, susceptibility to injury accrues with age, but the relationship is not monotonic. It appears that there is a period of maximal susceptibility at about 20-30 days of age, with RONs from older rats being somewhat more resistant to anoxia or aglycemia.[10] The mechanisms underlying this age-related vulnerability to injury are not well understood, but appear to parallel axonal myelination and associated reorganization of ion channel distributions on the axolemma.

Deregulation of Ionic Balance

One of the first and most dramatic consequences of energy failure in white matter is a marked deregulation of ionic homeostasis most pronounced in the axons *per se*, and to a lesser extent in glia. The latter elements appear more resistant, unless the insult is prolonged or severe, such as during combined anoxia-aglycemia.[13-15] Anoxia induces a substantial increase in $[K^+]_o$ as measured using ion sensitive microelec-

---

Figure 1. (continued) corresponding to the sudden loss of excitability (panel C). A second hyperpolarizing inflection typically precedes a sudden rate change (double arrow). The Ca^{2+}-dependent hyperpolarizations are much more pronounced with glycolytic failure than with anoxia. Glycolytic block with 2-deoxyglucose + aglycemia causes a more gradual initial hyperpolarization, which is absent with aglycemia alone.[7] The differences may reflect astrocytic glycogen metabolism and transfer of substrates to the axon which can proceed under aglycemic conditions, but not in the presence of inhibitors. All experiments were performed at 37 °C.

trodes in optic nerve *in vitro*. Within minutes, $[K^+]_o$ rises from a baseline of 3 mM to $\approx$14 mM.[16] While the increase is lower than in cortex, where values can reach 80 mM, this does not imply a restrained loss of intracellular K^+. Subsequent direct measurements of axoplasmic $[K^+]$ using electron probe x-ray microanalysis revealed a severe depletion of axoplasmic K^+ content to ~10% of normal, coupled with a parallel rise of $[Na^+]$ to ~ 100 mM;[17] influx into the axoplasm of the latter ion occurs largely through a non-inactivating subtype of TTX-blockable Na^+ channel.[18,19] Thus, with the available Na^+ and K^+ conductances present on the axolemma, these ions appear to flow down their electrochemical gradients during energy failure and exchange roughly in an electroneutral manner.

A curious phenomenon is observed when Na^+ channels are blocked with TTX in anoxic RON. On the one hand, net Na^+ accumulation is greatly reduced as expected, but K^+ efflux proceeds with the same vigor as seen without TTX.[19] Knowing that axonal resting membrane potential is heavily dependent on a healthy K^+ gradient, one might expect the anoxic depolarization to be similar whether TTX is present or not. Yet resting membrane potential is largely preserved during anoxia when TTX is present, despite a severe depletion of $[K^+]_i$. This contradiction can be explained by considering axoplasmic water content and the fact that x-ray microanalysis measures total, and not ionized, elements. In the presence of TTX, anoxia induces significant axonal water loss which will in turn concentrate the remaining K^+, raising the *free* concentration of this ion back up towards normal levels, thus maintaining a healthy membrane potential. If K^+ flowed out of the axon, without a compensatory electroneutral influx of Na^+, it follows that an anion must have accompanied the K^+ efflux. Indeed, x-microanalysis studies show that Cl^- is depleted, along with K^+, but only under conditions of Na^+ channel block.[19] This "anion paradox" induced by Na^+ conductance blockade is of more than academic interest, because the resultant water loss due to electroneutral efflux of K^+ and Cl^- (and probably of other organic anions such as amino acids that cannot be measured by x-ray microanalysis) will also concentrate remaining axoplasmic Na^+ which is deleterious by causing aberrant transport of dangerous substances such as Ca^{2+} and glutamate (see below). Recent data from our laboratory suggest that DIDS- and furosemide-sensitive anion transport is responsible for fluxing anions from the axoplasm under conditions of Na^+ channel inhibition.[20] Together, these observations suggest a role for adjunctive anion transport inhibition when Na^+ channel blockade is proposed as a neuroprotective strategy.

Excess Ca^{2+} entry into cells is thought to represent a "final common pathway" of cell death in many tissue types,[21] and white matter is no exception. Extracellular $[Ca^{2+}]$ in anoxic RON measured by ion-sensitive microelectrodes first *rises* modestly after anoxia onset, before falling well below baseline.[22] The initial increase is interpreted as being due to transient shrinkage of the extracellular space, which gives way to a sustained influx of Ca^{2+} into the intracellular compartment; this Ca^{2+} sink, together with the tight extracellular space of the adult RON, results in a sustained reduction in $[Ca^{2+}]_o$. Measurements of axoplasmic Ca^{2+} confirm a significant increase during the anoxic period. In fact, the time course of the fall in $[Ca^{2+}]_o$ (beginning about 20 min after onset of anoxia [22]) corresponds well to the accelerated rise of axoplasmic $[Ca^{2+}]$ as measured by x-ray microanalysis.[17] A recent *in vivo* study showed a very similar profile of $[Ca^{2+}]_o$ changes in subcortical white matter in anesthetized cats subjected to global cerebral ischemia, with a transient increase followed by a prolonged and substantial fall of $[Ca^{2+}]_o$ as ischemia is maintained.[23]

Glial cells have been shown to be more resistant to anoxia or aglycemia, compared to neurons or axons.[13,24-26] The relatively modest deregulation of ionic content in anoxic white matter glia is consistent with the relative resistance of these cells to injury. Optic nerve glia accumulate only modest amounts of Na^+ and lose modest amounts of K^+ at the end of a 60-minute anoxic exposure, far less than axons, whereas Ca^{2+} levels change very little. Changes in the myelin sheath however, do not parallel those in glial cell bodies or processes, suffering Na^+, K^+ and Ca^{2+} shifts that are more pronounced, but not as severe as the axoplasm.[17] After 60 minutes of anoxia, Ca^{2+} levels in the myelin sheath increase threefold above baseline, which indicates that this area has important Ca^{2+} uptake machinery and likely suffers Ca^{2+}-dependent injury much as the axon cylinder does (see below).

Ca-Mediated Injury:
Influx Pathways and Targets

While there is little question regarding the extent of Ca^{2+} changes in various intracellular compartments of white matter, three key questions need to be answered. 1) What is the correlation between cellular Ca^{2+} overload and functional injury in white matter? 2) If Ca^{2+} influx does cause injury, what are the precise mechanisms of aberrant Ca^{2+} transport during anoxia/ischemia? 3) What molecular targets are modulated by excessive Ca^{2+} levels to cause irreversible injury? The degree of irreversible injury in white matter depends on the length of exposure to anoxia or aglycemia.[10] In optic nerve for example, a 5-10 minute anoxic period causes complete loss of excitability yet is brief enough that the tissue can recover fully upon reoxygenation. Progressively longer exposure causes a gradually more severe injury, so that after 75 minutes or more of anoxia, no recovery is observed.[10] One might speculate that longer insults cause progressively larger intracellular Ca^{2+} loads, and initial electrophysiological studies appeared to support the idea that Ca^{2+} influx into anoxic RON is a gradual event.[27] Later experiments measuring total axoplasmic $[Ca^{2+}]$ directly confirmed that accumulation of this cation occurs progressively throughout a 60-minute anoxic challenge.[17] From these experiments therefore there is little doubt about the key role that Ca^{2+} overload plays in white matter damage, and that this Ca^{2+} excess occurs by influx from the extracellular space into the axoplasm and to a lesser extent the myelin sheath.

We also have evidence suggesting that the very first source of deleterious Ca^{2+} may not be from the exterior, but rather, as a result of release from intracellular stores. Axoplasm of white matter axons contains near-millimolar concentrations of total Ca^{2+}, most of which is likely bound to Ca^{2+}-binding proteins and sequestered in the endoplasmic reticulum.[28] Ca^{2+} retention in the latter compartment is energy dependent, and could be released in significant amounts should ATP levels fall. Confocal imaging of free Ca^{2+} in optic nerve axons reveals a prompt increase in axoplasmic $[Ca^{2+}]$ that precedes the increase in *total* (free + bound) Ca^{2+} levels as measured by x-ray microanalysis.[17,29] Moreover, this rise in free $[Ca^{2+}]$ is only slightly reduced in zero-external Ca^{2+}. Under conditions of glycolytic failure, a delayed Ca^{2+} increase is seen[29] that coincides very closely to a transient hyperpolarization in resting potential[7] and increase in CAP area (Fig. 1B and D); because this Ca^{2+} increase also persists in zero-Ca^{2+} solution it is highly likely that the source is from intracellular stores. Finally, excess release of Ca^{2+} from a caffeine-sensitive pool causes substantial functional injury in the RON even under normoxic conditions, which is reduced by prior depletion of stores of Ca^{2+} or block of caffeine-mediated Ca^{2+} release using procaine.[30] Taken together, these observations implicate Ca^{2+} release from internal stores as perhaps the first pathological translocation of this cation during anoxia or ischemia.

Whether intracellular Ca^{2+} stores play a major or minor role in white matter injury remains to be seen. What is certain is evidence of *net* Ca^{2+} entry during white matter anoxia shown by x-ray microanalysis, which undoubtedly plays a central role in the injury cascade. Being devoid of synapses, the mode of Ca^{2+} entry into anoxic myelinated axons is likley unique, compared to gray matter where overactivation of excitatory amino acid-gated channels is the most important route.[31-34] Figure 2 summarizes pharmacological experiments that have helped to characterize the mechanisms of Ca^{2+} entry into anoxic axons. Studies in rat optic nerve recorded *in vitro* have shown that removal of Ca^{2+} from the perfusate, with the addition of the Ca^{2+} chelator EGTA, allows

A.

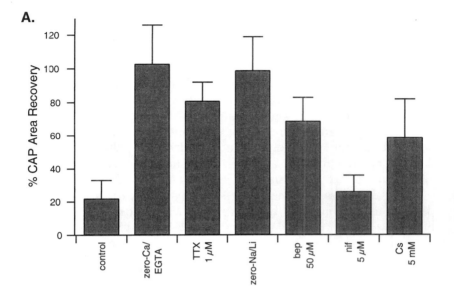

B.

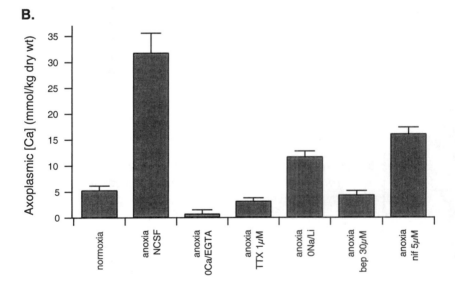

Figure 2. Bar graphs summarizing electrophysiological recovery of optic nerve compound action potential (CAP) after 60 minutes of anoxia (panel A) and accumulation of total (free + bound) axoplasmic Ca^{2+} measured by x-ray microanalysis (panel B) in normal CSF and during various ionic or pharmacological manipulations. In normal cerebro spinal fluid, CAP recovers to about 20%-30% of control after 60 minutes of anoxia followed by 60 minutes of reoxygenation, while axoplasmic $[Ca^{2+}]$ increases about six-fold at the end of the 60

(continued)

virtually complete recovery from one hour of anoxia.[27] Moreover, inhibition of voltage-gated Na$^+$ channels with TTX exerts a striking protective effect, as does removal of bath Na$^-$.[5] Taken together, these observations suggest that Ca^{2+} entry depends on Na$^+$ influx, the latter occurring to a large extent through TTX-blockable Na$^+$ channels. The Na$^+$-Ca^{2+} exchanger, a ubiquitous Ca^{2+} transporting protein,[35] would be an obvious candidate, operating in the reverse, Ca^{2+}-import mode under conditions of rising [Na$^+$]$_i$ and membrane depolarization. Direct inhibition of the Na$^+$-Ca^{2+} exchanger with benzamil or bepridil confirmed the very important role of this transporter in mediating Ca^{2+} overload in anoxic white matter.[4,5] Whether a component of Ca^{2+} influx occurs through voltage-gated Ca^{2+} channels remains controversial. An initial study using organic and inorganic inhibitors failed to show protective effects in the anoxic RON [36], although a subsequent report using the same model showed neuroprotective effects of L- and N-type Ca^{2+} channel antagonists.[37] A recent report where axoplasmic Ca^{2+} concentrations were directly measured using x-ray microanalysis failed to confirm a reduction of Ca^{2+} entry by the dihydropyridines nifedipine or nimodipine during *in vitro* optic nerve anoxia.[19] Thus the issue of voltage-gated Ca^{2+} channels in white matter anoxia remains unresolved.

The data on Ca^{2+} concentration changes presented above pertains mainly to the axonal cylinder. In contrast, very little is known about the response of the myelin sheath to injury. Myelin confers a crucial electrical property to axons by lowering transaxolemmal capacitance and raising the resistance thus facilitating rapid axial conduction of action currents. Well known examples of myelin damage in the CNS (eg, multiple sclerosis) or peripheral nervous system (eg, Guillain-Barré syndrome) illustrate how dependent white matter tracts are upon an intact myelin sheath. Conduction failure measured electrophysiologi-

---

Figure 2. *(continued)* minute anoxic exposure. Perfusing nerves in zero-Ca^{2+}/ 5 mM EGTA solution allows complete recovery of CAP area and completely prevents accumulation of axoplasmic Ca^{2-}. Blocking Na$^+$ channels with TTX, or preventing Na$^+$ accumulation by replacing this ion with Li$^+$ in the prefusate, both result in marked electrophysiological recovery and a parallel reduction in axoplasmic Ca^{2+} accumulation. The Na$^+$ dependency of Ca^{2+} influx indicates that reverse Na$^+$-Ca^{2+} exchange may be an important mechanism of Ca^{2+} entry during white matter anoxia, which is supported by the functional protection and Ca^{2+} sparing effect of the Na$^+$-Ca^{2+} exchange inhibitor bepridil. Cs$^+$ ions also displayed marked neuroprotective effects, possibly through a reduction of Na$^+$ entry via the mixed conductance inward rectifier channel. In panel B, the apparent reduction of Ca^{2+} accumulation with nifedipine, a blocker of L-type voltage gated Ca^{2+} channels, is artifactual as this effect was not statistically different from that seen with vehicle (0.01% DMSO) alone.[19]

cally is not able to reliably distinguish between damage to the axon cylinder or disruption of the myelin sheath, either or both of which can lead to conduction block and a reduction of amplitude of the compound propagated action potential. Measurement of myelin Ca^{2+} levels has shown that this region accumulates substantial amounts of this ion, although not as much as axoplasm. Pharmacological studies revealed some intriguing differences compared with the axon cylinder. For instance, as with axoplasm, the Na^+-Ca^{2+} exchange inhibitor bepridil inhibits Ca^{2+} accumulation in the myelin during anoxia, as does TTX. However, in contrast to axoplasm, TTX does not alter the degree of Na^+ gain (LoPachin and Stys, unpublished observations). Therefore, while the Na^+-Ca^{2+} exchanger appears to play a significant role in Ca^{2+} accumulation, and has been shown to be abundant in CNS myelin,[38] unlike the axon cylinder, the stimulus for reverse exchange does not depend on Na^+ influx through TTX-blockable Na^+ channels. A possible explanation is discussed in the section on white matter excitotoxicity below.

Central axons are critically dependent on oxidative phosphorylation for maintenance of electrochemical gradients, with only a small component of the energy requirement derived from glycolysis under normal conditions.[7] It follows that the well being of mitochondria is crucial for survival of white matter. On the one hand Ca^{2+} ions are known to stimulate mitochondrial energy production,[39] but excess accumulation in the mitochondrial matrix is detrimental. These organelles are generally thought to cycle Ca^{2+} across their inner membranes with influx mediated by electrophoretic transport by a Ca^{2+} uniporter driven by the steep membrane potential on the order of -160 mV established by proton pumping, and efflux occurring via a Na^+-Ca^{2+} exchanger, which is distinct from the plasmalemmal exchanger.[40] A substantial collapse of the mitochondrial membrane potential during anoxia will not only severely inhibit ATP synthesis, but at the same time will also limit the amount of Ca^{2+} influx. In fact x-ray microanalysis confirms a relatively modest four- to five-fold increase in mitochondrial Ca^{2+} levels accumulating *during* the anoxic period. With *reoxygenation* however, in the setting of elevated free axoplasmic [Ca^{2+}] as demonstrated by confocal Ca^{2+} imaging, mitochondria accumulate huge amounts of Ca^{2+} now that electron transport resumes in the presence of oxygen. Total mitochondrial Ca^{2+} levels can exceed baseline concentrations by several hundred-fold in reoxygenated organelles.[41] Such tremendous Ca^{2+} accumulation likely is very damaging for several reasons. First, charge influx will dissipate the newly reestablished proton gradient, thus impairing ATP synthesis, even to the point of *consuming* glycolytic ATP, the last source of energy potentially capable of rescuing the axon.[40,42] Second, triggering the mitochondrial pore transition which will further collapse the gradient for protons and other ions necessary for normal function.[43,44] Finally, formation of insoluble precipitates of Ca^{2+} and phosphate that is undoubtedly deleterious when excessive.[45] It is conceivable therefore that reoxygenated white matter suffers a "secondary chemical anoxia" during the reperfusion phase as mitchondria attempt to resume function, but fail as they are forced to wastefully cycle Ca^{2+} to the detriment of ATP production. This could explain the secondary deterioration of ionic homeostasis observed in most larger optic nerve fibers occurring later in the reoxygenation phase.[41]

Although more resistant than neurons, glial cells are also damaged by ischemia[15] and may cause serious disruption of the supportive role of astrocytes, or myelin disintegration when oligodentrocytes are injured. Astrocytes seem able to withstand anoxia or aglycemia alone for extended periods of time.[25] However, under conditions of combined glycolytic and mitochondrial inhibition *in vitro*, these cells have been shown to accumulate substantial amounts of Na^+ and Ca^{2+}; the former occurs through a TTX-insensitive pathway whereas Ca^{2+} enters largely through L- and T-type voltage-gated Ca^{2+} channels.[14,46-48] Even less is known about the mechanisms of injury in oligodendrocytes, though these cells are also vulnerable to oxidative stress and Ca^{2+}-dependent injury.[49,50] Recent information suggests a potential role for excitotoxic damage in these cells; this aspect will be discussed in greater detail in the following section.

While there is now little doubt that axonal Ca^{2+} overload is the key step in the sequence of events leading to anoxic/ischemic white matter injury, the important question still remains: exactly why is excessive Ca^{2+} toxic? A key metabolic regulator of many biochemical pathways, Ca^{2+} modulates many different enzymes such as calpain, phospholipases, endonucleases, protein kinase C and others in most cell types.[51] Overactivation of some or many of these enzyme systems could wreak havoc with the normal structure and operation of an excitable cell. We have begun to investigate some of the potential targets of Ca^{2+} overload in anoxic white matter. The Ca^{2+}-activated neutral protease calpain[52] breaks down a number of substrates, one of which being the structural protein spectrin. Using antiserum raised against calpain-cleaved breakdown fragments of spectrin,[53] we have recently shown that calpain is greatly activated in anoxic optic nerve. What was unexpected is that reoxygenation seems to greatly stimulate calpain activity; indeed the amount of calpain-mediated spectrin breakdown after 1 hour of *in vitro* anoxia followed by 1 hour of reoxygenation is far greater than 1 hour of anoxia alone, and is about the same as from a continuous, 2-hour anoxic exposure.[54] In other words, the act of reoxygenation seems to be just as damaging as maintaining the anoxic insult continuously. Treatments that reduce Ca^{2+} influx such as TTX or Ca^{2+}-depleted perfusate demonstrate the predicted reduction of spectrin breakdown, as does treatment with the calpain inhibitor MDL28170. Interestingly, if not unfortunately, in contrast to interventions that reduce net Ca^{2+} accumulation, pharmacological inhibition of calpain improves electrophysiological function in anoxic optic nerve very little, despite a greatly improved biochemical profile with respect to spectrin breakdown.[54] Whether this is a failure of calpain inhibition to provide functional protection in white matter, or a dependency on the timing of application of inhibitors as has been suggested in organotypic hippocampal slice cultures,[55] remains to be seen. These preliminary observations suggest that calpain inhibition may be necessary but not sufficient for neuroprotection of white matter, with other Ca^{2+}-dependent pathways contributing to the overall injury, as hypothesized in Figure 3.

White Matter Excitotoxicty: Fact or Fiction?

As the prototypical excitatory neurotransmitter in the mammalian CNS, glutamate could be expected to induce toxicity only in areas that possess glutamatergic synapses. It would be surprising if excitotoxic mechanisms were at play in areas without synaptic machinery, where glutamate release mechanisms and receptors would be expected to be lacking. Indeed, a study using the NMDA antagonist ketamine showed no protective effects in anoxic rat optic nerve at concentrations thought to be specific for NMDA receptor inhibition.[56] However, this would not rule out a possible contribution from non-NMDA ionotropic or metabotropic receptors.

Recent reports have raised the possibility of excitotoxic injury mechanisms in white matter, a tissue devoid of synapses. For instance, a modest protective effect was observed in isolated spinal cord white matter after traumatic injury in the presence of the AMPA-kainate antagonist NBQX.[57] Not only do astrocytes possess non-NMDA ionotropic glutamate receptors,[58] but recent reports indicate that oligodendroglia also are vulnerable to injury through activation of AMPA-kainate receptors.[59,60] By extension, this raises the possibility that the myelin sheath could express glutamate receptors as well and be vulnerable to such injury. We recently re-examined the issue of excitotoxic damage in the anoxic optic nerve model, and have found that kynurenic acid, a broad spectrum antagonist of ionotropic glutamate receptors, confers robust neuroprotection against a 60-minute anoxic exposure (Sakr & Stys, unpublished data). Coupled with the negative results using ketamine, it is likely that AMPA-kainate receptors are involved. This finding was confirmed and extended in anoxic spinal dorsal col-

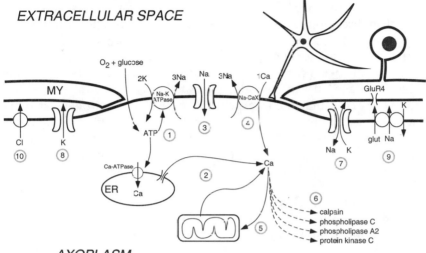

EXTRACELLULAR SPACE

AXOPLASM

Figure 3. Diagram illustrating sequence of interrelated events leading to anoxic injury of a central myelinated axon. Interruption of energy supply leads to failure of ATP-dependent pumps such as axolemmal Na^+-K^+-ATPase (1). Perhaps the first source of raised axonal $[Ca^{2+}]$ is from internal stores such as endoplasmic reticulum and mitochondria (2). Reduction of Na^+ pumping across the axolemma leads to accumulation of axoplasmic Na^+ mainly via non-inactivating Na^+ channels (3). The rise in $[Na^+]_i$, coupled with depolarization caused by K^+ efflux through a variety of K^+ channels (8) stimulates the Na^+-Ca^{2+} exchanger to operate in the Ca^{2+} import mode, overloading the axon with damaging amounts of this cation (4). The accumulation of axonal Ca^{2+} in turn leads to mitochondrial injury, especially during reoxygenation (5), and to activation of a number of Ca^{2+}-dependent enzyme systems that result in irreversible structural and functional injury to the fiber (6). A significant component of pathological Na^+ entry may also occur through Cs^+-sensitive inward rectifier channels (7). Glial injury, particularly involving oligodentrocytes and the myelin sheath (MY), is exacerbated by glutamate export via the Na^+-K^+-glutamate transporter (9), which will be stimulated to release this transmitter under conditions of axoplasmic Na^+ loading and depolarization. AMPA receptors on myelin may mediate direct damage to this structure. Cl^- efflux through DIDS-sensitive pathway(s), plays a significant role, but only under conditions of Na^+ conductance blockade (10). The locations of the various channels and transporters are drawn for convenience and do not necessarily reflect their real distributions in central axons. Modified from Stys.[8]

umn. Here too AMPA-kainate receptors are implicated, with the AMPA subtype playing a major role because the relatively selective inhibitor GYKI 52466[61] is very neuroprotective.[62]

The intriguing questions raised by these observations are: 1) what is the source of glutamate, 2) how is it released in a tissue without synapses, and 3) which cells and subcellular regions are targets for excitotoxicity? These important questions are far from being conclusively answered, but recent data have provided some clues. Glutamate is known to be present in the axoplasm in millimolar concentrations,[63,64] and, coupled with the rise in $[Na^+]_i$, decrease in $[K^+]_i$ and depolarization during white matter anoxia/ischemia, glutamate could be released by reverse Na^+-dependent glutamate transport.[65,66] Using immunohistochemistry, we have recently demonstrated the presence of several isoforms of Na^+-glutamate transporter in central and peripheral myelinated axons.[62] Moreover, the competitive inhibitor of Na^+-glutamate transport L-*trans*-pyrollidine-2,4-dicarboxylic acid[67] was found to be highly neuroprotective in anoxic dorsal columns.[62] Using antibodies raised against calpain-mediated breakdown products of spectrin[68] and myelin basic protein,[69] we have evidence that glutamate-dependent injury is mainly localized to astrocytes, oligodendrocytes, and the myelin sheath itself, with axon cylinders unaffected.[70] Indeed, we have recently demonstrated the presence of GluR4 (but not GluR2) receptor subunits in myelin of dorsal column myelinated axons, raising the intriguing notion that myelin may be directly vulnerable to excitotoxic damage by activation of Ca^{2+}-permeable AMPA receptors.[70] Taken together, these preliminary observations are consistent with the notion that glutamate is released from a cytosolic compartment by reversal of the Na^+-dependent glutamate transporter, inducing excitotoxic damage in glia and myelin by either allowing Ca^{2+} to permeate directly through Ca^{2+}-permeable AMPA receptors, stimulating reverse Na^+-Ca^{2+} exchange (by causing Na^+ entry and depolarization), or both. Careful dissection of this novel white matter injury mechanism will provide a wealth of information with important implications for optimal neuroprotection of this tissue.

Neuroprotection of Injured White Matter

Figure 3 summarizes the various signal transduction pathways thought to play a role in white matter injury. With a thorough understanding of the various steps involved in the injury cascade, logical selection of which molecular targets to modulate in order to confer neuroprotection becomes more straightforward. Nonspecific downregulation of many of these steps can be achieved by hypothermia; cooling optic nerves by even a modest amount (2.5° or 5° C) is highly neuroprotective [71] as it is in gray matter.[72] Drug therapy may be more practical in the clinical setting however. Selection of a step that is common to several events in the injury cascade could be advantageous as this might interfere with several downstream pathways. For instance, inhibition of Na^+ channels, leading to a reduction of Na^+ influx and depolarization, might at the same time reduce Na^+-Ca^{2+} exchange-mediated Ca^{2+} entry

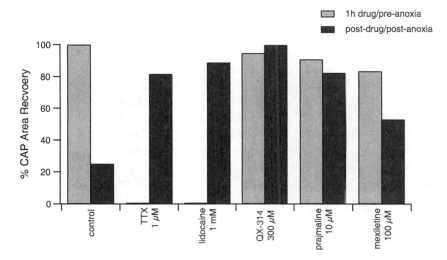

Figure 4. Bar graph depicting recovery of rat optic nerve compound action potential (CAP) area after anoxia in the presence of various Na^+ channel blocking agents. Drugs were applied beginning one hour before anoxia, continued during the 60-minute anoxic exposure, then washed for 1 to 3 hours after reoxygenation. Light bars show degree of suppression of activity by drug alone (before anoxia), and dark bars show recovery after 60-minute anoxia/wash. In normal CSF ('control'), there is no suppression pre-anoxia and CAP area recovers to ~ 20%-30% of pre-anoxic area. TTX, a state-independent Na^+ channel blocker, and lidocaine, a "use-dependent" local anesthetic, are both highly neuroprotective, but are potent anesthetics, completely abolishing normal electrogenesis. In contrast, the permanently charged quaternary amine derivative of lidocaine QX-314, as well as the the charged anti-arrhythmic prajmaline (N-propyl-ajmaline), are both very effective neuroprotectants at concentrations that show little depression of pre-anoxic activity. Mexiletine, a use-dependent anti-arrhythmic Na^+ channel blocker, is also quite effective. The advantage of this agent is that because it is a primary amine and exists in both neutral and charged, protonated forms, it is able to penetrate across the blood brain barrier and confer protection after systemic administration, whereas QX-314 and prajmaline are ineffective *in vivo*.[5,76-78]

and Na^+-glutamate transport-mediated release of this neurotransmitter.

We have studied a number of voltage-gated Na^+ channel blockers for their neuroprotective efficacy and have found surprising variability in their efficacy.[8] An additional constraint with this class of agent is the tendency to interfere with normal electrogenesis, an issue that will be very important from the point of view of clinical toxicity. For example, as shown in Figure 4, TTX is a very effective neuroprotectant in anoxic white matter, but interferes with normal conduction and would therefore not be useful clinically. There exists a variety of "use-dependent" Na^+ channel blockers from the local anesthetic and anti-arrhythmic classes that are preferentially active at the open conformation of the voltage-gated Na^+ channel,[73-75] and would therefore be relatively selective for the non-inactivating Na^+ channel subtype implicated in axonal injury.[18] As shown in Figure 4, these "use-dependent" blockers such as QX-314 are highly effective neuroprotectants, even at concentrations that only minimally inhibit normal axonal excitability.[76,77] Although very effective *in vitro*, agents such as QX-314 are completely ineffective after systemic administration *in vivo* because the permanently charged nature of this quaternary amine prevents it from crossing the blood brain barrier (Stys, unpublished data). Therefore an additional requirement is the ability to penetrate into the CNS at concentrations sufficient to confer neuroprotection. The feasibility of this approach was demonstrated with mexiletine, a primary amine antiarrhythmic Na^+ channel blocker. Not only is this agent reasonably effective *in vitro* against optic nerve anoxia, but after intra-peritoneal injection, mexiletine was found to penetrate into the CNS at concentrations sufficient to significantly protect optic nerves from *in situ* ischemia.[78] The structure of mexiletine allows it to exist in both neutral and protonated forms, with the former able to penetrate the blood brain barrier, and the charged form probably a more efficient blocker of non-inactivating Na^+ channels.

Whereas voltage-gated Na^+ channels occupy a prominent position in the injury cascade, modulation of additional pathways may provide additional benefit. For example, if the transporter(s) responsible for Cl^- movement during the "anion paradox" (see above) are identified, concomitant block of Cl^- efflux will not only reduce mechanical damage induced by volume changes, but will prevent the concentration of remaining cytosolic Na^+ ions and further inhibit the deleterious operation of Na^+-Ca^{2+} exchange and Na^+-glutamate transport. Complementary sparing of the integrity of the myelin sheath may best be achieved with glutamate transport blockers or AMPA antagonists, as TTX does not reduce the Na^+ load in this region during anoxia (LoPachin & Stys, unpublished). Another intriguing possibility is modulation of intrinsic "autoprotective" mechanisms recently identified in white matter. GABA-B receptor activation in adult rat optic nerves is partially protective against anoxic injury, and is due to endogenously released transmitter, since it can be reproduced with nipecotic acid, an inhibitor of GABA uptake. This signal transduction pathway appears to involve a G-protein/protein kinase C-mediated mechanism, although neither the final phosphorylation targets nor the source (axonal and/or glial) of the transmitter have been conclusively identified.[79] Another neuromodulator, adenosine, is also released during white matter anoxia and confers partial neuroprotection via a protein kinase C-dependent pathway.[80] Pharmacological modulation of these intrinsic signal transduction pathways may prove to be a useful adjunct in a multipronged neuroprotective strategy.

Conclusions

Given the important functional role of CNS white matter tracts, it is important to address this region when devising therapeutic strategies for brain and spinal cord injury, be it from ischemic, traumatic or other causes. While Na$^+$ channel inhibitors initially appear to be useful agents, potentially any of the pathways illustrated in Figure 3, and others yet to be discovered, could be useful targets for modulation in order to confer neuroprotection in white matter. Even in such a seemingly simple tissue, it may be that a combination approach may be better than intervention at any single step in the cascade. In such a case, a thorough understanding of the fundamental mechanisms will be even more important, in order to devise treatments that address parallel rather than sequential steps, thus avoiding unnecessary redundancy and maximizing the expected additive benefit.

References

1. American Heart Association. 2000 Heart and Stroke Statistical Update. Dallas, TX., 1999. http://www.americanheart.org/statistics/05stroke.html.
2. Hildebrand C, Waxman SG. Postnatal differentiation of rat optic nerve fibers: Electron microscopic observations on the development of nodes of ranvier and axoglial relations. *J Comp Neurol* 1984;224:25-37.
3. Foster RE, Connors BW, Waxman SG. Rat optic nerve: Electrophysiological, pharmacological and anatomical studies during development. *Dev Brain Res* 1982;3:371-386.
4. Imaizumi T, Kocsis JD, Waxman SG. Anoxic injury in the rat spinal cord - pharmacological evidence for multiple steps in Ca2+-dependent injury of the dorsal columns. *J Neurotrauma* 1997;14:299-311.
5. Stys PK, Waxman SG, Ransom BR. Ionic mechanisms of anoxic injury in mammalian CNS white matter: Role of Na$^+$ channels and Na$^+$-Ca^{2+} exchanger. *J Neurosci* 1992;12:430-439.
6. Clarke DD, Sokoloff L. Circulation and energy metabolism of the brain. In Siegel GJ, Agranoff BW, Albers RW, Molinoff PB (eds): *Basic Neurochemistry.* New York: Raven Press; 1994:645-680.
7. Leppanen LL, Stys PK. Ion transport and membrane potential in CNS myelinated axons. II: Effects of metabolic inhibition. *J Neurophysiol* 1997;78:2095-2107.
8. Stys PK. Anoxic and ischemic injury of myelinated axons in CNS white matter: From mechanistic concepts to therapeutics. *J Cereb Blood Flow Metab* 1998;18:2-25.
9. Stryer L. Biochemistry, New York, W. H. Freeman, 1988.

10. Fern R, Davis P, Waxman SG, et al. Axon conduction and survival in CNS white matter during energy deprivation: A developmental study. *J Neurophysiol* 1998;79:95-105.

11. Ransom BR, Fern R. Does astrocytic glycogen benefit axon function and survival in CNS white matter during glucose deprivation? *GLIA* 1997;21:134-141.

12. Swanson RA. Physiologic coupling of glial glycogen metabolism to neuronal activity in brain. *Can J Physiol Pharmacol* 1992;70:S138-S144.

13. Silver IA, Deas J, Erecinska M. Ion homeostasis in brain cells: Differences in intracellular ion responses to energy limitation between cultured neurons and glial cells. *Neuroscience* 1997;78:589-601.

14. Fern R. Intracellular calcium and cell death during ischemia in neonatal rat white matter astrocytes in situ. *J Neurosci* 1998;18:7232-7243.

15. Ransom BR, Fern R. Anoxic-ischemic glial cell injury: Mechanisms and consequences. In Haddad GG, Lister G (eds): *Tissue Oxygen Deprivation* . New York: Marcel Dekker; 1996: 617-652.

16. Ransom BR, Walz W, Davis PK, et al. Anoxia-induced changes in extracellular K^+ and pH in mammalian central white matter. *J Cereb Blood Flow Metab* 1992;12:593-602.

17. LoPachin RM, Stys PK. Elemental composition and water content of rat optic nerve myelinated axons and glial cells: Effects of in vitro anoxia and reoxygenation. *J Neurosci* 1995;15:6735-6746.

18. Stys PK, Sontheimer H, Ransom BR, et al. Non-inactivating, TTX-sensitive Na^+ conductance in rat optic nerve axons. *Proc Natl Acad Sci USA* 1993;90:6976-6980.

19. Stys PK, LoPachin RM. Mechanisms of ion flux in anoxic myelinated CNS axons. *Neuroscience* 1998;82:21-32.

20. Malek S, Stys PK. Role of anion transport in axonal depolarization in anoxic rat optic nerve. *Soc Neurosci Abstr* 2000.

21. Schanne FA, Kane AB, Young EE, et al. Calcium-dependence of toxic cell death: A final common pathway. *Science* 1979;206:700-702.

22. Brown AM, Fern R, Jarvinen JP, et al. Changes in $[Ca^{2+}]_o$ during anoxia in CNS white matter. *Neuroreport* 1998;9:1997-2000.

23. Kumura E, Graf R, Dohmen C, et al. Breakdown of calcium homeostasis in relation to tissue depolarization: Comparison between gray and white matter ischemia. *J Cereb Blood Flow Metab* 1999;19(7):788-793.

24. Goldberg MP, Choi DW. Combined oxygen and glucose deprivation in cortical cell culture: calcium-dependent and calcium-independent mechanisms of neuronal injury. *J Neurosci* 1993;13:3510-3524.

25. Harold DE, Walz W. Metabolic inhibition and electrical properties of type-1-like cortical astrocytes. *Neuroscience* 1992;47:203-211.

26. Swanson RA, Choi DW. Glial glycogen stores affect neuronal survival during glucose deprivation in vitro. *J Cereb Blood Flow Metab* 1993;13:162-169.

27. Stys PK, Ransom BR, Waxman SG, et al. Role of extracellular calcium in anoxic injury of mammalian central white matter. *Proc Natl Acad Sci USA* 1990;87:4212-4216.

28. Kostyuk P, Verkhratsky A. Calcium stores in neurons and glia. *Neurosci* 1994;63:381-404.

29. Ren Y, Brown A, Ransom BR, et al. Confocal calcium imaging in live CNS myelinated axons in vitro: Role of internal calcium release during metabolic inhibition. *Soc Neurosci Abstr* 2000;in press:.

30. Steffensen I, Stys PK. Intracellular calcium dynamics in CNS myelinated axons. *Soc Neurosci Abstr* 1996;22:341.

31. Siesjo BK, Wieloch T: *Cellular and Molecular Mechanisms of Ischemic Brain Damage*, New York, Raven Press, 1996.

32. Siesjö BK. Calcium and ischemic brain damage. *Eur Neurol* 1986;25:45-56.

33. Choi DW. Cerebral hypoxia: Some new approaches and unanswered questions. *J Neurosci* 1990;10:2493-2501.

34. Haddad GG, Jiang C. O_2 deprivation in the central nervous system: On mechanisms of neuronal response, differential sensitivity and injury. *Prog Neurobiol* 1993;40:277-318.

35. Steffensen I, Stys PK. The Na^+-Ca^{2+} exchanger in neurons and glial cells. *The Neuroscientist* 1996;2:162-171.

36. Stys PK, Ransom BR, Waxman SG. Effects of polyvalent cations and dihydropyridine calcium channel blockers on recovery of CNS white matter from anoxia. *Neurosci Lett* 1990;115:293-299.

37. Fern R, Ransom BR, Waxman SG. Voltage-gated calcium channels in CNS white matter: Role in anoxic injury. *J Neurophysiol* 1995;74:369-377.

38. Steffensen I, Waxman SG, Mills L, et al. Immunohistochemical localization of the Na^+-Ca^{2+} exchanger in rat central and peripheral myelinated axons. *Brain Res* 1997;776:1-9.

39. Duchen MR. Ca(2+)-dependent changes in the mitochondrial energetics in single dissociated mouse sensory neurons. *Biochem J* 1992;283:41-50.

40. Nicholls DG. A role for the mitochondrion in the protection of cells against calcium overload? In Kogure K, Hossmann K-A, Siesjo BK, Welsh FA (eds): *Progress in Brain Research*. Elsevier; 1985: 97-106.

41. Stys PK, LoPachin RM. Elemental composition and water content of rat optic nerve myelinated axons during in vitro post-anoxia reoxygenation. *Neuroscience* 1996;73:1081-1090.

42. Nicholls DG. Calcium transport and proton electrochemical potential gradient in mitochondria from guinea-pig cerebral cortex and rat heart. *Biochem J* 1978;170:511-522.

43. Gunter TE, Pfeiffer DR. Mechanisms by which mitochondria transport calcium. *Am J Physiol* 1990;258:C755-786.

44. Crompton M, Andreeva L. On the involvement of a mitochondrial pore in reperfusion injury. *Basic Res Cardiol* 1993;88:513-523.

45. Carafoli E. Mitochondrial pathology: An overview. *Ann NY Acad Sci* 1986;488:1-18.

46. Rose CR, Waxman SG, Ransom BR. Effects of glucose deprivation, chemical hypoxia, and simulated ischemia on Na^+ homeostasis in rat spinal cord astrocytes. *J Neurosci* 1998;18:3554-3562.

47. Yu ACH, Gregory GA, Chan PH. Hypoxia-induced dysfunctions and injury of astrocytes in primary cell cultures. *J Cereb Blood Flow Metab* 1989;9:20-28.

48. Duffy S, MacVicar BA. In vitro ischemia promotes calcium influx and intracellular calcium release in hippocampal astrocytes. *J Neurosci* 1996;16:71-81.

49. Scolding NJ, Morgan BP, Campbell AK, et al. The role of calcium in rat oligodendrocyte injury and repair. *Neurosci Lett* 1992;135:95-98.

50. Juurlink BH. Response of glial cells to ischemia: Roles of reactive oxygen species and glutathione. *Neurosci Biobehav Rev* 1997;21:151-166.

51. Orrenius S, Nicotera P. Mechanisms of calcium-related cell death. In Siesjo BK, Wieloch T (eds): *Cellular and Molecular Mechanisms of Ischemic Brain Damage.* New York: Raven Press; 1996:137-152.

52. Suzuki K, Sorimachi H, Yoshizawa T, et al. Calpain: Novel family members, activation, and physiologic function. *Biol Chem* 1995;376:523-529.

53. Roberts-Lewis JM, Savage MJ, Marcy VR, et al. Immunolocalization of calpain I-mediated spectrin degradation to vulnerable neurons in the ischemic gerbil brain. *J Neurosci* 1994;14:3934-3944.

54. Jiang Q, Stys PK. Calpain inhibitors confer biochemical, but not electrophysiological, protection against anoxia in rat optic nerves. *J Neurochem* 2000;74:2101-2107.

55. Brana C, Benham CD, Evans M, et al. Protective and toxic consequences of inhibition of calpain activation by oxygen-glucose deprivation in organotypic hippocampal slice cultures. *Soc Neurosci* (Abstr) 1998;24:1227.

56. Ransom BR, Waxman SG, Davis PK. Anoxic injury of CNS white matter: Protective effect of ketamine. *Neurology* 1990;40:1399-1403.

57. Agrawal SK, Fehlings MG. Role of NMDA and non-NMDA ionotropic glutamate receptors in traumatic spinal cord axonal injury. *J Neurosci* 1997;17:1055-1063.

58. Chiu SY, Kriegler S. Neurotransmitter-mediated signaling between axons and glial cells. *GLIA* 1994;11:191-200.

59. Matute C, Sanchez-Gomez MV, Martinez-Millan L, et al. Glutamate receptor-mediated toxicity in optic nerve oligodendrocytes. *Proc Natl Acad Sci USA* 1997;94:8830-8835.

60. McDonald JW, Althomsons SP, Hyrc KL, et al. Oligodendrocytes from forebrain are highly vulnerable to AMPA/kainate receptor-mediated excitotoxicity. *Nat Med* 1998;4:291-297.

61. Paternain AV, Morales M, Lerma J. Selective antagonism of AMPA receptors unmasks kainate receptor- mediated responses in hippocampal neurons. *Neuron* 1995;14:185-189.

62. Li S, Mealing GA, Morley P, et al. Novel injury mechanism in anoxia and trauma of spinal cord white matter: Glutamate release via reverse Na+-dependent glutamate transport. *J Neurosci* 1999;19:RC16.

63. Battistin L, Grynbaum A, Lajtha A. The uptake of various amino acids by the mouse brain in vivo. *Brain Res* 1971;29:85-99.

64. Fonnum F. Glutamate: A neurotransmitter in mammalian brain. *J Neurochem* 1984;42:1-11.

65. Taylor CP, Geer JJ, Burke SP. Endogenous extracellular glutamate accumulation in rat neocortical cultures by reversal of the transmembrane sodium gradient. *Neurosci Lett* 1992;145:197-200.

66. Roettger V, Lipton P. Mechanism of glutamate release from rat hippocampal slices during in vitro ischemia. *Neuroscience* 1996;75:677-685.

67. Vornov JJ, Tasker RC, Park J. Neurotoxicity of acute glutamate transport blockade depends on coactivation of both NMDA and AMPA/Kainate receptors in organotypic hippocampal cultures. *Exp Neurol* 1995;133:7-17.

68. Hewitt KE, Lesiuk HJ, Tauskela JS, et al. Selective coupling of μ-calpain activation with the NMDA receptor is independent of translocation and autolysis in primary cortical neurons. *J Neurosci Res* 1998;54:223-232.

69. Matsuo A, Lee GC, Terai K, et al. Unmasking of an unusual myelin basic protein epitope during the process of myelin degeneration in humans: A potential mechanism for the generation of autoantigens. *Am J Pathol* 1997;150:1253-1266.

70. Li S, Stys PK. Mechanisms of ionotropic glutamate receptor-mediated excitotoxicity in isolated spinal cord white matter. *J Neurosci* 2000;20:1190-1198.

71. Stys PK, Waxman SG, Ransom BR. Effects of temperature on evoked electrical activity and anoxic injury in CNS white matter. *J Cereb Blood Flow Metab* 1992;12:977-986.

72. Ginsberg MD, Globus MY, Dietrich WD, et al. Temperature modulation of ischemic brain injury--a synthesis of recent advances. *Prog Brain Res* 1993;96:13-22.

73. Yeh JZ, Tanguy J. Na channel activation gate modulates slow recovery from use-dependent block by local anesthetics in squid giant axons. *Biophys J* 1985;47:685-694.

74. Wang GK, Brodwick MS, Eaton DC, et al. Inhibition of sodium currents by local anesthetics in chloramine-T-treated squid axons. The role of channel activation. *J Gen Physiol* 1987;89:645-667.

75. Khodorov BI. Role of inactivation in local anesthetic action. *Ann NY Acad Sci* 1991;625:224-248.

76. Stys PK, Ransom BR, Waxman SG. Tertiary and quaternary local anesthetics protect CNS white matter from anoxic injury at concentrations that do not block excitability. *J Neurophysiol* 1992;67:236-240.

77. Stys PK. Protective effects of antiarrhythmic agents against anoxic injury in CNS white matter. *J Cereb Blood Flow Metab* 1995;15:425-432.

78. Stys PK, Lesiuk H. Correlation between electrophysiological effects of mexiletine and ischemic protection of CNS white matter. *Neuroscience* 1996;71:27-36.

79. Fern R, Waxman SG, Ransom BR. Endogenous GABA attenuates CNS white matter dysfunction following anoxia. *J Neurosci* 1995;15:699-708.

80. Fern R, Waxman SG, Ransom BR. Modulation of anoxic injury in CNS white matter by adenosine and interaction between adenosine and GABA. *J Neurophysiol* 1994;72:2609-2616.

81. Stys PK, Lehning EJ, Sauberman AJ, et al. Intracellular concentrations of major ions in rat myelinated axons and glia: Calculations based on electron probe X-ray microanalyses. *J Neurochem* 1997;68:1920-1928.

82. Leppanen LL, Stys PK. Ion transport and membrane potential in CNS myelinated axons. I: normoxic conditions. *J Neurophysiol* 1997;78:2086-2094.

Chapter 12

CADASIL, What Can We Learn About White Matter Stroke?

Marie-Germaine Bousser, MD, Hugues Chabriat, MD, Anne Joutel, MD, and Elizabeth Tournier-Lasserve, MD

Introduction

CADASIL (Cerebal Autosomal Dominant Arteriopathy with Subcortical Infarcts and Leukoencephalopathy) is the acronym we suggested in 1993[1] to designate a familial condition which had already received at least 6 different names[2] since its probable first description by van Bogaert in 1955 as "Binswanger's disease"in two sisters.[3] CADASIL was chosen to emphasize the four main characteristics of this disease: it is a small artery disease of the brain, with an autosomal dominant pattern of transmission characterized by recurrent small deep infarcts and a more or less extensive white matter disorder.

The CADASIL story started in 1976 when we were able to examine a 50-year-old man with no vascular risk factor who recently had a minor stroke with dysarthria and a clumsy right hand. His brain computed tomography (CT) scan was very abnormal with a diffuse leukoaraiosis and areas of more marked hypodensities suggestive of small deep infarcts (later confirmed by magnetic resonance imaging [MRI]). Multiple investigations were performed including blood tests, cerebrospinal fluid (CSF) studies, four-vessel angiography, echocardiography, muscle biopsy, mitochondrial studies, and no cause was found.[4,5] The patient recovered completely. In 1977, he started to have migraine attacks,

From: Choi D, Dacey RG, Hsu CY, Powers WJ. *Cerebrovascular Disease: Momentum at the End of the Second Millennium.* Armonk, NY: Futura Publishing Company, Inc., © 2002.

but otherwise he was well until 1983, when he had another small subcortical infarct with a left sensory deficit. From then on, he progressively deteriorated with a pseudo-bulbar palsy and subcortical dementia. He became bed-ridden, totally dependent, and he died in 1996, 20 years after his first symptoms.

There was no known family history of stroke until, in 1984, his 33-year-old daughter came to see us with a 2-year history of multiple transient episodes of dysphasia, one pure motor stroke and attacks of migraine with and without aura. She had no vascular risk factors except for smoking, and again all investigations were normal. Around the same time we were able to see her 30-year-old brother who had experienced in 1982 a 5-day episode of dysarthria; the striking fact was that both of them had major MRI abnormalities with hyposignals on T1WI suggestive of small, deep infarcts and hypersignals on T2WI indicating a white matter disorder.[5]

It was then obvious that this condition was familial and, to cut a very long story short, we were able to analyze clinically, with MRI, and genetically almost all adult members of this large family. Among the 57 subjects examined, 11 (6 males and 5 females; mean age of 43 years) had already presented subcortical ischemic events, despite the absence of vascular risk factors. Three of them had subcortical dementia with pseudo-bulbar palsy. Four had migraine and one had epilepsy and a manic-depressive syndrome. All had severe MRI abnormalities, again suggestive of small, deep infarcts and white matter disorder. Men and women were equally affected and could equally transmit the disease, so that the transmission of this condition was obviously autosomal dominant.[1,4,5]

The patient who had seizures and manic depressive episodes later suffered recurrent strokes and dementia and she died of intra-cerebral hemorrhage.[6] Autopsy confirmed the presence of multiple small deep infarcts and of an extensive white matter abnormality with palor and loss of myelin. It revealed the presence of small artery disease that was different from amyloid and arteriosclerotic angiopathies. Though widely distributed, it affected predominantly small lepto-meningeal arteries as well as brain arteries that had a thickened eosinophilic media. On electron microscopy, there was a very unusual osmiophilic granular deposit situated within the basal lamina of the smooth muscle cells, which were themselves very abnormal, decreased in number with an enlarged endoplasmic reticulum and a thickened basal membrane.

One of the most striking findings in the study of this family was that eight totally asymptomatic subjects also had white matter abnormalities of variable severity on MRI T2WI. The presence of these abnormalities was used to define the status of the subjects for the genetic study:[1] all subjects with an abnormal MRI were defined as affected whereas all subjects above 35 years of age with a normal MRI were considered as nonaffected. Subjects below the age of 35 with a normal MRI had an unknown status. A systematic screening of the whole genome was undertaken and nearly halfway through Lod scores > 6 were obtained with several markers on chromosome 19.[1] This location was rapidly confirmed on a second family which, interestingly, had long been considered to be affected by familial multiple sclerosis. This was the situation in 1993, but things have evolved very rapidly since, in 1996, positional cloning allowed us to identify the responsible gene as Notch 3, a gene present and highly conserved in different species from the drosophilia to humans.[7] Further studies have shown over 30 different mutations, which are all located in the extra-cellular domain of the gene which contains 34 epidermal-growth-factor-like repeats.[8] These numerous mutations are highly stereotyped: they are mis-sense mutations leading to the creation or substitution of a cysteine residue within an epidermal growth factor (EGF) leading to 7 or 5 cysteines instead of the normal 6.

This is where we stand now: CADASIL is a familial small artery disease of the brain which is not so rare, since over 250 families have been identified worldwide.[8,9] This condition is remarkable in that, firstly, its gene is known and is expressed in the vessel wall and, secondly the arterial lesion has specific features with these abnormal smooth muscle cells and this mysterious granular osmiophilic deposit. CADASIL can thus be an excellent model to study small artery diseases of the brain and in particular to better understand the pathogenesis of small deep infarcts and white matter ischemia. The study of this condition has already taught us a number of things.

Firstly, this arterial wall disease is a systemic condition. Although the symptoms are purely cerebral and although no infarcts have so far been oberved in other organs, the same vascular lesion, in particular the granular osmiophilic deposit, is found in other arteries such as kidney, muscle or skin arteries (this has led to the possibility of diagnosing CADASIL on a simple skin biopsy.[10-12]

As regards the brain infarcts on MRI T1WI, they are indeed small subcortical infarcts which predominantly involve the periventricular and deep white matter, less frequently the basal ganglia, and most unusually (< 2 %) the cortex.[13,14] It is not astonishing that with such a distribution, the clinical presentation is that of the classic lacunar syndromes: in a study of 53 CADASIL patients with stroke, the main signs were pure motor stroke in 35%, hemiplegia and dysarthria in 18%, isolated dysarthria or dysphasia in 16%, pure sensory stroke in 9%, sensori-motor stroke in 9%. Other signs such as hemianopia, vertigo, cerebellar signs or facial palsy were extremely rare (≥ 3 %).[9] In a CADASIL population of any age, these small, deep infarcts are inconsistent, presenting in around 75% of cases. The reason is that infarcts occur late in the disease and dramatically increase in frequency with age. This increase is particularly marked for the deep white matter, basal ganglia and brainstem. Although these infarcts are indeed subcortical, CADASIL allowed us to confirm the well-known secondary cortical dysfunction related to subcortical lesions. Positron-emission tomography (PET) was performed in our first patient at a stage when he was already demented.[15] It showed a 50% matched reduction in cerebral blood flow (CBF) and oxygen metabolism ($CMRO_2$) not only in the white matter, but also in the cortex, indicating a diffuse metabolic depression which probably played a major role in the pathogenesis of dementia in this patient.

A similar PET study was performed in a 57-year-old, totally asymptomatic subject (a cousin of the previous subject) who had a diffuse white matter abnormality on MRI T2WI. It showed a 40% decrease in CBF, an increase in oxygen extraction fraction and a normal $CMRO_2$.[14] This oligemic pattern is consistent with the classical view that chronic ischemia in the long penetrating arteries is the underlying mechanism both for the leukoencephalopathy and for the small deep infarcts which thus appear as distal field infarcts. Recent SPECT data are in keeping with this presumed mechanism.[16]

The leukoencephalopathy is a key feature of CADASIL and it is crucial to its diagnosis. However it is in no way specific and it is extremely variable both in severity and distribution. The severity of T2 white matter hypersignals increases with age: in a study of 75 affected subjects,[14] we showed that under the age of 30, nearly half the subjects still had a normal MRI while the other half had only a very mild leukoaraiosis. By contast, after the age of 30, all affected subjects had abnormal T2WI and after the age of 60, they all had diffuse and severe white matter abnormalities, particularly marked in demented subjects. As regards the location, CADASIL again illustrates the selective vulnerability of some subcortical regions so that, after the age of 55, hypersignals are almost constant in periventricular areas, deep white matter and basal ganglia. There is no good correlation between the location of lesions and the various clinical patterns but the cognitive deterioration appears more linked to involvement of basal ganglia than to the white matter lesions themselves.

Thus, as any other small artery disease of the brain, CADASIL is mainly characterized by recurrent small, deep infarcts often leading to subcortical dementia, and by white matter abnormalities, both being most likely due to chronic ischemia in the long penetrating arteries. But one of the most fascinating lesion of CADASIL is that there are other symptoms (which can even occur in the absence of ischemic events) such as severe mood disorders, present in arond 15% of affected subjects, migraine with aura present in 40% and progressive subcortical dementia in the absence of stroke in 8%.[1,2,4,5,9,16-23] Moreover subtle cognitive (mainly frontal) alterations can be found early in the disease in the absence of major vascular events.[19]

In some families[16-18] migraine is the leading symptom, as in one of our patients, a 60-year-old man who had attacks of migraine with aura (1 to 5 per month) since the age of 42.[17] His attacks were typical: the aura started by a left blurring of vision which lasted 15 to 30 minutes and was followed by uni-or bilateral tingling of the fingers going up the arm and then affecting the tongue and the lips, occasionally associated with dysphasia. The aura lasted less than 1 hour and was followed by a severe headache with nausea, vomiting, photo- and phonophobia. Besides these typical attacks, he had twice suffered very atypical attacks with agitation, confusion, and fever during 24 hours. His MRI showed on T2WI diffuse white matter abnormalities but no infarction on T1WI. The family study showed that six other members also had migraine attacks, usually with typical aura, but sometimes with unusual symptoms such as confusion or fever. None had a history of stroke. Interestingly within this family, there was one subject who had a completely different presentation with isolated progressive subcortical dementia. Cognitive impairment started around the age of 45 and progressively worsened with bilateral pyramidal signs, pseudobulbar palsy, bedridden state, and death about 10 years after the onset of the first symptoms. She had a most extensive white matter disorder and, at autopsy, there were numerous deep infarcts despite the absence of clinical history of stroke.[11] Other families have been reported with migraine and sometimes dementia dominating the clinical presentation.[15,18] It will be interesting to see if they have the same mutations as families with the usual stroke pattern of presentation.

To summarize what we have learned so far from CADASIL, we would say that it is a unique example of a small artery disease of the brain with a known gene expressed in the vessel wall, a disease that we can follow from the very early stages of asymptomatic white matter abnormalities to death 30 to 40 years later. Migraine, when it is present, starts at the mean age of 30, the first subcortical ischemic events occur around 45 years, mood disorders around 50, subcortical dementia around 60 and death arond 65. However, what we have learned from this disease is still very little compared to what is left to discover: the exact nature of this granular eosinophilic deposit in the arterial wall, the precise alteration of the smooth muscle cells, the phenotype-genotype correlations, the pathophysiology of the white matter disorder and the potential relationships with the white matter abnormalities that sometimes exist in Alzheimers'disease, the pathogenesis of migraine attacks and the relationships with the "usual" migraine with and without aura, the pathogenesis of the mood disorders and the possible links with manic depressive illness. Furthermore, with the gene identification, it should now be possible to assess the exact prevalence of the disease and to determine whether sporadic cases exist or not. Last, but not least, a treatment for this dreadful condition remains to be found. The fact that all mutations are all located in the extra-cellular domain of the gene points to this region as a good target for drug development.

Beyond the fact that CADASIL is a unique model of small artery diseases of the brain, it is also of major importance because it is the first human disease related to Notch 3, a gene involved in the development of the drosophilia embryo now found responsible for a cerebral arteriopathy in human adults. The identification of Notch 3 as a gene causing CADASIL has revealed the importance and previously completely unknown role of the Notch signalling pathway both in the adult life and in the physiology of the vessels. Beyond that, CADASIL gives us insight into other conditions such as migraine, manic depressive illness, vascular dementia, and possibly also Alzheimer's disease, because of the homology between another Notch pathway gene, Sel 12, and the presenilin gene involved in early onset familial Alzheimer's disease.

References

1. Tournier-Lasserve E, Joutel A, Melki J, et al. Cerebral autosomal dominant arteriopathy with subcortical infarcts and leukoencephalopathy maps on chromosome 19q12. *Nature Genetics* 1993;3:256-259.

2. Bousser M.G, Tournier-Lasserve E. Summary of the first International workshop on CADASIL. *Stroke* 1994;25:704-707.

3. Van Bogaert L. Encéphalopathie sous-corticale progressive (Binswanger) à évolution rapide chez deux soeurs. *Med Hellen* 1955;24:961-972.

4. Bousser MG, Tournier-Lasserve E, Aylward R, et al. Reccurent strokes in a family with diffuse white-matter abnormalities - a new mitochondrial cytopathy. *J Neurol* 1988;235 (suppl. 1) : S4-S5

5. Tournier-Lasserve E, Iba-Zizen MT, Romero N, et al. Autosomal dominant syndrome with stroke-like episodes and leukoencephalopathy. *Stroke* 1991;22:1297-1302.

6. Baudrimont M, Dubas F, Joutel A, et al. Autosomal dominant leukoencephalopathy and subcortical ischemic strokes: A clinicopathological study. *Stroke* 1993;24:122-125.

7. Joutel A, Corpechot C, Ducros A, et al. Notch3 mutations in CADASIL, a hereditary adult-onset condition causing stroke and dementia. *Nature* 1996;383:707-710.

8. Joutel A, Vahedi K, Corpechot C, et al. Strong clustering and stereotyped nature of Notch3 mutations in CADASIL patients. *Lancet* 1997;350:1511-1515.

9. Chabriat H, Vahedi K, Iba-Zizen MT, et al. Clinical spectrum of CADASIL: A study of 7 families. *Lancet* 1995;346:934-939.

10. Ruchoux MM, Chabriat H, Bousser MG, et al. Presence of ultrastructural arterial lesions in muscle and skin vessels of patients with CADASIL. *Stroke* 1994;25:2291-2292.

11. Ruchoux MM, Guerrouaou D, Vandenhaute B, et al. Systemic vascular smooth muscle cell impairment in Cerebral Autosomal Dominant Arteriopathy with Subcortical Infarcts and Leukoencephalopathy. *Acta Neuropathol* 1995;89:500-512.

12. Schroder JM, Sellhaus B, Jorg J. Identification of the characteristic vascular changes in a sural nerve biopsy of a case with cerebral autosomal dominant arteriopathy with subcortical infarct and leukoencephalopathy. (CADASIL). *Acta Neuropathol* 1995;89:116-121.

13. Chabriat H, Taillia H, Iba-Zizen MT, et al. MRI features of Cerebral Autosomal Dominant Arteriopathy with Subcortical Infarcts and Leukoencephalopathy. *Neurology* 1996;46:A212.

14. Chabriat H, Levy C, Taillia H, et al. Patterns of MRI lesions in CADASIL. *Neurology*. 1998;51(2):452-457.

15. Chabriat H, Bousser MG, Pappata S. Cerebral autosomal dominant arteriopathy with subcortical infarcts and leukoencephalopathy: A positron emission tomography study in two affected family members. *Stroke* 1995;26:1729-1730.

16. Mellies JK, Bäumer T, Müller JA, et al. SPECT study of a German CADASIL family: A phenotype with migraine and progressive dementia only. *Neurology* 1998;50:1715-1721.

17. Chabriat H, Tournier-Lasserve E, Vahedi K, et al. Autosomal Dominant migraine with MRI abnormalities mapping to the CADASIL locus. *Neurology* 1995;45:1086 - 1091.

18. Verin M, Rolland Y, Landgraf F, et al. New phenotype of CADASIL with migraine as prominent clinical feature. *J Neurol Neurosurg Psychiat* 1995;59:579-585.

19. Taillia H, Chabriat H, Kurtz A, et al. Cognitive alterations in non-demented CADASIL patients. *Cerebrovascular Dis* 1998;8:97-101.

20. Vahedi K, Chabriat H, Ducros A, et al. Analysis of CADASIL clinical natural history in a series of 134 patients belonging to 17 families linked to chromosome 19. *Neurology* 1996;46:A211.

21. Wielaard R, Bornebroek M, Ophoff RA, et al. A four generation family with Cerebral Autosomal Dominant Arteriopathy with Subcortical Infarcts and Leukoencephalopathy (CADASIL) linked to chromosome 19q13. *Clin Neurol Neurosurg* 1995;97:307-313.

22. Ragno M, Tournier-Lasserve E, Fiori M, et al. An italian kindred with Cerebral Autosomal Dominant Arteriopathy with Subcortical Infarcts and Leukoencephalopathy (CADASIL). *Ann Neurol* 1995;38:231-236.

23. Sabbadini G, Francia A, Calandreillo L, et al. Cerebral Autosomal Dominant Arteriopathy with Subcortical Infarcts and Leukoencephalopathy (CADASIL). Clinical, neuroimaging, pathological and genetic study of a large Italian family. *Brain* 1995;118:207-215.

Section IV.

Inflammation

Chapter 13

Introduction

John M. Hallenbeck, MD

The following is a general framework with some background for the section on inflammation. A serviceable definition for inflammation would be a complex multifactorial process that occurs as a response of living, vascularized tissues to injury.[1] Defined in this way, it is no surprise that inflammatory mechanisms participate in ischemic brain damage. The essential question is whether inflammatory mediators serve only as a garbage detail, clearing out the debris and preparing injured tissue for healing, or whether the inflammatory mediators actually participate in progression of injury acutely, and promote healing and plasticity during the chronic recovery phase. Mediators of inflammation would include the following: endothelial cell activation, inflammatory cells including (granulocytes, monocytes, and lymphocytes) complement, reactive oxygen species, arachidionic acid metabolites and platelet activating factor, cytokines, vasoactive amines (eg, adenosine, serotonin, histamine), nitric oxide, endothelins, the contact activation system (factor XII, prekallikrein, high molecular weight kininogen, factor XI) coagulation and fibrinolysis, and proteinases.

We can pick up the thread of interest in inflammatory mediator participation in the progression of acute ischemic brain damage in the 1970s when there was interest and debate related to such concepts of microcirculatory perfusion impairment as the "no-reflow phenomenon" and "delayed post-ischemic hypoperfusion." In general, the mechanisms that impaired post-ischemic perfusion were attributed to changes in fluid mechanics, and increase in resistance due to swelling of perivascular astrocytes and endothelial cells and an increase in blood viscosity due to an increase in vascular permeability with a movement

From: Choi D, Dacey RG, Hsu CY, Powers WJ. *Cerebrovascular Disease: Momentum at the End of the Second Millennium.* Armonk, NY: Futura Publishing Company, Inc., © 2002.

of fluid from the bloodstream into the tissues. A minority view was that in addition to these mechanical factors, the highly reactive tissue, blood, could undergo a multifactorial interaction with damaged tissue that could contribute to progressive impairment of microvascular perfusion and ongoing cellular damage. Initial studies of inflammatory mediators focused on the phospholipase A^2 cascade mediators such as prostaglandins, leukotrienes, thromboxane A^2, prostacyclin and platelet activating factor. For a time, the interest in the relevance of these inflammatory mediators and microcirculatory flow problems to progressive brain damage in an acute ischemic injury zone were of sufficient interest to generate debate, but in 1981 a signal event occurred. Bo Siesjö seemed to say "may I play through," and he produced his classic article, "Cell damage in the brain: a speculative synthesis."[2] The compelling logic of these treatise ratcheted the stroke field around almost overnight so that virtually every stroke research laboratory was working on some aspect of calcium-induced neuronal injury. As the 1980s wore on, this interest evolved into a focus on excitotoxic nerve damage due to activation of NMDA channels by glutamate. Dennis Choi lit the way for this massive migration of interest among stroke researchers.[3] By the late 1980s, the emphasis on direct neurotoxic mechanisms was so strong that it was difficult to introduce the concept of ischemia into a discussion of stroke. Workers in the field would generally concede that (by definition) some vessel had to have become obstructed in order to set the stroke process into motion, but would regard things as really becoming interesting after that. At this stage, the mechanistic formulation that glutamate-mediated cytotoxicity led to accumulation of calcium in the cytosol was very clean and logical and the therapeutic targets seemed obvious. The only difficulty with sustaining this tidy and attractive concept as a unitary mechanism of ischemic damage was that somebody forgot to shoot the investigators. They kept on identifying new mediators of ischemic injury. Among these were inflammatory mediators.

Several converging influences have led to a resurgence of interest in inflammatory mechanisms in stroke.[4] Advances in endothelial cell biology and leukocyte biology along with the development of new tools to study the reactions of these cells were important factors. In addition, work continued to show participation of reactive oxygen species in acute ischemic brain damage. The identification and characterization of cytokines and the availability of tools to manipulate the cytokine system has also attracted attention and most recently interest in proteinases that can attack matrix proteins has begun to develop.

As any field matures, there are inconsistencies and questions that arise. With respect to inflammatory mediators in stroke, one example is the recent Enlimomab Trial in which a murine IgG_1 antibody to

ICAM-1 had unexpected outcome. The trial was not negative. It was robustly positive in the wrong direction. This outcome is heuristic and raises questions about introducing a heterologous protein into acutely ischemic brain.

A number of excellent laboratories have produced convincing evidence that inflammatory mediators participate in the evolution of stroke. At present, there is support for participation of such mediators in the initiation of stroke and in the progress of brain damage during the early hours of a stroke. There is a developing interest in the possibility that inflammation not only permits healing by clearing out tissue debris, but also promotes healing and plasticity. There is also some evidence that inflammatory cytokines are involved in the signaling pathways that regulate the development of tolerance to ischemia.

One challenge presented by inflammation is that any serious possibility that inflammatory mediators participate in the progression of ischemic brain damage leads to a step change in the number of candidate factors and the potential complexity of the process. Such multifactoriality imposes on investigators the need to be more integrative in their mechanistic concepts and in their experimental designs.

References

1. Cotran RS, Kumar V, Robbins SL, et al. Chapter 3. In Robbins SL (ed): *Pathologic basis of disease*, 5th Edition. Philadelphia, W.B. Saunders, 1994:51-92.
2. Siesjö BK. Cell damage in the brain: A speculative synthesis. *J Cereb Blood Flow Metab* 1981;1:155-185.
3. Choi DW. Glutamate neurotoxicity and diseases of the nervous system. *Neuron* 1988;1:623-634.
4. Hallenbeck JM. Inflammatory reactions at the blood-endothelial interface in acute stroke. In Siesjö BK, Wieloch T (eds): *Advances in Neurology, Vol 71; Cellular and molecular mechanisms of ischemic brain damage*. Philadelphia, Lippincott-Raven, 1996 pp281-300.

Chapter 14

Infection and Stroke Risk

Mark Fisher, MD

Introduction

Ischemic stroke is viewed as a clinical event largely occurring in a population with well-defined, classic risk factors (eg, hypertension, diabetes, and smoking). These risk factors are linked to stroke etiologies that are typically classified as large vessel occlusive disease, small vessel disease, and cardiogenic processes. While the at-risk population has been reasonably well defined, the timing of stroke is viewed as erratic and unpredictable.

There is substantial evidence questioning the adequacy of both of these views, ie, our ability to classify ischemic stroke and our inability to predict time of stroke occurrence. Large-scale stroke studies have repeatedly demonstrated that a large proportion of stroke patients cannot be classified by etiology. This proportion varies between 30% and 40%.[1-2] It is remarkable that this proportion has shown little variation over the past decade. Note that during this period, our ability to image the brain (by magnetic resonance imaging), the brain's vasculature (by magnetic resonance angiograpy), and the heart (by transesophageal echocardiography) have shown striking improvement. The differences between stroke and coronary artery disease in this regard (wherein "myocardial infarction of unknown etiology" is rarely encountered) could not be more striking.

The notion that stroke occurs at an unpredictable time has been also called into question. Epidemiologic studies have repeatedly shown that ischemic stroke onset tends to cluster in the early morning

From: Choi D, Dacey RG, Hsu CY, Powers WJ. *Cerebrovascular Disease: Momentum at the End of the Second Millennium.* Armonk, NY: Futura Publishing Company, Inc., © 2002.

hours.[3-4] Moreover, seasonal rates of stroke show variation, with the peak risk period being during the winter months.[4-6]

These observations imply that new ways are needed to conceptualize stroke mechanisms. The adequacy of any such new direction may be determined by a resultant improved classification ability that also addresses the issue of timing of stroke onset. A promising avenue for investigation of this issue is the relationship between stroke and infections. The importance of this approach is emphasized in the epidemiologic observation that elevations of C-reactive protein, a nonspecific indicator of inflammation, predicts ischemic stroke in healthy men.[7]

Epidemiology of Infections and Stroke

Syrjanen et al. are responsible for initial systematic observations of a possible relationship between "incidental" infections and stroke in adults.[8-9] Their first report documented serological abnormalities of bacterial infection (either stable high titers or four-fold increased titers in paired specimens) in 44% (15/34) of young (< 45 years) ischemic stroke patients versus only 9% (6/68) of controls. They found no evidence of viral infection, and there was no predominant bacterial organism.[8]

A second study of Syrjanen et al. surveyed young (< 50 years) ischemic stroke patients for febrile infection during the month prior to the stroke. A substantial proportion of the cases (19/54, or 35%) had a history of febrile illness during the prior month believed to be infection, compared to only 6% (3/54) of controls. Serological studies once again suggested a bacterial origin for infections in the stroke group (19/54 vs. 7/54 controls), and there was little serological evidence of viral infection. After controlling for classic stroke risk factors, relative risk for infections prior to stroke was 14.5. Notably, 80% of the infections were respiratory tract in origin.[9]

A study of Ameriso et al.[10] seemed to largely confirm the Finish studies. This study surveyed 50 consecutive ischemic stroke patients of all ages in an inner-city population. Fully one-third (17/50, 34%) had symptoms of febrile infections during the month prior to their stroke. Once again, respiratory tract infections predominated; they comprised 11 of 17 infectious illnesses reported.

In the first of a series of publications, Grau et al. reported a case-control study of 197 ischemic stroke patients of all ages.[11] They surveyed subjects for symptoms of infections, both febrile and nonfebrile, and found higher prevalence of infection in cases for the 1 month prior to the stroke (48/197, 24%) compared to control subjects (17/197); the latter consisted of age-, gender-, and residence-matched nonhospitalized subjects enrolled concurrent with stroke patients. The increased prevalence of infections during the 4-week period could be explained by the excess prevalence among cases during the 1-week period before the stroke (38/197 [19%] vs. 10/197 [5%]) for controls. Bacterial infections were common in the stroke group (23/38 infections, 61%), with no predominant organism. The vast majority (27/38, 71%) of infections among stroke patients were respiratory of the tract. Thus, during the one week prior to the stroke, approximately 14% more stroke patients experienced infections (for an odds ratio of 4.5).

Macko et al. reported similar findings.[12] They reported that fully 43% (16/37) of their stroke group had either an acute infectious or systemic inflammatory process (the latter associated with signs of immune system activation), compared to outpatient controls (32%, 15/47) or hospitalized controls (18%, 6/34). The increased prevalence in the stroke group could be explained by infection/inflammation occuring during the one week period prior to the stroke: 35% (13/37) for the stroke patients versus 9%-13% for the controls. Once again, respiratory tract illnesses predominated, accounting for 62% (3/13) of all infection/inflammation episodes occuring in the stroke group during the 1-week period.

Bova et al. reported a survey of infections occurring during the 2-month period prior to an acute ischemic stroke.[13] They found that 44/182 (24%) stroke patients had infections during this period, with 41/44 (93%) of the infections occuring during the 1-week period prior to the stroke. Ten percent (19/194) of their control group, consisting of patients sustaining ischemic stroke at least 6 months previously, had symptoms of infections during the prior two months.[13]

Grau et al. published additional work analyzing acute infection risk in 166 consecutive cerebral ischemia patients (130 with stroke, 36 with transient ischemic attacks).[14] Infection within the prior week was more frequent in ischemia patients (22%, 37/166) versus control subjects (8%, 14/166, P = 0.001, odds ratio 2.9 to 3.1). Frequency for infections prior to this 1-week period was comparable. Respiratory tract infections accounted for 78% (29/37) of the infections among ischemia patients during the prior week. No predominant organism was identified, and bacterial and viral infections were thought to be approximately equally common.[14]

Grau et al. performed further studies of what was apparently the same cohort,[15] analyzing the presence of chronic and recurrent infections in patients with cerebral ischemia and control subjects. "Frequent or chronic bronchitis" was twice as common (20.4 vs. 10.3%, P < 0.05) in cerebral ischemia patients compared to controls. Stroke patients also tended to have worse dental status, with more periodontitis and periapical lesions (P < 0.05).

Most studies of acute infections as precipitant of vascular events have focused on stroke. Meier et al described the relationship between acute respiratory tract infections and coronary artery disease.[16] They showed that patients with acute myocardial infarctions had a significant excess of respiratory tract infections within 10 days of the acute event, 2.8 versus 0.9% for controls (odds ratio of 2.7 to 3.6). Their findings thus implicate respiratory tract infections in approximately 2% of patients with acute myocardial infarction. It is interesting to note that this percentage increase, smaller than that reported in stroke patients, is associated with an odds ratio virtually identical to that reported by Grau et al. for stroke associated with infection during the prior week.[14]

Specific Infectious
Organisms Associated with Stroke

Mounting evidence has implicated several specific infectious organisms in the pathogenesis of clinical vascular disease. Clamydia pneumoniae (C pneumoniae) has received most of the attention. Helicobacter pylori and cytomegalovirus have also been studied extensively. Reports of these organisms have generally focused on the relation between chronic infection and the vascular event, usually myocardial ischemia.

C pneumoniae, a gram-negative bacterium, is an obligate intracellular organism linked to inflammatory vascular disease and atherosclerosis.[17] C pneumoniae is the defined pathogen in a small but significant subset of respiratory tract disoders. Among middle-aged and older adults, C pneumoniae accounts for 3% of cases of pneumonia, 5% of bronchitis, 5% of sinusitis, and 2% of pharyngitis.[18] Moreover, serological evidence of acute infection by C pneumoniae is found in 20% of patients presenting in emergency rooms with persistent cough.[19]

Extensive in vitro and animal work emphasizes the importance of C pneumoniae in vascular disease. C pneumonia infects endothelial cells, smooth muscle cells, and macrophages in vitro; all three cell types are important components of atherosclerotic lesions.[20] Intranasal innoculation of rabbits with C pneumoniae produces atherosclerotic changes, which are accelerated when combined with a diet high in cholesterol.[17,21]

Most clinical studies of C pneumoniae have focused on coronary artery disease. There appears to be at least a two-fold odds ratio associating C pneumoniae infection and coronary heart disease.[22]

Serological evidence of C pneumoniae infection has been reported to be present in an astounding 90% of patients presenting with acute myocardial infarction.[23] Most studies report lower prevalence, eg, C pneumoniae immune complexes found in 41% of patients with chronic coronary artery disease.[24] Coronary artery strains of C pneumoniae have been identified.[25] Pathologic analyses have shown viable C pneumoniae recoverable from coronary artery specimens (16%), with approximately 30% of coronary atheromas positive for C pneumoniae by polymerase chain reaction.[26]

These epidemiology and pathology reports have directly led to clinical trials of anti-Chlamydial agents. The macrolide antibiotic azithromycin, given for 3 to 6 days in myocardial infarction patients with C pneumoniae seropositivity, produced a four-fold reduced risk of coronary artery adverse events.[27] Thirty-day treatment of coronary artery disease patients with the macrolide roxithromycin produced a four- to five-fold reduced risk of coronary artery disease endpoints after 6 months.[28]

These provocative findings in the cardiology literature have been partially reproduced in cerebrovascular studies. Immunohistochemical studies demonstrate C pneumoniae in 55%-71% of carotid endarterectomy specimens.[29,30] C pneumoniae is found in endothelial cells, macrophages, and smooth muscle cells of carotid plaques, and infection is more common in plaques with thrombosis.[29,30] An initial study of C pneumoniae showed 24% of 58 patients with acute stroke or transient ischemic attack (TIA) (vs. 8% of controls) with specific IgG antibodies.[31] A larger study showed serological evidence of acute C pneumoniae infection in 14% of 176 stroke/TIA patients (vs. 6% of control subjects); 32% of stroke/TIA patients had evidence of prior C pneumoniae infection, compared to 13% of controls subjects.[32] These initial observations are of obvious importance, and demand further study.

A number of studies have also linked both Helicobacter pylori and cytomegalovirus to various vascular disorders, particularly coronary artery disease.[22] The findings of these investigations have generally not been as compelling as the studies of C pneumoniae.[33] Nevertheless, cytomegalovirus has been detected in carotid artery plaques by immunocytochemistry.[29]

Mechanisms of Stroke
Risk Associated with Infection

There are at least three mechanisms that plausibly link infections with risk for cerebrovascular disease: infections as atherogenic events, infections as procoagulant events, and infections producing the acute phase reaction. These three linked mechanisms view inflammation as both the consequence and mediator of clinical ischemic events. A continuing conceptual difficulty is distinguishing between those processes that may acutely and transiently raise stroke risk, versus those processes that appear more likely to have a subacute or even chronic effect on stroke risk.

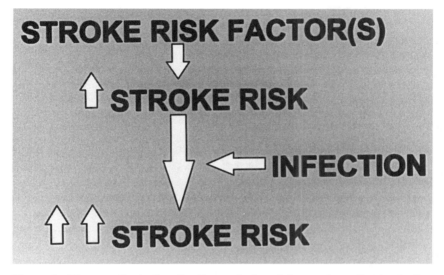

Figure 1. Diagram illustrating the theory that an inflammatory stimulus in the presence of a "classic" stroke risk factor substantially raises stroke risk beyond that of the stroke risk factor itself.

The now-classic experiments of Hallenbeck and coworkers demonstrated the importance of inflammation as a precipitant of stroke. This work analyzed the effects of endotoxin (also known as lipopolysaccharide or LPS), isolated from the cell wall of gram-negative bacteria and a key mediator of gram-negative sepsis. They found that endotoxin (given intrathecal) produced stroke in rats but only in the presence of stroke risk factors such as hypertension and diabetes.[34] Moreover, intravenous endotoxin resulted in enhanced production of the inflammatory and procoagulant cytokine tumor necrosis factor in hypertensive rats.[35,36] These findings have led to the provocative theory that an inflammatory stimulus in the presence of a "classic" stroke risk factor substantially raises stroke risk beyond that of the stroke risk factor itself (Figure 1). More recent work has emphasized the complex relationship between endotoxin, classic stroke risk factors, and infarction.[37] Nevertheless, the original theory remains potent. Indirect corroboration has come from evidence that hypertensive patients have increased likelihood of C pneumoniae infection.[38] Importantly, C pneumonia is an endotoxin-containing organism; chronic infection may produce chronic, subclinical inflammation.

Recent pathologic work has emphasized the importance of inflammation in atherosclerosis. Plaque rupture, which appears to be the defining event in the initiation of myocardial infarction and some forms of stroke, is associated with local infiltration of lymphocytes within the atherosclerotic lesion.[39] Upregulation of adhesion molecules is more prevalent in symptomatic versus asymptomatic carotid artery plaques.[40] The presence of C pneumoniae and perhaps other infectious organisms in carotid plaques,[29,30] with resulting local inflammation, may promote proliferation of the atheromatous lesion (with a prolonged effect on stroke risk) and provoke rupture of the atherosclerotic plaque (with transient, acute effects on stroke risk).

Studies of endothelial cells in culture have convincingly demonstrated critical procoagulant effects of endotoxin and other inflammatory mediators.[41,42] Inflammation produces reduction of endothelial endogenous anticoagulant function, ie, reduced fibrinolysis (downregulation of tissue plasminogen activator and enhanced plasminogen activator inhibitor-1) as well as reduction of the antithrombotic thrombomodulin/activated protein C axis.[41,42] Macko and colleagues demonstrated evidence of such processes in infection-associated stroke.[43] They reported reduced activity of tissue plasminogen activator and reduced circulating activated protein C in venous blood of patients with stroke preceded by recent infection or systemic inflammatory processes. These findings support the likelihood that acute infection has procoagulant effects, transiently adding incrementally to stroke risk from "classic" stroke risk factors.

The acute phase reaction is a non-specific response to injury, inflammation, and infection mediated by interleukin-6.[44] A variety of proteins are increased during the acute phase, notably C-reactive protein and fibrinogen. Importantly, elevations of C-reactive protein and fibrinogen predict stroke in longitudinal studies.[7,45-47] Elevated C-reactive protein and fibrinogen have been reported in infection-associated stroke.[10,48] Consequences of hyperfibrinogenemia include reduction of cerebral blood flow or blood flow velocity[49,50] and enhanced progression of carotid atherosclerosis.[51] Thus, hyperfibrinogenemia, a consequence of acute or chronic infection, may itself contribute to stroke risk. However, this effect is not likely to be acute.

There are a number of additional mechanisms potentially linking infection and stroke. Prolonged impairment of endothelial-dependent relaxation has been reported after brief vascular exposure to endotoxin;[52] impairment of cerebral vasodilation, particularly in the collateral circulation, could contribute to stroke risk. Several case reports link carotid dissection to respiratory infections.[53] These are provocative observations, and confirmatory studies are awaited.

Conclusions

Recent infection apppears to transiently increase risk for acute ischemic stroke, with an odds ratio of 3-4. These data suggest that as many as 10%-20% of acute ischemic strokes may be linked to systemic infections. These infections are overwhelmingly found in the respiratory tract. While no definite organism has been shown to provoke stroke, evidence from the cardiology literature suggests that Clamydia pneumoniae deserves serious consideration as a likely culprit. Inflammatory consequences of infection include procoagulant and atherogenic effects, suggesting that an infection-stroke mechanistic linkage is likely to be indirect and mediated by inflammatory factors.

References

1. Sacco RL, Ellenberg JH, Mohr JP, et al. Infarcts of undetermined cause: The NINDS Stroke Data Bank. *Ann Neurol* 1989;25:382-390.
2. Publications Committee for TOAST. Low molecular weight heparinoid, ORG 10172 (Danaparoid), and outcome after acute ischemic stroke. *JAMA* 1998;279:1265-1272.
3. Argentino C, Toni D, Rasura M, et al. Circadian variation in the frequency of ischemic stroke. *Stroke* 1990;21:387-389.
4. Kelly-Hayes M, Wolf PA, Kase CS, et al. Temporal patterns of stroke onset: The Framingham study. *Stroke* 1995;26:1343-1347.
5. Ricci S, Celani MG, Vitali R, et al. Diurnal and seasonal variations in the occurrence of stroke in a community-based study. *Neuroepidemiology* 1992;11:59-64.
6. Sobel E, Zhang Z, Alter M, et al. Stroke in the Lehigh Valley: seasonal variation in incidence rates. *Stroke* 1987;18:38-42.
7. Ridker PM, Cushman M, Stampfer MJ, et al. Inflammation, aspirin, and the risk of cardiovascular disease in apparently healthy men. *N Engl J Med* 1997;336:973-979.
8. Syrjanen J, Valtonen VV, Iivanainen M, et al. Association between cerebral infarction and increased bacterial antibody levels in young adults. *Acta Neurol Scand* 1986;73:273-278.
9. Syrjanen J, Valtonen VV, Iivanainen M, et al. Preceding infection as an important risk factor for ischaemic brain infarction in young and middle aged patients. *Br Med J* 1988;296:1156-1160.
10. Ameriso SF, Wong VLY, Quismorio FP, et al. Immunohematologic characteristics of infection-associated cerebral infarction. *Stroke* 1991;22:1004-1009.
11. Grau AJ, Buggle F, Heindl S, et al. Recent infection as a risk factor for cerebrovascular ischemia. *Stroke* 1995;26:373-379.
12. Macko RF, Ameriso SF, Barndt R, et al. Precipitants of brain infarction: Roles of preceding infection/inflammation and recent psychological stress. *Stroke* 1996;27:1999-2004.
13. Bova IY, Bornstein NM, Korczyn AD. Acute infection as a risk factor for ischemic stroke. *Stroke* 1996;27:2204-2206.
14. Grau AJ, Buggle F, Becher H, et al. Recent bacterial and viral infection is a risk factor for cerebrovascular ischemia: Clinical and biochemical studies. *Neurology* 1998;50:196-203.

15. Grau AJ, Buggle F, Ziegler C, et al. Association between acute cerebrovascular ischemia and chronic and recurrent infection. *Stroke* 1997;28:1724-1729.
16. Meier CR, Jick SS, Derby LE, et al. Acute respiratory-tract infections and risk of first-time acute myocardial infarction. *Lancet* 1998;351:1467-1471.
17. Laitinen K, Laurila A, Pyhala L, et al. Chlamydia penumoniae infection induces inflammatory changes in the aortas of rabbits. *Infection and Immunity* 1997;65:4832-4835. 18. Thom DH, Grayston JT, Campbell LA, et al. Respiratory infection with Chlamydia pneumoniae in middle-aged and older adult outpatients. *Eur J Clin Microbiol Infect Dis* 1994;13:785-792.
19. Wright SW, Edwards KM, Decker MD, et al. Prevalence of positive serology for acute Clamydia pneumoniae infection in emergency department patients with persistent cough. *Acad Emerg Med* 1997;4:179-183.
20. Godzik KL, O'Brien ER, Wang SK, et al. In vitro susceptbility of human vascular wall cells to infection with Chlamydia pneumoniae. *J Clin Microbio* 1995;33:2411-2414.
21. Muhlestein JB, Anderson JL, Hammond EH, et al. Infection with Chlamydia pneumoniae accelerates the development of atherosclerosis and treatment with azithromycin prevents it in a rabbit model. *Circulation* 1998;97:633-636.
22. Danesh J, Collins R, Peto R. Chronic infections and coronary artery disease: Is there a link? *Lancet* 1997;350:430-436.
23. Mazzoli S, Tofani N, Fantini A, et al. Chlamydia pneumoniae antibody response in patients with acute myocardial infarction and their follow-up. *Am Heart J* 1998;135:15-20.
24. Linnanmaki E, Leinonen M, Mattila K, et al. Chlamydia pneumoniae-specific circulating immune complexes in patients with chronic coronary heart disease. *Circulation* 1993;87:1130-1134.
25. Molestina RE, Dean D, Miller RD, et al. Characterization of a strain of C pneumoniae isolated from a coronary atheroma by analysis of the omp1 gene and biological activity in human endothelial cells. *Infection and Immunity* 1998;66:1370-1376.
26. Maass M, Bartels C, Engel PM, et al. Endovascular presence of viable Chlamydia pneumoniae is a common phenomenon in coronary artery disease. *J Am Coll Cardiol* 1998;31:827-832.
27. Gupta S, Leatham EW, Carrington D, et al. Elevated Chlamydia pneumoniae antibodies, cardiovascular events, and azithromycin in male survivors of myocardial infarction. *Circulation* 1997;96:404-407.
28. Gurfinkel E, Bozovich G, Daroca A, et al. Randomized trial fo roxithromycin in non-Q wave coroanry syndromes: ROXIS pilot study. *Lancet* 1997;350:404-407.
29. Chiu B, Viira E, Tucker W, et al. Chlamydia pneumoniae, cytomegalovirus, and herpes simplex virus in atherosclerosis of the carotid artery. *Circulation* 1997;96:2144-2148.
30. Yamashita K, Ouchi K, Shirai M, et al. Distribution of Chlamydia pneumoniae infection in the atherosclerotic carotid artery. *Stroke* 1998;29:773-778.
31. Wimmer MLJ, Sandmann-Strupp R, Saikku P, et al. Association of Chlamydia infection with cerebrovascular disease. *Stroke* 1996;27:2207-2210.
32. Cook PJ, Honeybourne D, Lip GYH, et al. Chalmydia pneumoniae antibody titers are significantly associated with acute stroke and transient cerebral ischemia: The West Birmingham Stroke Project. *Stroke* 1998;29:404-410.

33. Ossewaarde JM, Feskens EJ, DeVries A, et al. Chlamydia pneumoniae is a risk factor for coronary heart disease in symptom-free elderly men, but Helicobacater pylori and cytomegalovirus are not. *Epidemiology and Infection* 1998;120:93-99.

34. Hallenbeck JM, Dutka AJ, Kochanek PM, et al. Stroke risk factors prepare rat brainstem tissues for modified local Shwartzman reaction. *Stroke* 1988;19:863-869.

35. Hallenbeck JM, Dutka AJ, Vogel SN, et al. Lipopolysaccharide-induced production of tumor necrosis factor activity in rats with and without risk factors for stroke. *Brain Research* 1991;541:115-120.

36. Siren AL, Heldman E, Doron D, et al. Release of proinflammatory and prothrombotic mediators in the brain and peripheral circulation in spontaneously hypertensive and normotensive Wistar-Kyoto rats. *Stroke* 1992;23:1643-1651.

37. Tasaki K, Ruetzler CA, Ohtsuki T, et al. Lipopolysaccharide pre-treatment induces resistance against subsequent focal cerebral ischemic damage in spontaneously hypertensive rats. *Brain Research* 1997;748:267-270.

38. Cook PJ, Lip GY, Davies P, et al. Chlamydia pneumoniae antibodies in severe essential hypertension. *Hypertension* 1998;31:589-594.

39. van der Wal AC, Becker AE, van de Loos CM, Das PK. Site of intimal rupture or erosion of thrombosed coronary atherosclerotic plaques is characterized by an inflammatory process irrespective of the dominant plaque morphology. *Circulation* 1994;89:36-44.

40. DeGraba TJ, Siren AL, Penix L, et al. Increased endothelial expression of intercellular adhesion molecule-1 in symptomatic versus asymptomatic human carotid atherosclerotic plaque. *Stroke* 1998;29:1405-1410.

41. Schleef RR, Bevilacqua MP, Sawdey M, et al. Cytokine activation of vascular endothelium: Effects on tissue type plasminogen activator and type 1 plasminogen activator inhibitor. *J Biol Chem* 1988;263:5797-5803.

42. Esmon CT, Taylor FB, Snow TR. Inflammation and coagulation: Linked processes potentially regulated through a common pathway mediated by protein C. *Thromb Haemost* 1991;66:160-165.

43. Macko RF, Ameriso SF, Gruber A, et al. Impairments of the protein C system and fibrinolysis in infection-associated stroke. *Stroke* 1996;27:2005-2011.

44. Gershenwald JE, Fong Y, Fahey TJ, et al. Interleukin 1 receptor blockade attenuates the host inflammatory response. *Proc Natl Acad Sci USA* 1990;87:4966-4970.

45. Wilhelmsen L, Svardsudd K, Korsan-Bengsten K, et al. Fibrinogen as a risk factor for stroke and myocardial infarction. *New Engl J Med* 1984;311:501-505.

46. Kannel WB, Wolf PA, Castelli WP, et al. Fibrinogen and risk of cardiovascular disease: The Framingham Study. *JAMA* 1987;258:1183-1186.

47. Beamer NB, Coull BM, Clark WM, et al. Persistent inflammatory response in stroke survivors. *Neurology* 1998;50:1722-1728.

48. Grau AJ, Buggle F, Steichen-Wiehn, et al. Clinical and biochemical analysis of infection-associated stroke. *Stroke* 1995;26:1520-1526.

49. Grotta J, Ackerman R, Correia J, et al. Whole blood viscosity parameters and cerebral blood flow. *Stroke* 1982;13:296-301.

50. Ameriso SF, Paganini-Hill A, Meiselman HJ, et al. Correlates of middle cerebral artery blood flow velocity in the elderly. *Stroke* 1990;21:1579-1583.
51. Grotta JC, Yatsu FM, Pettigrew LC. Prediction of carotid stenosis by lipid and hematologic measurements. *Neurology* 1989;39:1325-1331.
52. Bhagat K, Moss R, Collier J, et al. Endothelial "stunning" following a brief exposure to endotoxin: A mechanism to link infection and infarction? *Cardiovascular Research* 1996;32:822-829.
53. Grau AJ, Brandt T, Forsting M, et al. Infection-associated cervical artery dissection. *Stroke* 1997;28:453-455.

Chapter 15

The Extracellular Matrix and Focal Cerebral Ischemia

Gregory J. del Zoppo, MD

Introduction

There is surprisingly little information available regarding the effects of focal ischemia, let alone global ischemia, on the most important structural constituent of the central nervous system (CNS): the matrix. Rather than a static scaffolding for the cellular components of cerebral tissue, the matrix represents a complex, dynamic and responsive fabric. Emerging impressions suggest multiple roles for the matrix in CNS diseases. The matrix appears to be important to 1) the integrated functioning of the brain, 2) the development of cerebral and cerebrovascular tissue, and 3) manifestations of inflammatory illnesses of the CNS.[1,2] Observations from other organ systems, including the lung and integument,[3-6] suggest complex responses of matrix in the CNS to injury and intervention.

The matrix components and their responses to tissue injury must be considered in relationship to their cellular receptors, the synthetic apparatus that generates the matrix components, and the enzyme systems responsible for the alterations in matrix architecture. With these four elements in mind, there is evidence that matrix components and their receptors participate actively in 1) the embryological development of the brain, 2) the binding of vascular cellular components to one another, 3) the delimitation of the vascular lumen from the surrounding brain parenchyma, 4) brain vascular and parenchymal injury, and 5)

This work was supported in part by grant RO1 NS 26945 of the National Institute of Neurological Disorders and Stroke.

From: Choi D, Dacey RG, Hsu CY, Powers WJ. *Cerebrovascular Disease: Momentum at the End of the Second Millennium.* Armonk, NY: Futura Publishing Company, Inc., © 2002.

Table 1

Extracellular Matrix Components in Central Nervous System

Basal Laminin*	Intercellular
Laminins	Proteoglycans
Collagen IV	Cat301pg
Fibronectin	pgT1
Heparin Sulfates	Versican
Entactin	Hyaluronan
Nidogen	Heparan Sulfates
Thrombospondin	

*Vascular sources

processes of angiogenesis and neogenesis. Matrix components may also be important to maintaining distances between neurons and neighboring cells, and hence their functional integrity. The potential importance of the matrix to focal ischemia derives from changes in the matrix that participate in vascular and tissue "remodelling"[7] and the hemorrhagic transformation that accompanies ischemic injury.[8,9]

The Extracellular Matrix of the Central Nervous System

In the adult brain, the extracellular matrix (ECM) allows organization of the parenchymal cell and vascular cell components (Table 1). Generally, the basal lamina portion of the ECM holds cells of the microvasculature and large vessels together and places boundaries between tissue cell groups, in the brain most particularly between the endothelium and the astrocyte compartments. The basal lamina is a fabric of laminins, type IV collagen, fibrinonectin, glycosaminoglycans, chondroitin sulfate, and heparin sulfates studded with entactin, thrombospondin, and nidogen (Table 1).[2] These components are commonly found in the basal lamina of cerebral microvessels of all diameters. They interact with each other in a highly ordered manner.[10-12] Of note, sheets of laminin are generated by spontaneous self-assembly of individual laminin molecules into a fabric with a repetitive weave.[2,11] To these sheets individual entactin and nidogen molecules adhere, allowing interactions with type IV collagen. The laminin backbone also allows local variations in composition and thickness placed upon the matrix arrays. Implied is a dynamic relationship between basal lamina composition and environmental requirements. This is most evident in the need for rapid synthesis of basal lamina during angiogenesis and neogenesis.[13,14]

Interaction among neurons and glia, and maintenance of the extracellular spaces of the neuropil involve other constituents of the ECM. Although less well appreciated, in the adult brain selected proteoglycans have been identified between neurons and their neighboring cells.[1] Among those matrix components are glycosaminoglycans, including hyaluronan/proteoglycan, which maintain extracellular volume and distance between cells via solvation of the glycosaminoglycan side chains (Table 1).[15] Additionally, versican, a hyaluronan-binding proteoglycan, and tenascin/cytotactin have been isolated from adult brain.[16-19] Two other proteoglycans, Cat-301 proteoglycan (Cat-301pg) and proteoglycan T1 (pgT1) have been associated with the extracellular matrix of adult brain of several mammalian species.[20,21] pgT1/hyaluronan complexes contribute to the insoluble intercellular matrix within the adult brain, while Cat-301pg is associated with certain neuron subpopulations.[22,23] Their synthesis, maintenance, and functional characteristics within the CNS are under study.

Components of the ECM are required for vasculogenesis and for neurite adhesion and extension *in vitro*, as suggested by the transient and ordered appearance of fibronectin and laminin in the developing cerebral cortex.[1,24] Depending on its composition, the matrix of the adult CNS serves to bind and delimit the microvascular endothelial cell and astrocyte end-feet compartments while maintaining their close apposition, and to separate neurons from adjacent non-neuronal cells. Each function requires a distinct group of matrix constituents, which provide structural support, but must allow involution or growth of vascular structures, as well as alteration of dendritic growth and synaptic interactions. Furthermore, as indicated below, receptors for specific matrix constituents may serve a signalling function, which may also be transmitted through the matrix itself. These interactions of the ECM allow flexibility in response while maintaining close relationships to their cells of origin.

Derivation Of The Microvascular Extracellular Matrix

The anatomic and functional relationships of microvascular endothelial cells to the basal lamina, and to astrocyte end-feet support their consideration as a complex.[25,26] The proximity of the endothelium to neighboring astrocytes in cerebral capillaries suggests a close functional relationship for communication and nutrient supply.[26] During development, the endothelium is derived from the mesenchyme, while astrocytes originate from ectoderm. In the adult brain, the laminins and collagen are found almost exclusively as the basal lamina in microvessels and as the meninges.[1] Generated by endothelial cells and astrocytes in concert during development, the basal lamina forms a biologically active connection between these two cell compartments. Organotypic tissue cultures (eg, murine spinal cord/pia-arachnoid explants) have shown that intact basal lamina requires the juxtaposition of microvascular endothelium and astrocytes.[27,28] Microvascular endothelial cells and astrocytes also may play reciprocal roles in the generation of matrix proteins. In culture, astrocytes secrete laminin, fibronectin, and chondroitin sulfate proteoglycan, while collagens stimulate astrocyte-induced endothelial cell maturation.[29-31] Conversely, endothelial cell-derived ECM components stimulate astrocyte growth and function (eg, glutamine synthetase activity).[32,33] These developmental interrelationships highlight the close functional association of endothelial cells and astrocytes, and their interaction with the basal lamina. In noncapillary microvessels, individual smooth muscle cells are encased in ECM, which is continuous with the basal lamina.[26] This suggests that smooth muscle cell-matrix interactions may be important in vascular responses to injury.

The basal lamina is also one important barrier to the transmigration of circulating blood cells.[8,9] The primary barrier, derived in part from intact interendothelial tight junctions, prevents contact of plasma constituents with the extravascular compartment.[34] This blood-brain barrier also relies upon the interdependence of endothelial cells and astrocytes, as elegantly shown in chick-quail adrenal vascular tissue/ brain tissue xenograft[35] and fetal-adult hippocampal/neocortex allograft preparations.[36] Astrocytes promote many microvascular blood-brain barrier properties including the development of endothelial cell tight junctions, Evan's blue exclusion, and HT7/neurothelin generation.[37-39] Soluble factor(s) generated by astrocytes are necessary to maintain endothelial blood-brain barrier characteristics including the induction of tight junctions, transendothelial resistance, and glucose/amino acid transport polarity.[36,40,41] The basal lamina and blood-brain barriers, then, depend exquisitely upon cooperation between these two unrelated cell types. Disruption of both barriers, as during ischemic stroke, contributes to edema formation and hemorrhagic transformation.[9]

Integrins: Receptors for Matrix Ligands

When considering the fate of the matrix (eg, basal lamina) ligands, it is necessary to examine together their respective individual cellular matrix receptors (eg, integrins), and the proteases which modify the receptor-matrix relationships. Integrins are heterodimeric transmembrane glycoproteins consisting of two noncovalently linked subunits, α and β, which act as cellular receptors for adhesion to ECM.[42] The noncovalent linkages between the α and β subunits allow the generation of a functional receptor. Both subunits consist of a cytoplasmic domain important for intracellular signalling, a transmembrane domain, and an NH_2-terminal extracellular domain which supplies the receptor function. The associations of α subunit subtypes with β subunit subtypes is conserved, but allows for redundancy in matrix ligand specificity.[43]

Specific integrins have also been shown to act as transducers of intracellular signals. This is best illustrated by the fate of integrin $\alpha_{IIb}\beta_3$ during platelet activation.[44,45] Here regulation of integrin function occurs by ligand occupancy of the NH_2-terminal receptor site, conformational change of the receptor, and exposure of the unique COOH-terminal cytoplasmic domain to phosphorylation. Tyrosine phosphorylation of a number of membrane-associated proteins accompany cellular activation, so that the integrin cytoplasmic tail is an important participant in the "outside-in" signaling that accompanies platelet cytoskeletal reorganization.[45]

Examples of well-defined integrin-matrix interactions are found in specific extracerebral cell systems. For instance, upon activation platelets expose integrin $\alpha_{IIb}\beta_3$ which interacts specifically with fibrin(o-gen) and von Willebrand factor, while integrin $\alpha_2\beta_1$ interacts with subendothelial collagen upon exposure of the vascular basal lamina. Integrin $\alpha_V\beta_3$ on smooth muscle cells interacts with many ligands, including fibrinonectin, vitronectin, fibrinogen, von Willebrand factor, osteopontin, and thrombospondin. Integrin $\alpha_1\beta_1$ on endothelial cells mediates adhesion to collagen IV and laminins, while integrin $\alpha_6\beta_4$ allows the binding of cutaneous basal cells specifically to laminin-5 in the basement membrane.[46] Through interactions of this sort, integrins participate in vascular processes central to tissue development, vascular structural integrity, cell-cell adhesion, and intercellular communication.[47,48]

Matrix attachments of individual cells are specialized complexes, which when in culture occur at focal contact points.[49] It is now clear that metalloproteinases (MMPs), which degrade matrix, and integrin receptors can interact together at focal contact points between cells and matrix.[50,51] For instance, MMP-2 colocalizes with the integrins $\alpha_3\beta_1$ and $\alpha_V\beta_3$ on transformed tumor cells,[50,52] and MMP-9 interacts with β_1-integrins in focal contacts of cells with matrix *in vitro*.[51] In one formulation, when cells attach to matrix via integrin receptors, the respective MMP is not secreted; but with detachment, the MMP is secreted and the receptor is not expressed at the contact point. Hence, conditions that increase MMP expression and decrease integrin expression may lead to cellular detachment. Reciprocal relationships between specific MMPs and integrin receptors for their matrix ligands appear to play a role in certain cell-matrix interactions.

Distribution of ECM and Integrin Receptors in the Cerebral Microvasculature

Immunocytochemical studies have shown that matrix ligands within the basal lamina, and selected integrin heterodimers and their subunits are distributed together within cerebral microvessels of the nonhuman primate.[53] The intermediate filaments laminin-1 and laminin-5, together with collagen type IV, and fibronectin (of cellular origin) codistribute in all cerebral microvessels.[8,54,55] These basal lamina antigens also codistribute with smooth muscle α-actin in arterioles and precapillary arterioles, consistent with the interdigitation of basal lamina among smooth muscle cells of the vascular media.[26]

Under nonischemic conditions, cerebral microvessels in the nonhuman primate have been shown to express selected α and β integrin subunits.[53,56] Integrin $\alpha_1\beta_1$ antigens colocalize with the endothelium, lying interior to the basal lamina in all microvessels and to vascular medial smooth muscle in arterioles; while, integrin $\alpha_6\beta_4$ colocalizes with GFAP-expressing astrocytes at their end-feet.[8,54,57,58] Integrin $\alpha_1\beta_1$ has also been associated with endothelial cells of all microvessels in postmortem human brain.[48] Interestingly, integrin $\alpha_6\beta_4$ is not expressed on all microvessels.[54] Integrin subunit α_3, also associated with $\alpha_6\beta_4$ in other noncerebral sites (eg, basal layer of the cutis) is found on an overlapping subset of microvessels (J.H. Heo and G.J. del Zoppo, unpublished data).[53] The constitutive expression of integrin $\alpha_1\beta_1$ on microvascular endothelial cells and integrin $\alpha_6\beta_4$ on astrocyte end-feet, together with the co-expression of their respective known ligands in the basal lamina is consistent with the premise that integrins $\alpha_1\beta_1$ and $\alpha_6\beta_4$ link their respective cells to the basal lamina.[46,59] In this way, under nonischemic conditions, the endothelium and astrocyte end-feet are brought into close apposition with each other. However, under conditions of focal cerebral ischemia, these relationships are significantly disturbed.

Alterations in Matrix Integrity

Profound local changes in matrix integrity and brain architecture accompany focal cerebral ischemia,[8,54] multiple sclerosis,[60-62] tumorigenesis,[63-67] and other disorders. MMPs, plasminogen activators (PAs), and serine proteases secreted by endothelial cells, astrocytes, microglia, and other cells within the CNS in response to these conditions can alter the basal lamina, and thereby change endothelial cell-astrocyte relationships, and promote remodelling of blood vessels. Disruption of the basal lamina during ischemia may result from shutdown of matrix protein synthesis or from proteolysis of individual matrix components. There is very little information about vascular matrix turnover in the CNS under normal conditions. Based on analogy from noncerebral tissues,[3,4,6] tumor reactivity,[63-65] and limited studies in cerebral ischemia,[68-70] matrix degradation may be achieved by secretion of MMPs, generation of plasmin by PAs, activation of serine proteases (eg, thrombin), or release of polymorphonuclear (PMN) leukocyte-specific granule enzymes. Of these, proteolysis by secreted MMPs, PAs, or serine proteases is likely to be most rapid, and to cause the most significant local vascular injury.

MMPs are Zn^{+2} endopeptidases which degrade specific components of the matrix.[71,72] They assist in migration of normal and transformed cells,[72] and participate in vascular remodelling.[51] The MMPs are secreted as inactive precursors which are activated either by specific circulating proteases (eg, pro-MMP-9 by plasmin) or by membrane-associated MMPs on cells (eg, pro-MMP-2 by MT-MMP-1). Gelatinases A (MMP-2) and B (MMP-9), the most well-characterized of the matrix metalloproteinases, are constitutively present in plasma (Table 2).[73] MMP-2 or MMP-9 are also released from vascular endothelium, vascular smooth muscle, and leukocytes during inflammation and cleave collagen IV and laminin to promote vascular remodelling.[74,75]

The activity of secreted MMPs is restricted by their natural inhibitors, which are designated the tissue inhibitors of metalloproteinases (TIMPs).[76] TIMP-2 is a specific inhibitor of MMP-2, while TIMP-1 inhibits most other MMPs.[71,76] By inhibiting the activities of MMPs, they play an important role in maintaining the balance between degradation and formation of the matrix.

In the cadaveric human brain, MMP-1, MMP-2, and MMP-9 have been identified with microglia and MMP-3 with microvessels.[77] In isolated cell systems, in contrast, MMP-9 is associated with microvascular endothelial cells, while MMP-2, MMP-3, and MMP-9 have been found on quiescent and LPS-stimulated astrocytes.[78-80] Transcription of MMP-1, MMP-3, and MMP-9 in microvascular endothelial cells is stimulated by the inflammatory cytokines IL-1β and TNF-α *in vitro*.[81]

Separately, PAs secreted by endothelial cells affect matrix components directly, and indirectly by generating plasmin. Laminin is a substrate for plasmin.[82,83] But, plasmin also activates MMP-1, MMP-3, and MMP-9.[72,84] We have shown that cerebral microvascular endothelial

Table 2

Characteristics of the Metalloproteinases MMP-2 and MMP-9*

Protease	Cell Source(s)	Ligands	Activator(s)	Inhibitor(s)	Integrin(s)†
MMP-2	Endothelium Astrocytes Microglia Neurons	Laminin Collagens I, IV, V Fibronectin Vitronectin Gelatin Aggrecan Elastin	MT-MMP-1 MT-MMP-3	TIMP-2	Subunit α_3
MMP-9	Endothelium Microglia Neurons [PMN Leukocytes]	Collagens IV, V Fibronectin Vitronectin Gelatin Elastin	Plasmin MMP-1 MMP-2 MMP-3 MMP-7 Trypsin Chymotrypsin Cathepsin G	TIMP-1	Subunit β_1

*In relation to central nervous system presestation
†Associated with focal contacts in isolated cell culture systems[50-52]

cells express t-PA antigen *in situ*, consistent with the known secretory properties of these cells.[85,86] Additionally, astrocytes produce t-PA and urokinase in response to specific mitogens.[87] Nonischemic rodent brain tissues also generate PA activity.[88]

Two other sources of matrix proteolysis may be important. Among serine proteases, thrombin is interesting because it has multiple actions. It is generated very early (within 1-2 hours) during MCA:O as shown by the appearance of fibrin in ischemic microvessels in the primate basal ganglia.[89] Thrombin stimulates MMP-2 and MMP-9 secretion by vascular smooth muscle cells.[90,91] Also, upon activation PMN leukocytes release granule enzymes, including collagenase (MMP-8), gelatinase B (MMP-9), elastase, and cathepsin G during the inflammatory phase following ischemia, which can degrade laminins and collagens of the vascular basal lamina.[92-95] This allows egress of cells from the blood circulation into the perivascular tissues.

Focal Cerebral Ischemia: The Fate of the Matrix and Its Receptors

The complex relationships among the basal lamina components, their cellular integrin receptors, and the endogenous enzyme systems responsible for their synthesis and degradation are exposed during focal cerebral ischemia. Following MCA:O, cerebral microvascular basal lamina is lost. Our group has shown recently that the basal lamina antigens laminin-1, laminin-5, collagen IV, and cellular fibronectin disappear together during sustained MCA:O and subsequent reperfusion (Figure 1).[8,54] For instance, the fraction of microvessels in the basal ganglia displaying laminin-1 antigen decreases from 0.98 ± 0.04 to 0.55 ± 0.27 (2p < 0.0001) within 24 hours following MCA:O.[8] In the nonhuman primate, these changes are prominent in the region of most severe neuron injury within the ischemic territory. Hamann et al. have demonstrated that this loss of microvascular basal lamina is significantly associated with regions of hemorrhage within the ischemic region.[9]

Following MCA:O, microvascular integrin expression undergoes most rapid change in the region of severe neuron injury. Rapid significant loss of microvascular endothelial cell integrin $\alpha_1\beta_1$ expression, as early as two hours following MCA:O in this region (2p < 0.007), is accompanied by a highly significant simultaneous abrupt loss of subunit β_1 from select perivascular astrocyte fibres (Figure 2).[56] Electron microscopic studies confirm that the disappearance of the integrin $\alpha_1\beta_1$ loss is <u>not</u> due to loss of endothelial cells as these remain intact. Focal ischemia also alters the close relationship between the astrocyte end-

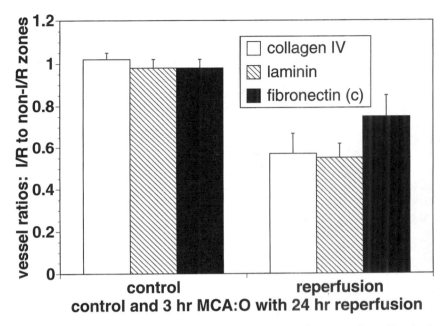

Figure 1. Reduction in number of microvessels displaying matrix (basal lamina) constituents following experimental focal ischemia.[8]

feet and the basal lamina.[25,26,40,54,96] Early following MCA:O, the number of microvessels expressing integrin $\alpha_6\beta_4$ also falls rapidly ($2p < 0.01$) in the region of severe neuron injury, exceeding the fall in expression of the ligand laminin-5 (Figure 3).[54]

The microvascular expressions of integrins $\alpha_1\beta_1$ and $\alpha_6\beta_4$ are, then, equally sensitive to ischemia. Their rapidly reduced expressions indicate substantial changes at the matrix-cell junction within the microvessels. Those changes are graded with respect to the degree of neuron injury, being most pronounced in the regions of severe ischemic neuron damage.[54,70,97,98] They accompany alterations in the vascular matrix. So far, the mechanisms responsible for these integrin-matrix alterations due to focal cerebral ischemia have not been elucidated.

Responses of Matrix-Modifying Enzymes to Focal Cerebral Ischemia

The disappearance of matrix proteins following focal cerebral ischemia may be due to proteolysis, blockade of transcription, inhibition of translation, or combinations of these. Of particular interest, hinted at by specific cell associations within the CNS, are the potential roles of activated proteolytic systems in matrix metabolism. Remodeling of

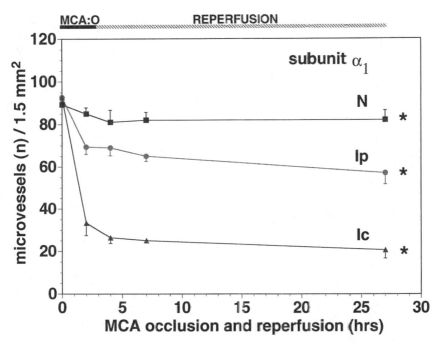

Figure 2. Rapid decrease in the expression number (n) of microvessels displaying immunoreactive integrin subunit α_1 during experimental MCA:O in the region of severe ischemic neuron injury (Ic), in the region peripheral thereto (Ip), and in the contralateral non-ischemic territory (N). *$2p < 0.05$ between pairs.

the microvascular basal lamina occurs when secreted proteases such as specific MMPs and PAs (through plasmin) degrade laminin, collagen, or fibronectin.[84,85,97] MMP expression within the brain changes during ischemic stroke. Anthony et al. reported the marked expression of MMP-9 by PMN leukocytes in human brain within 1 week of stroke, and MMP-2 from macrophages thereafter.[98] In anesthetized Wistar-Kyoto and spontaneously hypertensive rats (SHRs), Rosenberg et al. showed that latent MMP-9 increases by 12 to 24 hours and latent MMP-2 increases by 5 days after MCA:O.[69] But, in neither human nor rodent model studies was a direct association of MMP-2 or MMP-9 with neuron injury or hemorrhage demonstrated. Previously, Rosenberg et al. had clearly shown that bacterial collagenase (Type VII, Sigma) given stereotactically in large quantities could elicit hemorrhage in Sprague-Dawley rats.[68] Those studies suggested that the increased expressions of MMP-2 and MMP-9 occur late (>24 hours) during sustained ischemic stroke. There is limited evidence that the primary inhibitory system for MMPs is also upregulated. In one study, TIMP-1 mRNA was induced at 12 hours and reached a peak level at 2 days after MCA:O in the SHR.[99] Those findings suggest a potential role for MMPs in the development

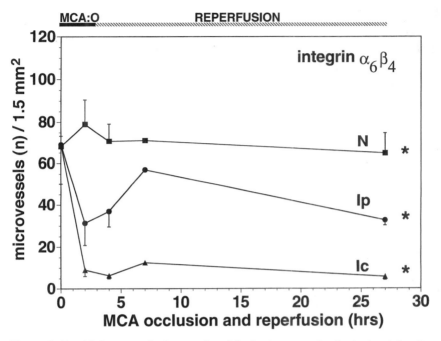

Figure 3. Rapid decrease in the number (n) of microvessels displaying integrin $\alpha_6\beta_4$ during experimental MCA:O in the Ic, Ip, and N regions (as in Figure 2). *2p<0.05 between pairs.

of ischemic cerebral tissue injury, however a relationship to matrix injury was not developed.

In separate recent experiments in the nonhuman primate, a significant increase in the expression of the latent forms of MMP-2 and MMP-9, and the active form of MMP-2 has been shown 1 to 2 hours after MCA:O in the ischemic basal ganglia (J.H. Heo and G.J. del Zoppo, unpublished data). Within the first 2 hours, a highly significant correlation with the number of severely injured neurons was seen (r = 0.9763, 2p < 0.0008). No increased expression of MMP-2 was seen in normal tissue, however. These results indicate the *de novo* synthesis of MMP-2 by cells within the ischemic zone in direct association with neuron injury, and in the same time and location as microvascular integrin and basal lamina loss. These findings are a significant refinement on observations made following MCA:O in rodent models.[69] Differences in species, model construct, mechanisms of neuron injury, and technical issues are probably involved.[57,69] Nonetheless, these early studies suggest that there is a highly significant temporal, spatial and associative congruence of microvascular injury, matrix degradation, MMP-2 expression, and neuron injury during focal cerebral ischemia, which appears clearest so far in the nonhuman primate.

The contributions of plasminogen activator release and the release of granule-associated proteases during PMN leukocyte to matrix degradation in the ischemic brain are also unexplored. Quantitating the microvascular presentation of MMPs and their TIMPs is essential to demonstrate their contributions to matrix degradation during ischemia, and to further support interventions which might maintain basal lamina integrity and neuron function.

Summary

There is a growing appreciation that processes which lead to vascular and parenchymal injury within the central nervous system, as in other organ systems, affect the integrity of the extracellular matrix. It is now well-established in a number of isolated systems (eg, in cell culture, and specific end-organs) that matrix components together with their integrin receptors are important in processes of embryological development, for structural integrity and cell viability, in signalling events, and maintenance of vascular permeability barriers and tissue demarcations. In the CNS the function of matrix components to maintain intercellular relationships between neurons and their neighbors is not well understood. However, many of the principal constituents have been determined. Experimental evidence so far supports the view that focal cerebral ischemia leads to microvascular injury which may contribute to perivascular hemorrhage, and may be directly involved with neuron injury. Disturbance of the integrin-matrix interactions appears to be particularly rapid following focal cerebral ischemia. Modulation of matrix integrity during focal cerebral ischemia is likely to involve endogenous secretion of a number of enzymes including metalloproteinases, plasminogen activators, and serine proteases, in addition to enzymes secreted from invading inflammatory cells, including PMN leukocytes. The identification of specific enzyme systems important to changes in the vascular matrix, for instance, may lead to new interventions that maintain microvascular structure and tissue integrity, and reduce neuron injury during focal ischemia. There is little doubt that these explorations will add to understanding other common processes in the CNS, including embryological development, intercellular communication, disseminated sclerosis, and Alzheimer's disease.

References

1. Carlson SS, Hockfield S. Central nervous system. In Comper WD (ed): *Extracellular Matrix, Volume 1.* Melbourne: Harwood Academic Publishers; 1996:1-23.

2. Yurchenko PD, Schittny JC. Molecular architecture of basement membranes. *J Biol Chem* 1986;261:1577-1590.

3. Shadzeidi S, Mulier B, de Crombrugghe B, et al. Enhanced type III collagen gene expression during bleomycin-induced lung fibrosis. *Thorax* 1993;48: 622-628.

4. Broekelmann TJ, Limper AH, Colby TV, et al. Transforming growth factor β1 is present at sites of extracellular matrix gene expression in human pulmonary fibrosis. *Proc Natl Acad Sci* 1991;88:6642-6646.

5. Briggaman RA. Biochemical composition of the epidermal-dermal junction and other basement membranes. *J Invest Dermatol* 1982;78:1-6.

6. Quaglino D, Nanney LB, Ditescheim JA, et al. Transforming growth factor-beta stimulates wound healing and modulates extracellular matrix gene expression in pig skin: Incisional wound model. *J Invest Dermatol* 1991;97: 34-42.

7. Gibbons GH, Dzau VJ. The emerging concept of vascular remodeling. *N Engl J Med* 1994;330:1431-1438.

8. Hamann CF, Okada Y, Fitridge R, et al. Microvascular basal lamina antigens disappear during cerebral ischemia and reperfusion. *Stroke* 1995;26:2120-2126.

9. Hamann GF, Okada Y, del Zoppo GJ. Hemorrhagic transformation and microvascular integrity during focal cerebral ischemia/reperfusion. *J Cereb Blood Flow Metab* 1996;16:1373-1378.

10. Yurchenco PD, Schittny JC. Molecular architecture of basement membranes. *FASEB J* 1990;4:1577-1590.

11. Yurchenco PD, O'Rear JJ. Basal lamina assembly. *Curr Opin Cell Biol* 1994;6: 674-681.

12. Aumailley M. Structure and supramolecular organization of basement membranes. *Kidney Int* 1995;47:S4-S7.

13. Mignatti P, Rifkin DB. Plasminogen activators and matrix metalloproteinases in angiogenesis. *Enzyme & Protein* 1996;49:117-137.

14. Aviezer D, Hecht D, Safran M, et al. Perlecan, basal lamina proteoglycan, promotes basic fibroblast growth factor-receptor binding, mitogenesis, and angiogenesis. *Cell* 1994;79:1005-1013.

15. Ransom BR, Sontheimer H. The neurophysiology of glial cells. *J Clinical Neurophys* 1992;9:224-251.

16. Bondareff W. An intracellular substance in rat cerebral cortex: Submicroscopic distribution of ruthenim red. *Anat Rec* 1967;157:527-536.

17. Castejon HV. Histochemical demonstration of sulphated polysaccharides at the coat of nerve cells in the mouse central nervous system. *Acta Histochemistry* 1970;38:55-64.

18. Perides G, Lane WS, Andrews D, et al. Isolation and partial characterization of a glial hyaluronate-binding protein. *J Biol Chem* 1989;264:5981-5987.

19. Perides G, Rahemtulla F, Lane WS, et al. Isolation of a large aggregating proteoglycan from human brain. *J Biol Chem* 1992;267:23883-23887.

20. Iwata M, Carlson SS. A large chondroitin sulfate proteoglycan has the characteristics of a general extracellular matrix component of adult brain. *J Neurosci* 1993;13:195-207.

21. Iwata M, Wight TN, Carlson SS. A brain extracellular matrix forms aggregates with hyaluronan. *J Biol Chem* 1993;268:15061-15069.

22. Zaremba S, Naegele JR, Barnstable CJ, et al. Neuronal subsets express multiple high-molecular weight cell-surface glyconjugates defined by monoclonal antibodies. *J Neurosci* 1990;10:2985-2995.

23. Hockfield S, Kalb RG, Zaremba S, et al. Expression of neural proteoglycans correlates with the acquisition of mature neuronal properties in the mammalian brain. *Cold Spring Harbor Symp Quant Biol* 1990;55:504-514.

24. Sanes JR. Extracellular matrix molecules that influence neural development. *Annu Rev Neurosci* 1989;12:491-516.

25. del Zoppo GJ. Microvascular changes during cerebral ischaemia and reperfusion. *Cerebrovasc Brain Metab Rev* 1994;6:47-96.

26. Peters A, Palay BL, Webster HD. *The Fine Structure of the Nervous System. Neurons and Their Supporting Cells, 3rd ed.* New York: Oxford University Press; 1991.

27. Bernstein JJ, Getz R, Jefferson M, et al. Astrocytes secrete basal lamina after hemisection of rat spinal cord. *Brain Res* 1985;327:135-141.

28. Kusaka H, Hirano A, Bornstein MB, et al. Basal lamina formation by astrocytes in organotypic cultures of mouse spinal cord tissue. *J Neuropathol Exp Neurol* 1985;44:295-303.

29. Tagami M, Yamagata K, Fujino H, et al. Morphological differentiation of endothelial cells co-cultured with astrocytes on type-I or type-IV collagen. *Cell Tissue Res* 1992;268:225-232.

30. Webersinke G, Bauer H, Amberger A, et al. Comparison of gene expression of extracellular matrix molecules in brain microvascular endothelial cells and astrocytes. *Biochem Biophys Res Commun* 1992;189:877-884.

31. Ard MD, Faissner A. Components of astrocytic extracellular matrix are regulated by contact with axons. *Ann N Y Acad Sci* 1991;633:566-569.

32. Kozlova M, Kentroti S, Vernadakis A. Influence of culture substrata on the differentiation of advanced passage glial cells in cultures from aged mouse cerebral hemispheres. *Int J Dev Neurosci* 1993;11:513-519.

33. Nagano N, Aoyagi M, Hirakawa K. Extracellular matrix modulates the proliferation of rat astrocytes in serum-free culture. *GLIA* 1993;8:71-76.

34. Risau W, Wolburg H. Development of the blood-brain barrier. *TINS* 1990;13:174-178.

35. Janzer RC, Raff MC. Astrocytes induce blood-brain barrier properties in endothelial cells (Letter). *Nature* 1987;325:353-355.

36. Hurwitz AA, Berman JW, Rashbaum WK, et al. Human fetal astrocytes induce the expression of blood-brain barrier specific proteins by autologous endothelial cells. *Brain Res* 1993;625:238-243.

37. Risau W, Hallmann R, Albrecht U, et al. Brain astrocytes induces the expression of an early cell surface marker for blood-brain barrier specific endothelium. *EMBO J* 1986;5:3179-3183.

38. Schlosshauer B, Herzog KH. Neurothelin: An inducible cell surface glycoprotein of blood-brain barrier specific endothelial cells and distinct neurons. *J Cell Biol* 1990;110:1261-1274.

39. Lobrinus JA, Juillerat-Jeanneret L, Darekar P, et al. Induction of the blood-brain barrier specific HT7 and neurothelin epitopes in endothelial cells of the chick chorioallantoic vessels by a soluble factor derived from astrocytes. *Dev Brain Res* 1992;70:207-211.

40. Minakawa T, Bready J, Berliner J, et al. In vitro interaction of astrocytes and pericyte with capillary-like structures of brain microvessel endothelium. *Lab Invest* 1991;65:32-40.

41. Estrada C, Bready JV, Berliner JA, et al. Astrocyte growth stimulation by a soluble factor produced by cerebral endothelial cells in vitro. *J Neuropathol Exp Neurol* 1990;49:539-549.

42. Ruoslahti E. Integrins. *J Clin Invest* 1991;87:1-5.

43. Hynes RO, Bader BL. Targeted mutations in integrins and their ligands: Their implications for vascular biology. *Thromb Haemost* 1997;78:83-87.

44. Du X, Ginsberg MH. Integrin $\alpha_{IIb}\beta_3$ and platelet function. *Thromb Haemost* 1997;78:96-100.

45. Shattil SJ, Gao J, Kashiwagi H. Not just another pretty face: Regulation of platelet function at the cytoplasmic face of integrin $\alpha_{IIb}\beta_3$. *Thromb Haemost* 1997;78:220-225.

46. Tamura RN, Rozzo C, Starr L, et al. Epithelial integrin $\alpha_6\beta_4$: Complete primary structure of α_6 and variant forms of β_4. *J Cell Biol* 1990;111:1593-1604.

47. Luscinskas FW, Lawler J. Integrins as dynamic regulators of vascular function. *FASEB J* 1994;8:929-938.

48. Albelda SM. Differential expression of integrin cell-substratum adhesion receptors on endothelium. In Steiner R, Weisz PB, Langer R (eds): *Angiogenesis: Key Principles--Science--Technology--Medicine.* Basel, Switzerland: Birkhäuser Verlag; 1992:188-192.

49. Pasqualini R, Hemler ME. Contrasting roles for integrin β_1 and β_5 cytoplasmic domains in subcellular localization, cell proliferation, and cell migration. *J Cell Biol* 1994;125:447-460.

50. Chintala SK, Sawaya R, Gokaslan ZL, et al. Modulation of matrix metalloprotease-2 and invasion in human glioma cells by $\alpha_3\beta_1$ integrin. *Cancer Lett* 1996;103:201-208.

51. Partridge CA, Phillips PG, Niedbala MJ, et al. Localization and activation of type IV collagenase/gelatinase at endothelial focal contacts. *Lung Cell Mol Physiol* 1997;16:L813-L822.

52. Brooks PC, Strömblad S, Sanders LC, et al. Localization of matrix metalloproteinase MMP-2 to the surface of invasive cells by interaction with integrin $\alpha_V\beta_3$. *Cell* 1996;85:683-693.

53. Haring H-P, Akamine P, Habermann R, et al. Distribution of the integrin-like immunoreactivity on primate brain microvasculature. *J Neuropathol Exp Neurol* 1996;55:236-245.

54. Wagner S, Tagaya M, Koziol JA, et al. Rapid disruption of an astrocyte interaction with the extracellular matrix mediated by $\alpha_6\beta_4$ during focal cerebral ischemia/reperfusion. *Stroke* 1997;28:858-865.

55. Fuchs E, Weber K. Intermediate filaments: Structure, dynamics, function, and disease. *Annu Rev Biochem* 1994;63:345-382.

56. del Zoppo GJ, Haring H, Tagaya M, et al. Loss of $\alpha_1\beta_1$ integrin immunoreactivity on cerebral microvessels and astrocytes following focal cerebral ischemia/reperfusion. *Cerebrovasc Dis* 1996;6:9

57. Tagaya M, Liu K-F, Copeland B, et al. DNA scission following focal brain ischemia: Temporal differences in two species. *Stroke* 1997;28:1245-1254.

58. Okada Y, Copeland BR, Hamann GF, et al. Integrin $\alpha_V\beta_3$ is expressed in selected microvessels following focal cerebral ischemia. *Am J Pathol* 1996;149:37-44.

59. Wegiel J, Wisniewski HM. Rosenthal fibers, eosinophilic inclusions, and anchorage densities with desmosome-like structures in astrocytes in Alzheimer's disease. *Acta Neuropathol (Berl)* 1994;87:335-361.

60. Sobel RA. The extracellular matrix in multiple sclerosis lesions. *Journal of Neuropathology & Experimental Neurology* 1998;57:205-217.

61. Previtali SD, Archelos JJ, Hartung HP. Modulation of the expression of integrins on glial cells during experimental autoimmune encephalomyelitis. A central role of TNF-alpha. *Am J Pathol* 1997;151:1425-1435.

62. Jackson DY, Quan C, Artis DR, et al. Potent alpha 4 beta 1 peptide antagonists as potential anti-inflammatory agents. *Journal of Medicinal Chemistry* 1997;40:3359-3368.

63. Liotta LA, Rao CN, Wewer UM. Biochemical interactions of tumor cells with the basement membrane. *Annu Rev Biochem* 1986;55:1037-1057.

64. Koukoulis GK, Howeedy AA, Korhonen M, et al. Distribution of tenascin, cellular fibronectins and integrins in the normal, hyperplastic and neoplastic breast. *J Submicrosc Cytol Pathol* 1993;25:285-295.

65. Koukoulis GK, Virtanen I, Korhonen M, et al. Immunohistochemical localization of integrins in the normal, hyperplastic, and neoplastic breast. Correlations with their functions as receptors and cell adhesion molecules. *Am J Pathol* 1991;139:787-799.

66. Khokha R, Denhardt DT. Matrix metalloproteinases and tissue inhibitor of metalloproteinases. A review of their role in tumorigenesis and tissue invasion. *Invasion Metastasis* 1989;9:391-405.

67. Stetler-Stevenson M, Mansoor A, Lim M, et al. Expression of matrix metalloproteinases and tissue inhibitors of metalloproteinases in reactive and neoplastic lymphoid cells. *Blood* 1997;89:1708-1715.

68. Rosenberg GA, Mun-Bryce S, Wesley M, et al. Collagenase-induced intracerebral hemorrhage in rats. *Stroke* 1990;21:801-807.

69. Rosenberg GA, Navratil M, Barone F, et al. Proteolytic cascade enzymes increase in focal cerebral ischemia in rat. *J Cereb Blood Flow Metab* 1996;16:360-366.

70. Rosenberg GA, Dencoff JE, Correa N Jr., et al. Effect of steroids on CSF matrix metalloproteinases in multiple sclerosis: Relation to blood-brain barrier injury. *Neurology* 1996;46:1626-1632.

71. Woessner JF Jr. Matrix metalloproteinases and their inhibitors in connective tissue remodeling. *FASEB J* 1991;5:2145-2154.

72. Nagase H. Activation mechanisms of matrix metalloproteinases. *Biol Chem* 1997;378:151-160.

73. Vortio T, Baumann M. Human gelatinase/type IV collagenase is a regular plasma component. *FEBS Lett* 1989;155:285-289.

74. Ueda Y, Imai K, Tsuchiya H, et al. Matrix metalloproteinase 9 (gelatinase B) is expressed in multinucleated giant cells of human giant cell tumor of bone and is associated with vascular invasion. *Am J Pathol* 1996;148:611-622.

75. Morodomi T, Ogata Y, Sasaguri Y, et al. Purification and characterization of matrix metalloproteinase 9 from U937 monocytic leukaemia and HT1080 fibrosarcoma cells. *Biochem J* 1992;285:603-611.

76. Gomez DE, Alonso DF, Yoshiji H, et al. Tissue inhibitors of metalloproteinases: Structure, regulation and biological functions. *Eur J Cell Biol* 1997;74:111-122.

77. Maeda A, Sobel RA. Matrix metalloproteinases in the normal human central nervous system, microglial nodules, and multiple sclerosis lesions. *J Neuropathol Exp Neurol* 1996;55:300-309.

78. Jackson CJ, Nguyen M. Human microvascular endothelial cells differ from macrovascular endothelial cells in their expression of matrix metalloproteinases. *Int J Biochem Cell Biol* 1997;29:1167-1177.

79. Gottschall PE, Deb S. Regulation of matrix metalloproteinase expressions in astrocytes, microglia and neurons. *Neuroimmunomodulation* 1996;3:69-75.

80. Wells GM, Catlin G, Cossins JA, et al. Quantitation of matrix metalloproteinases in cultured rat astrocytes using the polymerase chain reaction with a multi-competitor cDNA standard. *GLIA* 1996;18:332-340.

81. Hanemaaijer R, Koolwijk P, le Clercq L, et al. Regulation of matrix metalloproteinase expression in human vein and microvascular endothelial cells. Effects of tumour necrosis factor α, interleukin 1 and phorbol ester. *Biochem J* 1993;296:803-809.

82. Liotta LA, Goldfarb RH, Brundage R, et al. Effect of plasminogen activator (urokinase), plasmin, and thrombin on glycoprotein and collagenous components of basement membrane. *Cancer Res* 1981;41:4629-4636.

83. Liotta LA, Goldfarb RH, Terranova VP. Cleavage of laminin by thrombin and plasmin: Alpha-thrombin selectively cleaves the beta chain of laminin. *Thromb Res* 1981;21:663-673.

84. Krane SM. Clinical importance of metalloproteinases and their inhibitors. In: Inhibition of Matrix Metalloproteinases: Therapeutic Potential (Eds. R.A. Greenwald, L.M. Golub). *Ann N Y Acad Sci* 1994;732:1-10.

85. Levin EG, del Zoppo GJ. Localization of tissue plasminogen activator in the endothelium of a limited number of vessels. *Am J Pathol* 1994;144:855-861.

86. Levin EG, Loskutoff DJ. Cultured bovine endothelial cells produce both urokinase and tissue-type plasminogen activators. *J Cell Biol* 1982;94:631-636.

87. Tranque P, Robbins R, Naftolin F, et al. Regulation of plasminogen activators and type-1 plasminogen activator inhibitor by cyclic AMP and phorbol ester in rat astrocytes. *GLIA* 1992;6:163-171.

88. Sappino A-P, Madani R, Huarte J, et al. Extracellular proteolysis in the adult murine brain. *J Clin Invest* 1993;92:679-685.

89. Okada Y, Copeland BR, Fitridge R, et al. Fibrin contributes to microvascular obstructions and parenchymal changes during early focal cerebral ischemia and reperfusion. *Stroke* 1994;25:1847-1854.

90. Fabunmi RP, Baker AH, Murray EJ, et al. Divergent regulation by growth factors and cytokines of 95 kDa and 72 kDa gelatinases and tissue inhibitors of metalloproteinases-1, -2, and -3 in rabbit aortic smooth muscle cells. *Biochem J* 1996;315:335-342.

91. Galis ZS, Kranzhöfer R, Fenton JW II, et al. Thrombin promotes activation of matrix metalloproteinase-2 produced by cultured vascular smooth muscle cells. *Arterioscler Thromb Vasc Biol* 1997;17:483-489.

92. Murphy G, Reynolds JJ, Bretz U, et al. Collagenase is a component of the specific granules of human neutrophil leukocytes. *Biochem J* 1987;162:195-197.

93. Watanabe H, Hattori S, Katsuda S, et al. Human neutrophil elastase: Degradation of basement membrane components and immunolocalization in the tissue. *J Biochem* 1990;108:753-759.

94. Heck LW, Blackburn WD, Irwin MH, et al. Degradation of basement membrane laminin by human neutrophil elastase and cathepsin G. *Am J Pathol* 1990;136:1267-1274.

95. Pike MC, Wicha MS, Yoon P, et al. Laminin promotes the oxidative burst in human neutrophils via increased chemoattractant receptor expression. *J Immunol* 1989;142:2004-2011.

96. Chan PH, Chu L. Ketamine protects cultured astrocytes from glutamate-induced swelling. *Brain Res* 1989;487:380-383.

97. Woessner JF Jr. The family of matrix metalloproteinases. *Ann N Y Acad Sci* 1994;732:11-21.

98. Anthony DC, Ferguson B, Matyzak MK, et al. Differential matrix metalloproteinase expression in cases of multiple sclerosis and stroke. *Neuropathol Appl Neurobiol* 1997;23:406-415.

99. Wang X, Barone FC, White RF, et al. Subtractive cloning identifies tissue inhibitor of matrix metalloproteinase-1 (TIMP-1) increased gene expression following focal stroke. *Stroke* 1998;29:516-520.

Chapter 16

Some Principles of the Inflammatory Reaction to Brain Ischemia—Sense and Purpose

Julie A. Ellison, PhD, Frank C. Barone, PhD, and Giora Z. Feuerstein, MD

Introduction

Inflammation is a cellular response following injury to a vascularized tissue. After an ischemic insult to the brain the injured endothelium, glia, and neurons release cytokines and chemokines that recruit activated peripheral immune cells to the site of injury. Subsequently these immune cells secrete inflammatory mediators that generate the classic brain response to injury characterized by astrocytic gliosis[1-5] and microglial activation.[6,7] Investigations of inflammation after brain ischemia have focused upon the acute sequelae of inflammation documenting a cascade of novel gene expression associated with cell activation and recruitment to the site of injury. Little attention has been given to the initial inflammatory signals that are responsible for restoring the cellular homeostasis and tissue integrity. While the initial recruitment of leukocytes to the injured brain can be viewed negatively, in fact macrophages are critical for establishing the milieu necessary for debridement and repair of the injured tissue.[8] Thus it might be argued that the purpose of the inflammatory response after focal stroke is to activate and recruit cells to mediate the repair of brain injury by: 1) activation of glia in the peri-infarct region; 2) compartmentalization of the injured cells; 3) removal of the infarcted tissue debris by phagocytes;

From: Choi D, Dacey RG, Hsu CY, Powers WJ. *Cerebrovascular Disease: Momentum at the End of the Second Millennium.* Armonk, NY: Futura Publishing Company, Inc., © 2002.

4) stimulation of angiogenesis; and 5) establishment of a new glial-pial boundary if necessary.

Comparison of the inflammatory response in the brain with that seen in peripheral organs supports the idea that the brain inflammatory response uses the same effector molecules to generate the acute response. Studies have revealed that the *de novo* synthesis of cytokines, chemokines, and adhesion molecules occurs in the brain as in the periphery in response to injury.[9] However, very little work has been conducted to understand the late resolution phase of the inflammatory reaction. While attenuating the early inflammatory response appears to be important, it is the wound healing response that ultimately confines the injury, remodels the cellular and structural elements to restore homeostasis thus permitting an environment conducive to regeneration. Wound healing after injury to the central nervous system (CNS) is generally considered within the broad context of gliosis which for decades has been portrayed in an entirely negative context: gliosis is the barrier to regeneration. This focus solely upon astrocytes, gliosis, and scar formation as negative elements has skewed our perception of wound healing in the CNS. In fact recent studies present a much more complex picture of wound healing after brain injury as a cellular response that limits and contains the injury, and potentially can provide a positive environment for regeneration.[3,10-12]

In this chapter we will briefly present key aspects of the acute inflammatory response after focal brain ischemia. The cascade of new gene expression that unfolds following focal stroke will be outlined. Furthermore, the roles of two key cytokines, tumor necrosis factor alpha (TNFα and interleukin-1 beta (IL1β , and the cooperative actions of adhesion molecules in the acute inflammatory response will be discussed. The main focus will be upon the late matrix remodeling and wound healing process initiated in response to the ischemic insult. Although often considered as a single event, inflammation and wound healing can be considered as two responses to injury; the inflammation occurs early (hours, days) after the injury while the wound healing occurs later (days, weeks) after the insult. Recent data concerning the complex wound healing response of the brain will be presented with data from our lab illustrating the need to consider wound healing as a necessary aspect of restoring homeostasis after injury.

New Gene Expression After Focal Stroke

Focal ischemia is a powerful stimulus to elicit genomic responses in the brain. The pattern of gene expression induced by ischemia is exhibited as waves of sequential genes expressed over different time

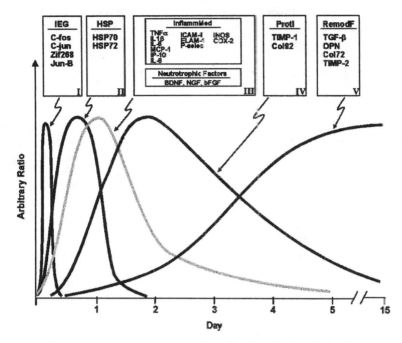

Figure 1. Time course of gene expression after focal ischemia in the rat cortex induced by middle cerebral artery occlusion. Five waves of gene expression include a broad range of upregulated transcription factors (phase 1); heat-shock proteins (phase 2); pro-inflammatory mediators including cytokines, chemokines, adhesion molecules, and growth factors (phase 3) and compensatory growth factors; protease and protease inhibitor gene expression (phase 4); and delayed remodeling of proteins involved in resolution of the tissue injury (phase 6).

points. Figure 1 illustrates that in response to ischemia many genes exhibit an increased expression. Transcription factors (immediate early genes; IEG) are the first "wave" as shown by members of the fos and jun families that are rapidly and transiently upregulated.[13-17] A second "wave" consists of the heat shock proteins (HSP). Heat shock protein mRNA is usually expressed within 1-2 hours and then down regulated by 1-2 days.[13,15] Of great interest is the third "wave" that initially was characterized by the initiation of the classic inflammatory gene expression cascade but has now been expanded to include expression of neurotrophic factors and cell death mediators. Genes induced in the inflammatory cascade include TNFα and IL1β [18-20] IL6,[17] IL8 and MCP-1.[21,22] This third wave is likely to play a significant role in the initiation of endothelial priming prior to neutrophil and monocyte infiltration. In addition to cytokine gene induction, adhesion molecule expression such as ICAM-1, ELAM-1 and P-selectin is also increased.[23-25] These adhesion molecules are crucial for leukocyte adhesion to the endothelium prior to infiltration. Several neurotrophic factor genes are induced after ischemia. In several models of ischemic insult to the brain-derived neurotrophic factor (BDNF), nerve growth factor (NGF), and basic fibroblast growth factor (bFGF) increase within the first 24 hours after injury.[16,26-29] More recently, we have identified a fourth "wave" of new gene expression that may well be associated with the acute inflammatory reaction to brain ischemia. This fourth "wave" includes proteolytic enzymes (metalloproteinases; Col92) implicated in damage to extracellular matrix,[30] and their endogenous protease inhibitors after focal stroke. The expression of these genes in stroke appears to be related to the influx of inflammatory cells and is associated with secondary brain injury and repair processes after stroke. The fifth "wave" of new gene expression includes mediators such as transforming growth factor-β and osteopontin that may be important in tissue remodeling.

Inflammation, TNFα, IL1β and Brain Ischemia

The response to injury in peripheral organs is manifested by the rapid production of a wide array of inflammatory mediators that initiate inflammatory processes. A key mediator of this response is TNFα, which may act as a pleiotropic peptide to elicit the production of other cytokines (eg, IL-1β, IL-6 and IL-8), endothelial cell adhesion molecules (eg, ELAM-1, ICAM-1, and VCAM-1), and surface adhesion ligands on neutrophils and monocytes (eg, VLA-4, LFA-1 and Mac-1 integrins).[31-34] The resultant activation of endothelial-cell adhesion molecules promotes neutrophil adherence to activated endothelium - a key event in the inflammatory reaction. The initiation of the inflammatory response in the brain is believed to be triggered by TNFα, the mRNA and protein both increasing after brain ischemia.[19,20,35] After middle cerebral artery occlusion (MCAO) TNFα mRNA is elevated in the infarcted zone as early as 1 hour postocclusion with peak expression at 12 hours and persistent expression for about 5 days. The early expression of TNFα mRNA prior to leukocyte infiltration suggests that TNFα may be involved in this response. TNFα has been localized to neurons and astrocytes.[19] The functional significance of TNFα expression in the brain was studied by microinjection of TNFα into the rat cortex; TNFα induced leukocyte adhesion to the capillary endothelium, but no evidence for neurotoxicity at the site of injection was found. Therefore, TNFα may exert a primary effect on microvascular inflammatory response as reflected by neutrophil adhesion to brain capillary endothelium. The injection of TNFα into the cerebroventricular space prior to injury exacerbated the ischemic injury.[36] Additional evidence for the effect of TNFα comes from in vitro studies demonstrating that addition of TNFα to endothelial cells cause a cytoskeletal rearrangement of endothelial cells such that a sheet of endothelial cells has long-lasting increases in permeability.[37] These data suggest that TNFα may prime the brain for subsequent damage by activating capillary endothelium to a "partial," pro-adhesive state possible through the upregulation of surface endothelial adhesion molecules, and by contributing to vascular leakiness essential for leukocyte diapedesis.[38]

The early accumulation of neutrophils after ischemic brain damage has been clearly demonstrated based upon histological,[3,39-44] biochemical (increased myeloperoxidase activity),[45-47] and ^{111}In-labeled leukocyte studies.[48] It is postulated that neutrophils induce tissue damage due to their vascular plugging and rheologic effects, and by their generation and release of oxygen radicals and cytotoxic products as they are activated in ischemic tissue.[44,49-52]

IL1β, like TNFα, is one of the initiating molecules in the inflammatory process. IL1β is a cytokine with multiple proinflammatory and cell-growth modulatory actions.[53] Like TNFα, IL1β modulates endothelial permeability.[31,37] After focal stroke, IL1β mRNA is rapidly upregulated within 3-6 hours, peaks at 12 hours, and returns to basal levels at 5 days, mimicking the profile of TNFα.[18,20] Evidence that IL1β may play a deleterious role after focal stroke is found in several studies utilizing overexpression of IL1β or its endogenous antagonist IL1 receptor antagonist (IL1ra). Intracerebroventricular (ICV) injections of IL1β enhances brain edema, increases the number of neutrophils in ischemic areas and increases neutrophil-endothelial cell adhesion.[54] Furthermore, ICV injections of IL1β exacerbate the degree of infarction after MCAO,[55] whereas injections of IL1ra and IL1β antagonists reduce infarct size.[55-58]

As stated previously a cascade of de novo gene expression manifests the inflammatory response. Prominent in this response is the induction of adhesion molecules required for leukocyte infiltration by cytokines. Temporally the in vivo expression of cytokines precedes the expression of adhesion molecules (see above). In vitro studies have directly demonstrated induction of adhesion molecule expression by both TNFα and IL1β. Endothelial cells exposed to TNFα and IL1β had increased expression of ICAM-1.[59] Astrocytes exposed to TNFα and IL1β increased expression of ICAM-1, VCAM-1, E-selectin.[60-62] Microglia exposed to TNFα and IL1β had increased expression of ICAM-1, VCAM-1, β1 and β2 integrins.[63] In vivo after MCAO ICAM-1 is upregulated in microvessels as early as 1 hour after injury.[24,64] At 24 hours when leukocytes are entering the brain in increasing numbers, these cell populations expressed ICAM-1 and continued to express this adhesion molecule for 7 days. In the non-human primate MCAO model P-selectin and ICAM-1 were shown to be upregulated and similarly localized to the endothelium.[23] While the expression of adhesion molecules associated with leukocyte trafficking into the brain after injury appears to be well documented, the expression of adhesion molecules and associated matrix molecules which mediate matrix remodeling and regeneration within the brain parenchyma is just beginning to be mapped out.

Wound Healing in the Brain

Following an ischemic insult to the CNS, a massive reorganization of cells and tissue takes place as the surrounding cells attempt to limit the injury, repair the damage and restore normal architecture of the brain. This tissue remodeling requires *de novo* synthesis of proteins (largely via gene transcription) which enable cells to actively change their relationship with the existing extracellular matrix (ECM) and with other cells to reorganize the damaged tissue. The induced genetic response to effect matrix remodeling falls into three general categories: matrix proteases, extracellular matrix molecules, and integrins. Together these three categories of molecules enable cells to initiate a classic wound healing response as dead cells are removed and the remaining tissue is remodeled to form scar tissue.

Both astrocytes and microglia must alter their association with the ECM as a precursor to changes in cell shape, proliferation and migration. This is accomplished by altering the presentation of integrin receptors coupled with synthesis and secretion of new ECM and matrix proteases to degrade and reformat existing cell-matrix associations. Integrin receptor couple intracellular cytoskeletal elements and associated signaling molecules such as those found at focal adhesion sites with ECM molecules. Once thought to simply anchor the cell to the matrix, recent studies have demonstrated a dynamic role for integrin receptors that transduce signals in both an outside-in and inside-out direction.[65] In addition to synthesizing a set of integrin receptors specifically for matrix remodeling, cells synthesize provisional extracellular matrix molecules which allow for the dynamic adherence and attachment required for changes in cell shape, proliferation and migration.

The CNS contains very few of the classic extracellular matrix molecules which are found in the peripheral tissues. Only two sites in the brain, the blood vessels and the glial limitans at the pial surface, have basal lamina containing classic basal lamina molecules,[66] such as collagen, thrombospondin, fibronectin, laminin and vitronectin.[67-69] Within the interstitial matrix of the adult brain the predominant ECM components are hyaluronan, hyaluronan-binding proteoglycans such as members of the aggrecan family, versican and brevican and glycoproteins such as member of the tenascin family.[70-72] During the development of the brain the molecular composition of the chondroitin-sulfate proteoglycans change dramatically to reflect the maturation of synaptic contacts[71] concomitant with a decreasing extracellular space that exists in the adult brain.[73,74] The extracellular space of the adult nervous system is not permissive for the type of proliferation and migration that occurs after an ischemic insult.[75] Thus after an insult to the adult nervous system the ECM must be modified through *de novo* synthesis of key matrix proteases, ECM components and integrin receptors to allow microglia, astrocytes, and exogenous leukocytes the space to migrate and repair the injured tissue.

Osteopontin, a Provisional Matrix Molecule

Many matrix molecules that are upregulated after brain injury are also expressed during the development of the nervous system.[10,76] Their expression after injury is presumed to recapitulate the remodeling processes that formed the cytoarchitecture initially. We have recently identified expression of matrix protein, osteopontin (OPN) that does not appear to be expressed as a matrix protein during nervous system development, but is upregulated after focal stroke.

Osteopontin, an integrin ligand, is an acidic, secreted 41 kDa phosphoprotein containing an arginine-glycine-aspartate (RGD) recognition site was originally identified as a bone matrix protein and was subsequently localized to kidney, placenta, and blood vessels.[77,78] OPN interacts with multiple integrin receptors to effect cell adhesion, migration, and phagocytosis depending upon the specific integrin receptor. The functions of OPN have been extensively studied in peripheral smooth muscle cells, endothelial cells and macrophages. Functionally, OPN has chemotactic activity for smooth muscle cells and endothelial cells[79,80] regulating cell adhesion and migration[81] by interacting with three different integrin receptors $\alpha_v\beta_1$, $\alpha_v\beta_3$, and $\alpha_v\beta_5$. Cell adhesion is mediated by integrin receptors $\alpha_v\beta_1$ and $\alpha_v\beta_5$,[82] while integrin receptor $\alpha_v\beta_3$ mediates cell migration.[81] Two inflammatory cytokines, IL1β and TNFα, upregulate expression of OPN in macrophages[83] and in osteoblasts[84] demonstrating that cytokine expression can initiate the wound healing process. OPN expression has been associated with a number of disease processes involving extensive matrix remodeling including neointima formation in carotid arteries subjected to balloon angioplasty;[85,86] human atherosclerotic plaques;[80,87] myocardial injury[88] and renal tubulointerstitial fibrosis.[89,90] Furthermore, mice lacking a functional OPN gene display significantly decreased levels of debridement and greater disorganization of matrix during healing of an incisional skin wound.[91] Since extensive matrix remodeling occurs after focal ischemia in the brain, we considered that OPN might be upregulated following this insult[12,92]

Our studies demonstrated that OPN mRNA was maximally expressed at 5 days postischemia (Figure 2). Initial expression was seen at 3 hours after stroke; and by *in situ* hybridization was localized to the ventral medial aspect of the peri-infarct border. With time OPN mRNA increased in the peri-infarct region such that by 24 hours the core infarct was delineated by the surrounding cells expressing this mRNA. At 24 hours OPN protein is initially seen in quiescent microglia at the infarct border (Figure 3) and during 2-5 days after injury is seen within activated macrophages and secreted into the extracellular space (Figure 3). OPN protein was expressed at very high levels by macrophages in the infarct core at 5 days after focal stroke, and by 15 days levels had decreased significantly with expression restricted to an area of tissue adjacent to the newly formed pial surface.

To establish a functional role for the secreted OPN we conducted a migration assay using OPN and found that OPN had the capacity to induce directed migration of astrocyte.[92] In other models[88,93] where OPN expression was seen in conjunction with matrix modeling, the integrin receptor $\alpha_v\beta_3$ appeared to be one of the receptors modulating cell-OPN interactions. Moreover upregulation of $\alpha_v\beta_3$ has been reported to be essential for endothelial transformation to an angiogenic phenotype[94] and for migration toward an OPN gradient.[78]

Expression of Integrin Receptors After Brain Ischemia

Integrins are a family of transmembrane glycoprotein receptors that couple intracellular cytoskeletal elements with extracellular matrix molecules. Integrins exist as $\alpha\beta$ heterodimers that associate at their extracellular domains. Both the α and β subunit contribute to the ligand binding domain. Integrin receptors can recognize more than one ligand and likewise individual ligands can recognize and bind more than one integrin. One of the classic recognition sites in ECMs such as fibronectin, vitronectin, osteopontin is the Arg-Gly-Asp (RGD) sequence.[65]

Research into integrin receptor and associated ligand expression after focal stroke is in its infancy. Most of the work to date has focused upon the role of integrin receptors in modulating early events associated with vascular changes after an ischemic insult. Two integrins receptors, $\alpha_v\beta_3$ and $\alpha_6\beta_4$ have been suggested to play a role in vascular integrity and remodeling following focal ischemia within the infarcted area.[95,96] In a nonhuman primate model of transient forebrain ischemia

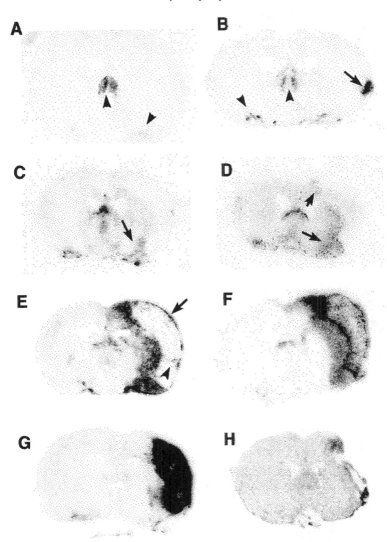

Figure 2. OPN gene expression after focal stroke. By in situ hybridization OPN mRNA expression is constitutively expressed in the septal nucleus and in ventral brain nuclei (**A**, arrowheads). In sham animals OPN mRNA was induced at the surgery site (**B**, arrow). At 3 hours (**C**) and 6 hours (**D**) OPN mRNA was induced in cells initially at the ventromedial aspect (**C**, arrow) and continuing to the dorsomedial aspect (**D**, arrows) of the infarct. At 24 hours cells expressing OPN mRNA are still largely confined to the peri-infarct region (**E**) with expression at the pial surface (arrow) and by a few cells in the infarct (arrowhead). At 48 hours (**F**) more cells within the infarct expressed OPN mRNA; by 5 days (**G**) the majority of cells expressing OPN mRNA are within the infarct with little expression in the peri-infarct region. At 15 days (**H**) mRNA levels returned to those found in naive rats.

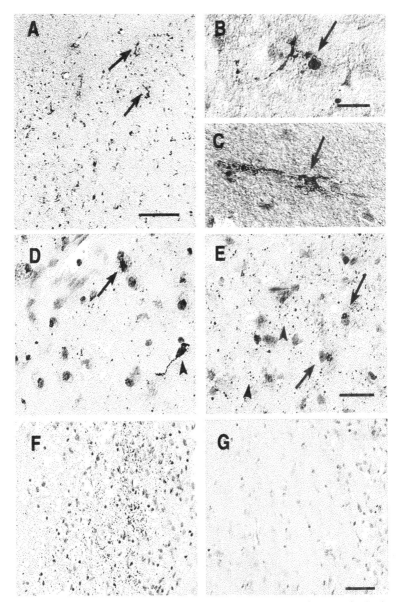

Figure 3. OPN protein expression in microglia and macrophages. At 24 hours OPN was expressed by microglia in the peri-infarct region (**A**, arrows); the microglia have a ramified appearance (**B**, **C**, arrows) and do not appear activated. At 48 hours, occasional microglia (**D**, arrowhead) expressing OPN are seen with the majority of OPN expressed by macrophages (**D**, arrow). By 5 days OPN was seen in a perinuclear location intracellularly (**E**, arrows) and in the extracellular matrix (**E**, arrowheads). At 15 days OPN expression was restricted to a thin area adjacent to the pial surface (**F**). No immunoperoxidase reaction was detected in the absence of primary antibody at any timepoint (**G**). Scale bar for **A** is 100 μm; **B,C** is 20 μm; **D,E** is 40 μm; **F,G** is 100 μm.

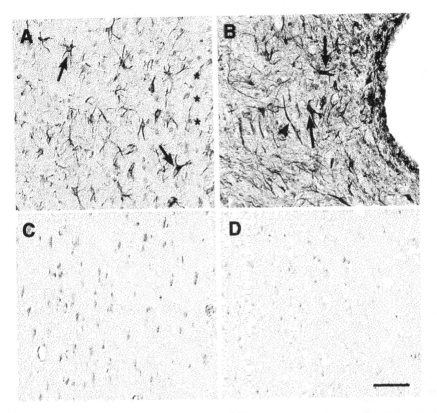

Figure 4. Integrin $\alpha_v\beta_3$ expression at 5 and 15 days post occlusion. The integrin $\alpha_v\beta_3$ was upregulated at 5 days in the ipsilateral cortex (**A**) as compared to the contralateral cortex (**C**). Integrin $\alpha_v\beta_3$ was expressed by cells (**A**, arrows) adjacent to the infarct (peri-infarct/infarct border identified by asterisks). By 15 days cells expressing integrin $\alpha_v\beta_3$ (**B**, arrows) had elongated cells processes (**B**, arrowhead) and were found adjacent to and at the glial-pial boundary (identified by asterisks). Scale bar for **A,B** is 100 μm; for C,D is 40 μm.

the integrin receptor $\alpha_v\beta_3$ was upregulated early (hours) in the ischemic event concomitant with an increase in one of its ligands, fibrinogen. Conversely in another study, the expression of integrin receptor $\alpha_6\beta_4$ and one of its ligands, laminin were both shown to decrease following ischemia.

Given the potential role of integrin receptors in matrix remodeling of the interstitial brain matrix at sites distal to the vasculature we undertook a study to determine the expression of integrin receptor $\alpha_v\beta_3$ after focal stroke.[12] The OPN receptor, integrin $\alpha_v\beta_3$ is expressed by astrocytes at 5 days and 15 days postischemia (Figure 4). These timepoints were chosen to identify potential cell populations that could interact with the OPN in the extracellular matrix. At 5 days postischemia astrocytes expressing integrin receptor $\alpha_v\beta_3$ are dispersed in the peri-infarct region; by 15 days these cells have reformed the glial limitans at the pial surface lost initially due to tissue injury following focal stroke. These data were intriguing as astrocytes in vitro express $\alpha_v\beta_3$[97] and radial glial of the developing nervous system have been reported to express integrin α_v.[98] Hirsch and colleagues[98] suggest that this integrin might be involved in the formation and orientation of the glial fibers that extend from the ventricular zone to the cortical plate. Similarly, the astrocytes expressing $\alpha_v\beta_3$ following focal ischemia reorganize from a stellate morphology to the more bipolar morphology characteristic of astrocytes of the glial limitans. These results presented demonstrate the diverse role integrin receptors might have in tissue remodeling. In addition to a role in vascular remodeling seen early following focal stroke[95,96] these findings suggest that integrin receptor $\alpha_v\beta_3$ participates in nonvascular remodeling associated with formation of a glial scar which occurs late in the resolution of the ischemic insult.

Interaction of Osteopontin with Integrin Receptor $\alpha_v\beta_3$

To explore potential functional aspects of the interaction between OPN and integrin receptor $\alpha_v\beta_3$ we established the timing of receptor-ligand interaction (Figure 5). The spatial-temporal interaction of extracellular OPN ligand and integrin receptor $\alpha_v\beta_3$ is at a distance at 5 days, however, by 15 days the astrocytes are localized within a matrix of OPN, suggesting that OPN may act as a chemotactic factor for astrocytes. This *in vivo* demonstration of an OPN gradient at a distance from astrocytes early in the formation of the glial scar followed by localization of astrocytes within an OPN-rich extracellular region suggests the findings of OPN as a chemotactic factor, an "astrokine," *in vitro* may also be true *in vivo*.

How might the interaction of OPN act to stimulate astrocyte process elongation and migration via the integrin receptor $\alpha_v\beta_3$? Ligation of integrin receptor $\alpha_v\beta_3$ by OPN ligand results in the rapid production of phosphoinositides.[99] Astrocytic hypertrophy and migration are dependent upon GFAP, the predominant intermediate filament expressed by these cells. The assembly/disassembly of GFAP is Ca^{2+} dependent[100] and IP3-induced Ca^{2+} release in astrocytes is directed by the type 3-inositol 1,4,5-trisphosphate receptor.[101] Thus OPN ligand binding to integrin receptor $\alpha_v\beta_3$ could stimulate release of intracellular Ca^{2+} stores causing a subsequent reorganization of the GFAP filament network.

Ligation of integrin receptors also mediates changes in gene expression. For instance, signaling through the fibronection and tenascin

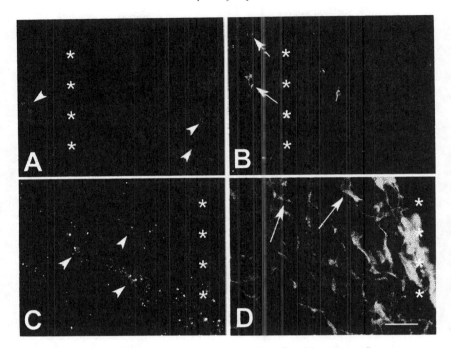

Figure 5. Timing of OPN-integrin $\alpha_v\beta_3$ interaction. Double immunofluorescence at 5 (**A,B**) and 15 (**C,D**) days demonstrated that at 5 days GFAP+ astrocytes (**B**, arrows) were at a distance from extracellular OPN (**A**, arrowheads) which was localized to the core infarct (to the right of the asterisks). By 15 days GFAP+ astrocytes (**C**, arrowheads) were found within a matrix of OPN (**D**, arrows). The medial peri-infarct/infarct border with a large infarct region to the right (**A,B**), and the glial-pial boundary (**C D**) are indicated by asterisks. Scale bar is 20 μm.

integrin receptors upregulated synthesis of matrix proteases in fibroblast.[102] In endothelial cells integrin ligation promoted cell survival by suppressing p53 activity, and by increasing the bcl-2/bax ratio.[103] Although no data exists regarding integrin-mediated gene induction in astrocytes, the activation of astrocytes, their transformation to migratory cells and subsequent acquisition of a pial astrocyte phenotype strongly suggests that a change in gene expression does occur.

Multifunctional Roles of Osteopontin After Ischemic Injury

The OPN gene is induced within 3 hours of an ischemic insult to the brain. This early gene expression suggests OPN might function as a stress response gene following focal ischemia. An acute phase response element has been identified within the promoter region of the OPN gene.[104] In vitro cells adhered to OPN have enhanced expression of heat shock proteins, and display a greater resistance to heat shock injury.[105] Furthermore, OPN confers cellular resistance to the damaging effects of nitric oxide and oxidative burst associated with inflammation by inhibiting induction of nitric oxide synthase[106] suggesting that in addition to mediating cell attachment and migration OPN has protective roles.[107] An inflammatory response after focal stroke has been clearly demonstrated,[9] thus it is not inconsistent that the cells responsible for clearing tissue debris and remodeling the matrix require protection from the toxic environment of the ischemic region.

Summary

The glial cell (astrocyte and microglia) response to brain injury is complex. One of the best understood responses is a classic wound healing response[3] with formation of a barrier between the injured and healthy tissue.[10,108,109] Historically the glial scar has been considered the singular barrier that must be prevented for restoration of normal brain function. However, many recent studies have suggested that the formation of a glial scar contribute to the walling off of the injury zone from the uninjured tissue thus protecting healthy cells from death as a result of the injury spreading.[10,12,108] Indeed in our model of focal stroke the glial scar formed in the early stages of an injury develops into a new glial limitans re-establishing the interface of the glial-pial boundary. Without this type of matrix remodeling the injury might increase in size, and the surface of the brain remain exposed.

These early events (hours, days) can probably be distinguished from later regenerative events (weeks, months) related to reestablishment of axonal connections and restoration of the normal cytoarchitecture of the brain. It is at this later time once the acute injury has been confined that these provisional matrix proteins, matrix enzymes and integrin receptors might possibly prevent the regeneration. Taken together, our data demonstrates profound changes in brain matrix remodeling following focal ischemic stroke, including the synthesis and release of matrix proteins alien to the normal brain, the expression of integrin receptors that ligate these proteins, and possibly a novel function for microglial-derived OPN in astrocyte migration following focal ischemia that may drive glial activation, organization and repair functions.

References

1. Perry VH, Gordon S. Macrophages and the nervous system. *Int Rev Cytol* 1991;125:203-244.

2. Petito CK, Morgello S, Felix JC, et al. The two patterns of reactive astrocytosis in postischemic rat brain. *J Cereb Blood Flow Metab* 1990;10:850-859.

3. Clark RK, Lee EV, Fish CJ, et al. Development of tissue damage, inflammation and resolution following stroke: An immunohistochemical and quantitative planimetric study. *Brain Res Bull* 1993;31:565-572.

4. Garcia JH, Yoshida Y, Chen H, et al. Progression from ischemic injury to infarct following middle cerebral artery occlusion in the rat. *Am J Pathol* 1993;142:623-635.

5. Li Y, Chopp M, Zhang ZG, et al. Expression of glial fibrillary acidic protein in areas of focal cerebral ischemia accompanies neuronal expression of 72-kDa heat shock protein. *J Neurol Sci* 1995;128:134-142.

6. Gehrmann J, Bonnekoh P, Miyazawa T, et al. Immunocytochemical study of an early microglial activation in ischemia. *J Cereb Blood Flow Metab* 1992;12(2):257-269.

7. Kato H, Kogure K, Araki T, et al. Graded expression of immunomolecules on activated microglia in the hippocampus following ischemia in a rat model of ischemic tolerance. *Brain Res* 1995;694:85-93.

8. Leibovich SJ, Ross R. The role of the macrophage in wound repair. *Am J Pathol* 1975;78:71-100.

9. Feuerstein GZ, Wang XK, Barone FC. Inflammation-related gene expression and stroke: Implications for new therapeutic targets. In Krieglestein J (ed): *Pharmacology of cerebral ischemia*. Stuttgart: MedPharm Scientific Publish. 1996;405-419.

10. Fitch MT, Silver J. Activated macrophages and the blood-brain barrier: Inflammation after CNS injury leads to increases in putative inhibitory molecules. *Exp Neurol* 1997;148:587-603.

11. Lehrmann E, Christensen T, Zimmer J, et al. Microglial and macrophage reactions mark progressive changes and define the penumbra in the rat neocortex and striatum after transient middle cerebral artery occlusion. *J Comp Neurol* 1997;386:461-476.

12. Ellison JA, Velier JJ, Spera P, et al. Osteopontin and its integrin receptor $\alpha v\beta 3$ are upregulated during formation of the glial scar after focal stroke. *Stroke* 1998;29:1698-1706.

13. Nowak TS Jr, Ikeda J, Nakajima T. 70 kDa heat shock protein and c-fox gene expression after transient ischemia. *Stroke* 1990;21(suppl III);107-111.

14. Uemura Y, Kowall NW, Moskowitz MA. Focal ischemia in rats causes time-dependent expression of c-fox protein immunoreactivity in widespread regions of ipsilateral cortex. *Brain Res* 1991;552:99-105.

15. Welsh FA, Moyer DJ, Harris VA. Regional expression of heat shock protein 70 mRNA and c-fos mRNA following focal ischemia in rat brain. *J Cereb Blood Flow Metab* 1992;12:204-212.

16. Hsu CY, An G, Liu JS, et al. Expression of immediate early gene and growth factor mRNAs in a focal cerebral ischemia model in the rat. *Stroke* 1993;24:I-78-81.

17. Wang XK, Yue T-L, Young PR, et al. Expression of interleukin-6, c-fox and zif268 mRNA in rat ischemic cortex. *J Cereb Blood Flow Metab* 1995;15:166-171.

18. Liu T, McDonnell PC, Young PR, et al. Interleukin-1β mRNA expression in ischemic rat cortex. *Stroke* 1993;24:125-128.

19. Liu T, Clark RF, McDonnell PC, et al. Tumor necrosis factor α expression in ischemia neurons. *Stroke* 1994;25:1481-1488.

20. Wang XK, Yue T-L, Barone FC, et al. Concommitant cortical expression of TNFα and IL-1β mRNA following transient focal ischemia. *Mol Chem Neuropathol* 1994;23:103-114.

21. Liu T, Young PR, McDonnell PC, et al. Cytokine-induced neutrophil chemoattractant mRNA expressed in cerebral ischemia. *Neurosci Lett* 1993;164:125-128.

22. Wang XK, Yue T-L, Barone FC, et al. Monocyte chemoattractant protein-1 (MCP-1) mRNA expression in rat ischemic cortex. *Stroke* 1995;26:661-666.

23. Okada Y, Copeland BR, Mori E, et al. P-selectin and intercellular adhesion molecule-1 expression after focal brain ischemia and reperfusion. *Stroke* 1994;25:202-211.

24. Wang X, Siren A-L, Liu Y, et al. Upregulation of intercellular adhesion molecule 1 (ICAM-1) on brain microvascular endothelial cells in rat ischemia cortex. *Mol Brain Res* 1994;26:61-68.

25. Wang XK, Yue T-L, Barone FC, et al. Demonstration of increased endothelial-leukocyte adhesion molecule 1 mRNA expression in rat ischemic cortex. *Stroke* 1995;26:1665-1669.

26. Lindvall O, Ernfors P, Bengzon J, et al. Differential regulation of mRNAs for nerve growth factor, brain-derived neurotrophic factor, and neurotrophin 3 in the adult rat brain following cerebral ischemia and hypoglycemic coma. *PNAS* 1992;89:648-652.

27. Takeda A, Onodera H, Sugimoto A, et al. Coordinated expression of messenger RNAs for nerve growth factor, brain-derived neurotrophic factor and neurotrophin-3 in the rat hippocampus following transient forebrain ischemia. *Neuroscience* 1993;55:23-31.

28. Lin TN, Te J, Lee M, Sun GY, et al. Induction of basic fibroblast growth factor (bFGF) expression following focal cerebral ischemia. *Brain Res Mol Brain Res* 1997;49:255-265.

29. Ferrer I, Lopez E, Pozas E, et al. Multiple neurotrophic signals converge in surviving CA1 neurons of the gerbil hippocampus following transient forebrain ischemia. *J Comp Neurol* 1998;394:416-430.

30. Rosenberg GA, Navratil M, Barone FC, et al. Proteolytic cascade enzymes increase in focal cerebral ischemia in rat. *J Cereb Blood Flow Metab* 1996;16:360-366.

31. Pober JS, Cotran RS. Cytokines and endothelial cell biology. *Physiol Rev* 1990;70:427-451.

32. Zimmerman GA, Prescott SM, McIntyre TM. Endothelial cell interaction with granulocytes: Tethering and signaling molecules. *Immunol Today* 1992;13:93-100.

33. Tracey KJ, Cerami A. Tumor necrosis factor, other cytokines and disease. *Ann Rev Cell Biol* 1993;9:317-343.

34. Hopkins SJ, Rothwell NJ. Cytokines and the nervous system. I: Expression and recognition. *Trends Neurosci* 1995;18:83-88.

35. Saito K, Suyama K, Nishida K, et al. Early increases in TNF-α and IL-1β levels following transient cerebral ischemia in gerbil brain. *Neurosci Lett* 1996;206:149-152.

36. Barone FC, Arvin B, White RF, et al. Tumor necrosis factor α: a mediator of focal ischemic brain injury. *Stroke* 1997;28(6):1233-1244.
37. Stolpen AH, Guinan EC, Fiers W, et al. Recombinant tumor necrosis factor and immune interferon act single and in combination to reorganize human vascular endothelial cell monolayers. *Am J Pathol* 1986;123:16-24.
38. Yi ES, Ulich TR. Endotoxin, interleukin-1 and tumor necrosis factor cause neutrophil dependent microvascular leakage in postcapillary venules. *Am J Pathol* 1992;140:659-663.
39. Garcia JH, Kamijyo. Cerebral infarction: Evolution of histopathological changes after occlusion of a middle cerebral artery in primates. *J Neuropathol Exp Neurol* 1997;33:409-421.
40. Pozzilli C, Lenzi GL, Argentino C, et al. Imaging of leukocytic infiltration in human cerebral infarcts. *Stroke* 1985;16:251-255.
41. Hallenbeck JM, Dutka AJ, Tanishima T, et al. Polymorphonuclear leukocyte accumulation in brain regions with low blood flow during the early post-ischemic period. *Stroke* 1986;17:246-253.
42. Chen H, Chopp M, Bodzin G. Neutropenia reduces the volume of cerebral infarct after transient middle cerebral artery occlusion in the rat. *Neurosci Res Commun* 1992;11:93-99.
43. Dereski MO, Chopp M, Knight RA, et al. Focal cerebral ischemia in the rat: Temporal profile of neutrophil responses. *Neurosci Res Comm* 1992;11:179-186.
44. Zhang RL, Chopp M, Chen H, et al. Temporal profile of ischemic tissue damage, neutrophil response, and vascular plugging following permanent and transient (2H) middle cerebral artery occlusion in the rat. *J Neurol Sci* 1994;125:3-10.
45. Barone FC, Hillegass LM, Price WJ, et al. Polymorphonuclear leukocyte infiltration into cerebral focal ischemic tissue: Myeloperoxidase activity assay and histologic verification. *J Neurosci Res* 1991;29:336-345.
46. Barone FC, Schmidt DB, Price WJ, et al. Reperfusion increases neutrophils and LTB4 receptor binding in rat focal ischemia. *Stroke* 1992;23:1337-1348.
47. Barone FC, Hillegass LM, Tzimas MN, et al. Time-related changes in mye-loperoxidase activity and leukotriene B4 receptor binding reflect leukocyte influx in cerebral focal stroke. *Molec Chem Neuropath* 1995;24:13-30.
48. Dutka AJ, Kochanek PM, Hallenbeck JM. Influences of granulocytopenia on canine cerebral ischemia induced by an embolism. *Stroke* 1989;20:390-395.
49. Hallenbeck JM, Dutka AJ. Background review and current concepts of reperfusion injury. *Arch Neurol* 1990;47:1245-1254.
50. del Zoppo GJ, Schmid-Schonbein GW, Mori E, et al. Polymorphonuclear leukocytes occlude capillaries following middle cerebral artery occlusion and reperfusion in baboons. *Stroke* 1991;22:1276-1283.
51. Grau AJ, Berger E, Sung K-L, et al. Granulocyte adhesion, deformability, and superoxide formation in acute stroke. *Stroke* 1992;23:33-39.
52. Kochanek PM, Hallenbeck JM. Polymorphonuclear leukocytes and monocytes/ macrophages in the pathogenesis of cerebral ischemia and stroke. *Stroke* 1992;23:1367-1379.
53. Dinarello CA. Biology of interleukin-1. *FASEB J* 1988;2:108-115.
54. Yamasaki Y, Matsuura N, Shozuhara H, et al. Interleukin-1 as a pathogenetic mediator of ischemic brain damage in rats. *Stroke* 1995;26:676-681.

55. Loddick SA, Rothwell NJ. Neuroprotective effects of human recombinant interleukin-1 receptor antagonist in focal cerebral ischemia in the rat. *J Cereb Blood Flow Metab* 1996;16:932-940.

56. Relton JK, Rothwell NJ. Interleukin-1 receptor antagonists inhibits ischemic and excitotoxic neuronal damage in the rat. *Brain Res Bull* 1992;29:243-246.

57. Relton JK, Martin D, Thompson RC, et al. Peripheral administration of interleukin-1 receptor antagonist inhibits brain damage after focal cerebral ischemia in the rat. *Exp Neurol* 1996;138:206-213.

58. Garcia JH, Liu K-F, Relton JK. Interleukin-1 receptor antagonist decreases the number of necrotic neurons in rats with middle cerebral artery occlusion. *Am J Pathol* 1995;147:1477-1486.

59. Fabry Z Waldschmidt MM, Hendrickson D, et al. Adhesion molecules on murine brain microvascular endothelial cells: Expression and regulation of ICAM-1 and LGp 55. *J Neuroimmunol* 1992;36:1-11.

60. Satoh J, Kastrukoff LF, Kim SU. Cytokine-induced expression of intercellular adhesion molecule-1 (ICAM-1) in cultured human oligodendrocytes and astrocytes. *J Neuropathol Exp Neurol* 1991;50:215-216.

61. Aloisi F, Borsellino G, Samoggia P, et al. Astrocytes cultures from human embryonic brain: Characterization and modulation of surface molecules by inflammatory cytokines. *J Neurosci Res* 1992;32:494-506.

62. Hurwitz AA, Lyman WD, Guida MP, et al. Tumor necrosis factor alpha induces adhesion molecule expression on human fetal astrocytes. *J Exp Med* 1992;176:1631-1636.

63. Sebire G, Hery C, Peudenier S, et al. Adhesion proteins on human microgial cells and modulation of their expression by IL-1a and TNFα. *Res Virol* 1993;144:47-52.

64. Clark WM, Lauten JD, Lessov N, et al. Time course of ICAM-1 expression and leukocyte subset infiltration in rat forebrain ischemia. *Mol Chem Neuropath* 1994;26:213-230.

65. Hynes, RO. Integrins: Versatility, modulation, and signaling in cell adhesion. *Cell* 1992;69:11-25.

66. Feringa ER, Kowalski TF, Vahlsing HL. Basal lamina formation at the site of spinal cord transection. *Ann Neurol* 1980;8:148-154.

67. Esiri MM, Morris CS. Immunocytochemical study of macrophages and microglial cells and extracellular matrix components in human CNS disease. 2.Non-neoplastic diseases. *J Neurol Sci* 1991;101:59-72.

68. Nag S. Immunohistochemical localization of extracellular matrix proteins in cerebral vessels in chronic hypertension. *J Neuropath Exp Neurol* 1996;55:381-388.

69. Seiffert D, Bordin GM, Loskutoff DJ. Evidence that extrahepatic cells express vitronectin mRNA at rates approaching those of hepatocytes. *Histochem Cell Biol* 1996;105:195-201.

70. Venstrom KA, Reichardt LF. Extracellular matrix 2: Role of extracellular matrix molecules and their receptors in the nervous system. *FASEB J* 1993;7:996-1003.

71. Koppe G, Bruckner G, Brauer K, et al. Developmental patterns of proteogly-can-containing extracelullar matrix in perineuronal nets and neuropil of the postnatal rat brain. *Cell Tiss Res* 1997;288:33-41.

72. Rauch U. Modeling an extracellular environment for axonal pathfinding and fasciculation in the central nervous system. *Cell Tiss Res* 1997;290:349-356.

73. van Harreveld A. The extracellular space in the vertebrate central nervous system. In Bourne GH (ed): *Structure and function of nervous tissue, vol IV.* New York: Academic Press. 1972;447-511.

74. Lehmenkuhler A, Sykova E, Svoboda J, et al. Extracellular space parameters in the rat neocortex and subcortical white matter during postnatal development determined by diffusion analysis. *Neuroscience* 1993;55:339-351.

75. Nicholson C, Sykova E. Extracellular space structure revealed by diffusion analysis. *Trends Neurosci* 1998;21:207-215.

76. Laywell ED, Dorries U, Bartsch U, et al. Enhanced expression of the developmentally regulated extracellular matrix molecule tenascin following adult brain injury. *Proc Natl Acad Sci USA* 1992;89:2634-2638.

77. Butler WT. The nature and significance of osteopontin. *Connect Tissue Res* 1989;23:123-126.

78. Giachelli CM, Liaw L, Murry CE, et al. Osteopontin expression in cardiovascular diseases. *Ann NY Acad Sci* 1995;760:109-126.

79. Liaw L, Almeida M, Hart CH, et al. Osteopontin promotes vascular cell adhesion and spreading and is chemotactic for smooth muscle cells in vitro. *Circ Res* 1994;74:214-224.

80. Yue T-L, McKenna PJ, Ohlstein EH, et al. Osteopontin-stimulated vascular smooth muscle cell migration is mediated by b3 integrin. *Exp Cell Res* 1994;214:459-464.

81. Weintraub AS, Giachelli CM, Krauss RS, et al. Autocrine secretion of osteopontin by vascular smooth muscle cells regulates their adhesion to collagen gels. *Am J Path* 1996;149:259-272.

82. Liaw L, Skinner MP, Raines EW, et al. The adhesive and migratory effects of osteopontin are mediated via distinct cell surface integrins: Role of smooth muscle cell migration to osteopontin in vitro. *J Clin Invest* 1995;95:713-724.

83. Miyazaki T, Tashiro T, Higuchi Y, et al. Expression of osteopontin in a macrophage cell line and in transgenic mice with pulmonary fibrosis resulting from the lung expression of a tumor necrosis factor-alpha transgene. *Ann NY Acad Sci* 1995;760:334-341.

84. Jin CH, Miyaura C, Ishimi Y, et al. Interleukin 1 regulates the expression of osteopontin mRNA by osteoblasts. *Mol Cell Endocrinol* 1990;74:221-228.

85. Giachelli CM, Bae N, Almeida M, et al. Osteopontin is elevated during neointima formation in rat arteries and is a novel component of human atherosclerotic plaques. *J Clin Invest* 1993;92:1686-1696.

86. Wang XK, Louden C, Ohlstein EH, et al. Osteopontin expression in platelet-derived growth factor stimulated vascular smooth muscle cells and carotid artery after balloon angioplasty. *Arter Thromb Vasc Biol* 1996;16:1365-1372.

87. O'Brien ER, Garvin MR, Stewart DK, et al. Osteopontin is synthesized by macrophage, smooth muscle, and endothelial cells in primary and restenotic human coronary atherosclerotic plaques. *Arterioscler Throm* 1994;14:1648-1656.

88. Murry CE, Giachelli CM, Schwartz SM, et al. Macrophages express osteopontin during repair of myocardial necrosis. *Am J Pathol* 1994;145:1450-1462.

89. Giachelli CM, Pichler R, Lombardi D, et al. Osteopontin expression in angiotensin II-induced tubulointerstitial nephritis. *Kidney Int* 1994;45:515-524.

90. Pichler R, Giachelli CM, Lombardi D, et al. Tubulointerstitial disease in glomerulonephritis: Potential role of osteopontin (uropontin). *Am J Pathol* 1994;144:915-926.

91. Liaw L, Birk DE, Ballas CB, et al. Altered wound healing in mice lacking a functional osteopontin gene (supp1). *J Clin Invest* 1998;101:1468-1478.

92. Wang XK, Louden C, Yue T-L, et al. Regulation of osteopontin expression in brain ischemia: Implication for matrix remodeling and astrocyte function. *J Neurosci* 1998;18:2075-2083.

93. Panda D, Kundu GC, Lee BI, et al. Potential roles of osteopontin and alphavbeta3 integrin in the development of coronary artery restenosis after angioplasty. *PNAS* 1997;94:9308-9813.

94. Brooks PC, Clark RAF, Cheresh DA. Requirement for vascular integrin alpha v beta 3 for angiogenesis. *Science* 1994;264:569-571.

95. Okada Y, Copeland BR, Hamann GF, et al. Integrin alphavbeta3 is expressed in selected microvessels after focal cerebral ischemia. *Am J Pathol* 1996;149:37-44.

96. Wagner S, Tagaya M, Koziol JA, et al. Rapid disruption of an astrocyte interaction with the extracellular matrix mediated by integrin alpha 6 beta 4 during focal cerebral ischemia/reperfusion. *Stroke* 1997;28:858-865.

97. Tawil NJ, Wilson P, Carbonetto S. Expression and distribution of functional integrins in rat CNS glia. *J Neurosci Res* 1994;39:436-447.

98. Hirsch Em Gullberg D, Balzac F, et al. α_v integrin subunit is predominantly located in nervous tissue and skeletal muscle during mouse development. *Dev Dyn* 1994;201:108-120.

99. Hruska KA, Rolnick F, Huskey M, et al. Engagement of the osteoclast integrin alpha v beta 3 by osteopontin stimulates phosphatidylinositol 3-hydroxyl kinase activity. *Endocrinol* 1995;136:2984-2992.

100. Bianchi R, Garbuglia M, Verzini M, et al. S-100 protein and annexin II2-p11(2) (calpactin I) act in concert to regulate the state of assembly of GFAP intermediate filaments. *Biochem Biophys Res Commun* 1995;208:910-918.

101. Yamamoto-Hino M, Miyawaki A, Kawano H, et al. Immunohistochemical study of inositol 1,4,5-trisphosphate receptor type 3 in rat central nervous system. *Neuroreport* 1995;6:273-276.

102. Tremble P, Chiquet-Ehrismann R, Werb Z. The extracellular matrix ligands fibronectin and tenascin collaborate in regulating collagenase gene expression in fibroblasts. *Mol Biol Cell* 1994;5:439-453.

103. Stromblad S, Becker JC, Yebra M, et al. Suppression of p53 activity and p21WAF1/IP1 expression by vascular cell integrin alphaVbeta3 during angiogenesis. *J Clin Inves* 1996;98:426-433.

104. Kimbro KS, Saavedra RA. The puerap motif in the promoter of the mouse osteopontin gene. *Ann NY Acad Sci* 1995;760:319-320.

105. Sauk JJ, Van Kampen CL, Norris K, et al. Expression of constitutive and inducible HSP70 and HSP47 is enhanced in cells persistently spread on opn or collagen. *Biochem Biophys Res Commun* 1990;2:135-142.

106. Hwang S-M, Lopez CA, Heck DE, et al. Osteopontin inhibits induction of nitric oxide synthase gene expression by inflammatory mediators in mouse kidney epithelial cells. *J Biol Chem* 1994;269:711-715.

107. Denhardt DT, Chambers AF. Overcoming obstacles to metastasis - defenses against host defenses: Osteopontin (opn) as a shield against attack by cytotoxic host cells. *J Cell Biochem* 1994;56:48-51

108. Ide CF, Scripter JL, Coltman BW, et al. Cellular and molecular correlates to plasticity during recovery from injury in the developing mammalian brain. *Prog Brain Res* 1996;108:365-377.

109. Reier PJ. Gliosis following CNS injury: the anatomy of astrocytic scars and their influences on axonal elongation. In Fedoroff S, Vernadakis A (eds): *Cell Biology and Pathology of Astrocytes*. New York: Academic Press. 1986;263-324.

Chapter 17

Reperfusion Damage in the Brain

Ping-An Li, MD, PhD, Tibor Kristián, PhD, Yi-Bing Ouyang, PhD, and Bo K. Siesjö MD, PhD

The term reperfusion damage is ambiguous. Thus, one intuitively feels that sustained ischemia, such as occurs after permanent occlusion of a middle cerebral artery (MCA), yields maximal tissue injury. What then, is reperfusion damage? A simple answer to that question would be: more extensive ischemic damage in reperfused animals. However, although reperfusion may occasionally aggravate damage by triggering fulminant tissue swelling, this is not usually the case since reperfusion after 2-3 hours of MCA occlusion seldom gives an infarction volume which is larger than that observed in sustained focal ischemia. For that reason, we have to define reperfusion damage as an aggravation of tissue injury which is triggered by mechanisms set in motion by reperfusion, ie, by the resupply of oxygen and glucose. In other words, the severity of tissue injury is enhanced by these mechanisms, and not by the reperfusion *per se*. It follows from this definition that, could these adverse reactions be blocked by therapeutic interventions, the severity of damage will be reduced.

This concept is illustrated in Figure 1, which schematically depicts infarct volumes in sustained focal ischemia, and following MCA occlusion periods of 0.5, 1, and 2 hours, as assessed by TTC staining after

The studies quoted in this chapter were supported by the Swedish Medical Research Council (14X-263), the Juvenile Diabetes Foundation International, the US Public Health Service via the NIH (5 R01NS07838), Centaur Pharmaceutical Company, US Navy, and the Queen Emma Foundation.

From: Choi D, Dacey RG, Hsu CY, Powers WJ. *Cerebrovascular Disease: Momentum at the End of the Second Millennium.* Armonk, NY: Futura Publishing Company, Inc., © 2002.

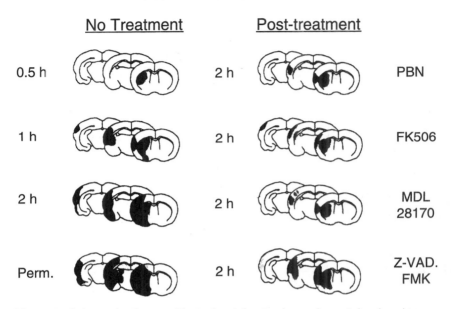

Figure 1. Schematic diagram illustrating infarct volumes in sustained and transient MCA occlusion of 0.5, 1, and 2 hours duration. The left panel shows that the infarct volume increases as the duration of ischemia is increased from 0.5 to 2 hours. The right panel illustrates how several pharmaceutical interventions during reperfusion, following 2 hours of MCA occlusion, can reduce the damage.

2 days of reperfusion. The scheme illustrates the increase in infarct volume when the duration of ischemia is increased from 30 minutes to 2 hours, also that the infarct volume at 2 hours is similar to that observed in permanent ischemia. As the right panel illustrates, though, several pharmacological agents, when given 1 hour or later after the start of reperfusion, following 2 hours of transient ischemia, markedly reduce infarct volume. These agents include the free radical spin trap α-phenyl-N-tert-butyl nitrone (PBN),[1] the immunosuppressant FK506,[2] the calpain inhibitor MDL28170 [3,4] and the caspase inhibitor Z-VAD.[5] Similar results have been obtained with an inhibitor of the nuclear enzyme poly (ADP-ribose) polymerase.[6,7] They all illustrate the fact that inhibition of reaction sequences set in motion by recirculation can decrease the extent of the tissue damage incurred. Clearly, most of the tissue injury observed after 2 hours of MCA occlusion can be classified as reperfusion injury.

Given these facts, we will probe into the mechanisms leading to reperfusion damage. We will first describe events occurring during ischemia, ie, those which "prime" the tissue for the cascade of reactions occurring during reperfusion. This is followed by a discussion of reperfusion events which have traditionally been thought to contribute to

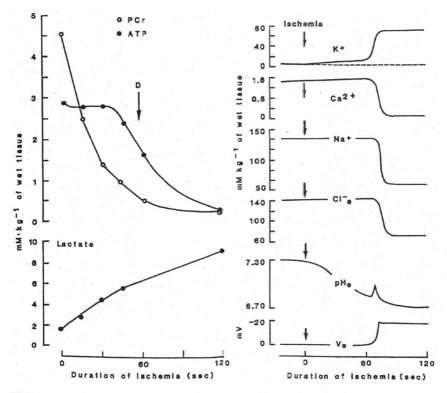

Figure 2. Left panel shows tissue concentrations of phosphocreatine (PCr), adenosine triphosphate (ATP), and lactate during the first 120 seconds of complete ischemia. D and arrow show the time of depolarization. Right panel depicts changes in extracellular concentrations of K^+, Ca^{2+}, Na^+, Cl^- (Cl^-_e) and pH (pH_e) and direct current potential (V_e). (Reproduced from Siesjö.[8])

reperfusion damage. The last part of the chapter is devoted to novel data and concepts which have materially altered our view on reperfusion events and on possibilities of ameliorating tissue damage caused by ischemia and reperfusion. For access to the original literature, the authors are referred to recent review articles.[8-14]

Bioenergetic Failure and Loss of Ion Homeostasis

Ischemia is accompanied by bioenergetic failure, this in turn leading to loss of ion homeostasis, the latter encompassing release of K^+ from cells and their uptake of Ca^{2+}, Na^+, and Cl^-. Indices of bioenergetic failure, as these are observed in dense global (forebrain) ischemia, are illustrated in Figure 2. The decrease in adenosine triphosphate (ATP) concentration is a major pathogenetic factor since it is accompanied by arrest of all energy-driven reactions, but it is not, *per se*, an event which predisposes the tissue to reperfusion damage. However, ATP is hydrolyzed to ADP and AMP, the latter being dephosphorylated and deaminated to nucleosides and bases, including hypoxanthine. As will be discussed below, hypoxanthine is a precursor in postischemic reactions leading to production of reactive oxygen species (ROS), notably $^{\cdot}O_2^-$ and H_2O_2.

Ischemia is accompanied by accumulation of lactate, and since lactate is released with a stoichiometrical amount of H^+, intra- and extracellular pH (pH_i and pH_e, respectively) are reduced. In complete ischemia, the amount of lactate accumulated corresponds to the preischemic stores of glucose and glycogen.[15] Therefore, the accumulation of lactate (and the severity of acidosis) varies directly with the plasma glucose concentration. If the ischemia is incomplete, allowing a continuous supply of glucose, hyperglycemic animals may become excessively acidotic. Such exaggerated acidosis during ischemia is known to aggravate ischemic damage, hasten its evolution, transform selective neuronal necrosis into infarction, and trigger postischemic seizures.[16,17] Following ischemia of brief to moderate duration, an adequate reperfusion leads to normalization of the bioenergetic state, as reflected in the energy charge of the adenine nucleotide pool, to normalization of the lactate concentration, and to resolution of the acidosis. Changes persisting during the early reperfusion period encompass a sustained reduction in the ATP concentration, reflecting slow resynthesis of adenine nucleotides, an increase in the PCr concentration above normal, and an alkaline shift in pH_i. The rise in pH_i above normal, which probably explains the rise in PCr concentration via a shift in the creatine kinase equilibrium, is of potential pathogenetic importance (see below).

Changes in extracellular calcium concentration ($[Ca^{2+}]_e$), and in the free, intracellular (cytosolic) calcium concentration ($[Ca^{2+}]_i$) are shown in Figure 3. Since influx of Na^+ and Cl^- is accompanied by osmotically obligated water, it leads to cellular ("cytotoxic") edema. This is probably not an important determinant of reperfusion events, though. Very likely, the most important event is the influx of calcium into cells through voltage-sensitive and agonist-operated channels. This influx leads to a rise in the free cytosolic calcium concentration $[Ca^{2+}]_i$ from about 0.1 mmol to values of 30-60 mmol. However, if ischemia is of brief to intermediate duration, reperfusion is followed by re-extrusion of the calcium accumulated, with normalization of $[Ca^{2+}]_i$ and $[Ca^{2+}]_e$.[18]

The results illustrated in Figures 2 and 3 pertain to dense global (forebrain) ischemia. In ischemia due to MCA occlusion, changes in ATP concentration are marked in the focus but less pronounced in the

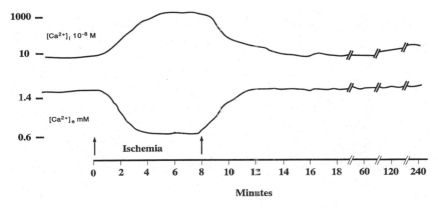

Figure 3. Simultaneous records of intra- and extracellular free calcium in area CA1 of the hippocampus of an anesthetized rat before, during, and after an ischemic episode lasting 8 minutes. Upper trace: Intracellular free calcium concentration recorded with a double barreled electrode (log scale 10-1,000 x 10^{-8} M). Lower trace: Record of extracellular free calcium (log scale 0.6-1.4 mM). Vertical arrows indicate beginning and end of ischemia. Oblique parallel line indicate breaks in the record as shown on the x-axis. (Retraced from Silver and Erecinska.[18])

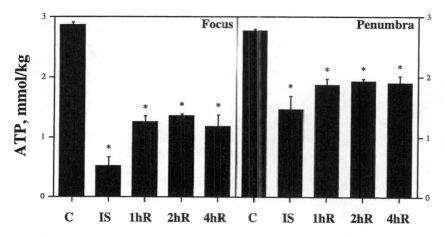

Figure 4. Changes in ATP contents of focal and penumbra tissues after 2 hours of middle cerebral artery (MCA) occlusion, as well as after 1, 2, and 4 hours of recirculation. Notice the secondary bioenergetic deterioration after 4 hours of recirculation in the focus. Data are presented as means ± SD. * P < 0.05 against control values. (Modified from Folbergrová et al.[20])

so called penumbra zone, ie, that part of the tissue which is "at risk" and which will be recruited in the infarction process, unless early reperfusion or pharmacological intervention is instituted.[19,20] Results obtained after 2 hours of MCA are illustrated in Figure 4. In the focus, the sum of adenine nucleotides is reduced to about half, demonstrating extensive breakdown of adenosine monophosphate (AMP). Again, penumbra changes are less dramatic.

Following reperfusion, the bioenergetic state is not normalized, as it is when animals are recirculated after brief to intermediate periods of forebrain ischemia. Thus, ATP concentrations are not normalized and PCr concentrations remain reduced. Since adenosine diphosphate (ADP) and AMP concentrations are not increased above normal, the reduced ATP concentration mostly reflects failure of cells to resynthesize adenine nucleotides. Sustained mitochondrial dysfunction is suggested by the abortive recovery of tissue lactate concentrations. The results of Figure 4 also demonstrate that the bioenergetic state shows a further compromise after 4 hours of recovery. Thus, when ischemia is of long duration (2 hours), recirculation fails to completely restore the bioenergetic state, and secondary energy failure is observed in spite of continued reflow. In other words, reperfusion damage is present already at the beginning of recirculation, and shows secondary aggravation.

Changes in the bioenergetic state during and after ischemia are reflected in $[Ca^{2+}]_e$ (values for $[Ca^{2+}]_i$ are not known). The penumbra shows the well-documented ischemic depolarization waves, resembling long-lasting spreading depressions.[21] In these areas, recirculation is followed by normalization of $[Ca^{2+}]_e$. In the focus, $[Ca^{2+}]_e$ is reduced to values similar to those observed in dense forebrain ischemia. However, recirculation fails to restore $[Ca^{2+}]_e$ to normal, suggesting continuous uptake of calcium by the energy-compromised cells.[22] It is tempting to speculate that this contributes to the delayed aggravation of the bioenergetic state.

Changes in Cerebral Blood Flow

Brain damage is incurred both after brief periods of global or forebrain ischemia, and after long periods of focal ischemia. In the former case, the damage matures after many hours, or days, and the delayed damage is preceded by a free interval in which the bioenergetic state and transmembrane ion gradients are restored to normal.[21-24] In the latter case, ie, after focal ischemia of long duration (eg, 2 hours) a free interval is observed only in the penumbra, while the focus shows only partial and short-lasting recovery.

Clearly, in both cases delayed or rapidly occurring bioenergetic compromise could reflect microvascular failure. However, there is little support for this possibility. For example, although brief periods of global or forebrain ischemia is followed by a delayed hypoperfusion (often preceded by a period of reactive hyperemia) this reduction in blood flow does not exceed the corresponding reduction in metabolic

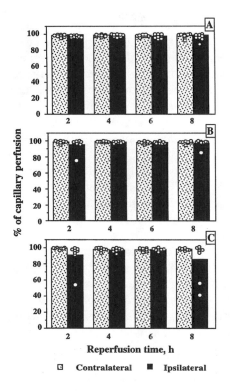

Figure 5. Percentage of capillary patency in normoglycemic animals subjected to 2 hours of MCA occlusion with 2, 4, 6, and 8 hours of recirculation. (**A**) neocortical penumbra, (**B**) neocortical focus, (**C**) striatal focus. Data are collected from 8 animals in each time point. Bars denote mean values and circles individual rats. No statistical significant differences could be found using either ANOVA plus post Scheffe's test for chronological data or unpaired *t*-test for ipsi- and contralateral comparison.

rate[25,26] and capillary patency, as assessed by markers of plasma flow, remains normal.[27] Furthermore, there is no evidence of a circulatory compromise during the first 4-6 hours of reflow following 2 hours of focal ischemia (Li et al., unpublished data). Thus, blood flow remains around normal values, erythrocyte velocity is not affected, the capillary patency is normal, and tissue PO_2 values rise above preischemic controls.[28,29] Similar results have been obtained in focal ischemia of 30 minute's duration, complicated by preischemic hyperglycemia.[30,31] Results on capillary patency after 2 hours of MCA occlusion are illustrated in Figure 5. Since bioenergetic failure develops in the absence of microcirculatory failure (2 hours ischemia in normoglycemic animals), and since 30 minutes of MCA occlusion in hyperglycemic animals gives rise to aggravation of damage, and to infarct development, with no evidence of gross microvascular dysfunction, it seems logical to incriminate mitochondrial function.

Function of Isolated Mitochondria

Ischemia is a mitochondrial disease in the sense that mitochondrial function is depressed, or ceased, when O_2 tensions are reduced, or fall to zero. However, even if the mitochondria are isolated and their respiratory activities are studied under optimal conditions *in vitro*, their function, as assessed by measurements of ADP- and uncoupler-stimulated oxygen consumption, is abnormal. This may reflect a respiratory block due to accumulation of free fatty acids. However, if the ischemia is of brief to intermediate duration, recirculation leads to normalization of mitochondrial function, as assessed *in vitro*. Clearly, this is an expected result, considering that the bioenergetic state is normalized.

We recall that neuronal damage after brief to intermediate periods of global or forebrain ischemia is delayed by hours or days. Such damage is accompanied by secondary mitochondrial dysfunction and bioenergetic failure.[24,32] Although this suggests that secondary mitochondrial failure may be the leading event, existing data do not make it clear whether mitochondrial dysfunction precedes bioenergetic compromise, the latter then causing cell death, or if such dysfunction is secondary to devitalization of cells by other mechanisms.

Results obtained with 2 hours of focal ischemia reveal a different pattern. Thus, the respiratory control ratio, as well as state 3 and uncoupler-stimulated respiration, is only partly normalized after 1 hour of recirculation, and then continuously falls (Figure 6). The results suggest that mitochondrial dysfunction is responsible both for the failure of cells to recover lactate (and PCr) concentrations at 1 hour of recirculation, and for the further deterioration of energy state at 4 hours. This raises the question about mechanisms which may be involved.

Mechanisms Causing Reperfusion Damage: Classical Concepts

It has been recognized for decades that ischemia triggers reactions which lead to degradation of cell structure. In fact, a fall in ATP concentration *per se* has this effect, simply because the spontaneous or enzyme-catalyzed degradation of structure is not matched by a corresponding resynthesis. However, most of the reactions involved are catalyzed by a rise in $[Ca^{2+}]_i$. These reactions encompass degradation of lipids by phospholipase A_2, breakdown of proteins by activation of proteases, and fragmentation of DNA by Ca^{2+}-dependent endonucleases. However, these reactions occur during ischemia, and do not necessarily qualify as mediators of reperfusion damage.

The most important event triggering reperfusion damage is the return of oxygen to the metabolically perturbed tissue. This is because oxygen is required for the generation of ROS, or of nitrous oxide (NO). Reactions in which ROS are generated encompass those in which hypo-

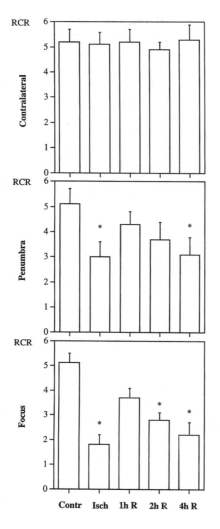

Figure 6. Changes in mitochondrial respiratory control ratio (RCR) in the contralateral cortex, as well as in ipsilateral penumbra and focus. Recirculation following 2 hours of MCA occlusion failed to fully restore the RCR, and secondary mitochondrial dysfunction was observed during the first 4 hours. * P < 0.05 against control values. (Modified from Kuroda and Sies.ö.[69])

xanthine and xanthine are degraded to uric acid by xanthine oxidase with the generation of $\cdot O_2^-$ and H_2O_2. This reaction, which may require the conversion of xanthine dehydrogenase to xanthine oxidase by Ca^{2+}-activated, limited proteolysis, could contribute to microvascular damage. Another series of reactions, probably of equal importance, is that leading to the production of prostaglandins and leucotrienes from accumulated arachidonic acid. This is because $\cdot O_2^-$ is released during the conversion of arachidonic acid to eicosanoids. A third cascade of events, one that probably plays a major role in the killing of cells, is that in which arginine is metabolized to NO by the constitutive or inducible forms of NO synthetase (NOS). Neither $\cdot O_2^-$, nor H_2O_2, or

NO, are particularly toxic. However, interactions among the three can yield the extremely toxic hydroxyl radical species ($\cdot$OH). This can either occur when $\cdot O_2^-$ and H_2O_2 react in the presence of pro-oxidant iron, or when $\cdot O_2^-$ and NO react to yield $\cdot$OH and peroxynitrate . The latter has a toxicity by itself, in part because it can cause nitrosylation of proteins.[33,34] It has been established beyond doubt that reperfusion following global/forebrain or focal ischemia is accompanied by enhanced production of $\cdot O_2^-$, H_2O_2, $\cdot$OH, NO, and peroxynitrate. This production, particularly of $\cdot$OH, is known to give rise to lipid peroxidation, protein oxidation, and oxidative damage to DNA.[35,36] This is the basis of the free radical hypothesis of reperfusion damage. The hypothesis is supported by elegant experiments in which either the superoxide dismutase or NOS was manipulated by gene knockout or overexpression.[37-46] These experiments have clearly shown that production of $\cdot O_2^-$, or of NO, influences infarct size after transient focal ischemia. However, less information exists for global or forebrain ischemia, and most free radical scavengers tested have had only moderate effects or none at all. It is also an unresolved issue how postischemic production of ROS, or of NO, can give rise to delayed brain damage. Finally, the targets of free radical attack have remained poorly defined, and the sequences of events leading to cell death await clarification.

Novel Aspects of Reperfusion Damage

The last 4 to 5 years of research have given novel insights into putative mechanisms of cell death following ischemia and reperfusion. A major part of the information amassed derives from *in vitro* experiments on non-neuronal cells, exposed to inducers of apoptotic cell death.[47-50] However, the concepts developed from such experiments seem to be generally valid and sufficient evidence exists that they apply to ischemia-reperfusion in the brain.[51]

Our own results on the effect of cyclosporin A (CsA) in experiments on forebrain ischemia of 7-10 minute duration provide a good starting point for discussing the novel concepts. In these experiments, a needle was inserted into the hippocampus on one side for the injection of genetically manipulated nerve growth factor-producing cells, and CsA was given to curb the immunological response.[52] It turned out that CsA, when combined with a needle lesion, dramatically ameliorated the ischemic damage, the needle lesion obviously having the effect of allowing CsA to be translocated across the blood-brain barrier. CsA was subsequently shown to ameliorate also the aggravated damage which is observed in hyperglycemic subjects, and to suppress postischemic seizures.[53]

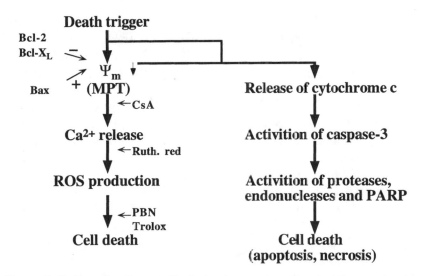

Figure 7. Schematic diagram illustrates how a decrease in $\Delta\Psi_m$ can lead to cell death. The left panel shows that mitochondrial depolarization due to an MPT may cause release of Ca^{2+} and production of ROS by mitochondria. Also shown are the sites of Bcl-2, Bcl-x_L, Bax, and of CsA, ruthenium red, and PBN or Trolox. The right panel illustrates how cytochrome c release can trigger activation of caspase-3 and of downstream enzymes whose activation is potentially detrimental.

The literature proved to contain abundant data on cellular effects of CsA. Apart from having an immunosuppressant effect, the drug is known to act as a more or less specific blocker of the mitochondrial permeability transition (MPT) pore which is assembled under adverse conditions, such as mitochondrial calcium accumulation, and oxidative stress. This was observed already in 1988 by Crompton et al.[54] who later suggested that pore opening played a role in reperfusion injury.[55-57] The characteristics of the MPT have been described in numerous articles.[55,58,59] The pore is a high conductance channel, permeable to all solutes with a molecular mass of < 1500 Daltons. It behaves as a Ca^{2+}-activated, voltage-modulated channel which, by its high conductance, allows Ca^{2+} to leave the mitochondria and other ions (including H^+) to equilibrate across the inner mitochondrial membrane. This leads to dissipation of the H^+ gradient with a collapse of the transmembrane potential ($\Delta\{\{Psi\}\}_m$) to cessation of ATP synthesis, and to uncoupling of oxidative phosphorylation. A result of this is a burst of production of ROS by the mitochondria.

Subsequent results obtained in thymocytes and other rapidly proliferating cells, committed to undergo apoptotic cell death by exposure to dexamethason, showed that the first event in the apoptotic cascade was a decrease in $\Delta\{\{Psi\}\}_m$ (Figure 7, left panel). This was followed by production of ROS, which preceded cell death. The first step, the fall in $\Delta\Psi_m$ was blocked by CsA and the second, the production of ROS, by ruthenium red, a blocker of mitochondrial Ca^{2+} uptake, while cell death was ameliorated by PBN and by the vitamin E analogue Trolox.

It was subsequently shown that a number of insults could trigger an MPT, and apoptotic cell death. These include exposure to dexamethasone, glutamate, and NO, the latter exerting its effect by being converted to peroxynitrate, deprivation of growth factors, and anoxia/ischemia. All of these "inducers" seemed to act on a common target, reducing $\Delta\Psi_m$ sufficiently to elicit an MPT. It could also be demonstrated that the protoncogene products Bcl-2 and Bcl-x_L "clamped" the mitochondrial membrane potential at its normal levels, thereby preventing a fall in $\Delta\Psi_m$ and apoptosis, and that Bax had an opposite effect, promoting apoptosis.[60,61]

Further studies revealed that the fall in $\Delta\Psi_m$ triggered a cascade of reactions which induced nuclear changes, characteristic of apoptosis, and cell death. The mediator molecules released from the mitochondria include an apoptosis-inducing factor (AIF), claimed to be a protease,[62] and cytochrome c.[63-65] Release of cytochrome c, which is not necessarily preceded by a fall in $\Delta\Psi_m$, leads to activation of caspase 3, one of a family of Interleukin β (2L-1β)-like proteases. Activation of caspase 3 is an intermediate step in a signal transduction chain which ends with the activation of proteases, endonucleases, and PARP.

The initiating step in this cascade is a perturbation of mitochondrial membrane function, leading to release of cytochrome c from the intermembraneous space. The mechanisms of this release are not known but suggestions range from a rupture of the outer membrane, secondary to mitochondrial swelling, to transport through channels created by upregulation of Bax. Whatever is the mechanisms of release of cytochrome c, it is inhibited by Bcl-2 and Bcl-x_L, antagonizing the effect of Bax. Clearly, changes in the expression of protoncogenes such as bcl-2 may modulate the release of cytochrome c and, therefore, do the activation of caspase 3 and downstream enzymes.

It has recently been suggested that the mitochondrial membrane perturbation, usually associated with an MPT, is a common initial step in pathways leading to both apoptosis and necrosis.[64,66] It has been proposed that the factor determining whether necrosis or apoptosis results is the class of proteases being activated; alternatively, necrosis results if the bioenergetic state deteriorates. This could conceivably occur by extensive loss of cytochrome c from mitochondria.

Reperfusion Damage in Ischemia of Brief or Long Duration: A Speculative Synthesis

Given the above facts, we can speculate on the likely mechanisms leading to delayed neuronal necrosis following ischemia of brief duration. We have previously proposed that calcium gradually accumulates in neurons in the postischemic period and, that once the Ca^{2+}_i values exceed the set point for net calcium accumulation by the mitochondria, they subsequently become overloaded with calcium.[67,68] This hypothesis is probably still valid since it is compatible with the delayed assembly of an MPT in response to mitochondrial calcium accumulation. If an MPT pore is opened during recirculation it could trigger secondary energetic compromise, and delayed neuronal damage, both because a burst of ROS production occurs, and because depolarized mitochondria cannot generate normal amounts of ATP.

It is not clear, though, if mitochondrial calcium accumulation is the dominating trigger of an MPT and, thereby, of secondary neuronal damage. However, it remains to be shown if a redox change, or intracellular alkalosis, modulate the assembly of an MPT pore. Thus, oxidative stress is known to be a major trigger of the MPT and alkalosis (if transmitted into the intramitochondrial space) is known to promote the assembly of an MPT pore. It also remains a possibility that the pore is assembled because Bcl-2 is downregulated, or Bax upregulated.

It is not clear what the role is of an MPT in ischemia of longer duration, as in MCA occlusion of 30 minute duration or longer. Thus, the possibility remains that mitochondrial dysfunction is due to extensive hydrolysis of mitochondrial membrane lipids, or inactivation of respiratory complexes. Clearly, although our primary hypothesis is that mitochondrial failure is a leading event in the pathogenesis of apoptotic and necrotic cell death, the validation of this hypothesis has to await an accurate assessment of the mitochondrial defects involved.

References

1. Zhao Q, Pahlmark K, Smith M-L, et al. Delayed treatment with the spin trap α-phenyl-N-tert-butyl nitrone (PBN) reduces infarct size following transient middle cerebral artery occlusion in rats. *Acta Physiol Scand* 1994;152:349-350.

2. Sharkey J, Butcher S. Immunophilins mediate the neuroprotective effects of FK 506 in focal cerebral ischemia. *Nature* 1994;371:336-339.

3. Markgraf CG, Velayo NL, Johnson MP, et al. Six-hour window of opportunity for calpain inhibition in focal cerebral ischemia in rats. *Stroke* 1997;29:152-158.

4. Bartus RT, Hayward NJ, Elliott PJ, et al. Calpain inhibitor AK295 protects neurons from focal brain ischemia. Effects of postocclusion intra-arterial administration. *Stroke* 1994;25:2267-2270.

5. Endres M, Namura S, Shimizu Sasamata M, et al. Attenuation of delayed neuronal death after mild focal ischemia in mice by inhibition of the caspase family. *J Cereb Blood Flow Metab* 1998;18:238-247.

6. Lo EH, Bosque-Hamilton P, Meng W. Inhibition of poly(ADP-ribose) polymerase: Reduction of ischemic injury and attenuation of N-methyl-D-aspartate-induced neurotransmitter dysregulation. *Stroke* 1998;29:830-836.

7. Eliasson MJ, Sampei K, Mandir AS, et al. Poly(ADP-ribose) polymerase gene disruption renders mice resistant to cerebral ischemia. *Nat Med* 1997;3:1089-1095.

8. Siesjö BK. Pathophysiology and treatment of focal cerebral ischemia. I. Pathophysiology. *J Neurosurg* 1992;77:169-184.

9. Siesjö BK. Pathophysiology and treatment of focal cerebral ischemia. II. Mechanisms of damage and treatment. *J Neurosurg* 1992;77:337-354.

10. Morley P, Hogan MJ, Hakim AM. Calcium-mediated mechanisms of ischemic injury and protection. *Brain Pathol* 1994;4:37-47.

11. Tymianski M, Tator CH. Normal and abnormal calcium homeostasis in neurons: A basis for the pathophysiology of traumatic and ischemic central nervous system injury. *Neurosurgery* 1996;38:1176-1195

12. Kristián T, Siesjö BK. Calcium in ischemic cell death. *Stroke* 1998;29:705-718.

13. Siesjö BK, Elmér E, Kristián T, et al. Role and mechanisms of secondary mitochondrial failure. *Acta Neurochir* 1999;73:7-13.

14. Siesjö BK, Ouyang Y, Kristián T, et al. Role of mitochondria in immediate and delayed reperfusion damage. In Ito U, Kirino T, Kuroiwa T, et al. (eds): *Maturation Phenomenon in Cerebral ischemia III*. Berlin: Springer-Verlag; 1998.

15. Ljunggren B, Norberg K, Siesjö BK. Influence of tissue acidosis upon restitution of brain energy metabolism following total ischemia. *Brain Res* 1974;77:173-186.

16. Siesjö BK. Acidosis and ischemic brain damage. *Neurochem Pathol* 1988;9:31-88

17. Li P-A, Siesjö BK. Role of hyperglycaemia-related acidosis in ischaemic brain damage. *Acta Physiol Scand* 1997;161:567-580.

18. Silver IA, Erecinska M. Ion homeostasis in rat brain in vivo: intra- and extracellular Ca^{2+} and H^+ in the hippocampus during recovery from short-term, transient ischemia. *J Cereb Blood Flow Metab* 1992;12:759-772.

19. Selman WR, VanDerVeer C, Whittingham TS, et al. Visually defined zones of focal ischemia in the rat brain. *Neurosurgery* 1987;21:825-830.

20. Folbergrová J, Zhao Q, Katsura K, et al. N-tert-butyl-α-phenylnitrone improves recovery of brain energy state in rats following transient focal ischemia. *Proc Natl Acad Sci* 1995;92:5057-5061.

21. Gido G, Kristián T, Siesjö BK. Extracellular potassium in a neocortical core area after transient focal ischemia. *Stroke* 1997;28:206-210.

22. Kristián T, Gido G, Siesjö BK. Calcium metabolism of focal and penumbra tissues in rats subjected to transient middle cerebral artery occlusion. *Exp Brain Res* 1998;120:503-509.

23. Erecinska M, Silver IA. Ions and energy in mammalian brain. *Prog Neurobiol* 1994;43:37-71.

24. Pulsinelli WA, Duffy TE. Regional energy balance in rat brain after transient forebrain ischemia. *J Neurochem* 1983;40:1500-1503.

25. Pulsinelli W, Levy D, Duffy T. Regional cerebral blood flow and glucose metabolism following transient forebrain ischemia. *Ann Neurol* 1982;11:499-509.

26. Kågström E, Smith M-L, Siesjö BK. Recirculation in the rat brain following incomplete ischemia. *J Cereb Blood Flow Metab* 1983;3:183-192.

27. Li P-A, Vogel J, He Q-P, et al. Preischemic hyperglycemia leads to rapidly developing brain damage with no change in capillary patency. *Brain Res* 1998;782:175-183.

28. Nakai A, Kuroda S, Kristián T, et al. The immunosuppressant drug FK506 ameliorates secondary mitochondrial dysfunction following transient focal cerebral ischemia in the rat. *Neurobiol Dis* 1997;4:288-300.

29. Tsuchidate R, He QP, Smith M-L, et al. Regional cerebral blood flow during and following 2 hour of middle cerebral artery occlusion in the rat. *J Cereb Blood Flow Metab* 1997;17:1066-1073.

30. Gisselsson L, Smith M-L, Siesjö BK. Hyperglycemia and focal brain ischemia. The influence of hyperglycemia on brain damage and blood flow in focal ischemia. *J Cereb Blood Flow Metab* 1999;19(3):288-297.

31. Li P-A, Gisselsson L, Keuker J, et al. Hyperglycemia-exaggerated ischemic brain damage following 30 min of middle cerebral artery occlusion is not due to capillary obstruction. *Brain Res* 1998;804(1):36-44.

32. Sims NR, Pulsinelli WA. Altered mitochondrial respiration in selectively vulnerable brain subregions following transient forebrain ischemia in the rat. *J Neurochem* 1987;49:1367-1374.

33. Beckman J, Beckman T, Chen J, et al. Apparent hydroxyl radical production by peroxynitrite: Implications for endothelial injury from nitric oxide and superoxide. *Proc Natl Acad Sci* 1990;87:1620-1624.

34. Beckman JS, Ye Y, Chen J, et al. The interactions of nitric oxide with oxygen radicals and scavengers in cerebral ischemic injury, In Siesjö BK, Wieloch T (eds): *Advances in Neurology: Cellular and Molecular Mechanisms of Ischemic Brain Damage*. Philadelphia: Lippincott-Raven Publishers; 1996;339-354.

35. Floyd RA, Carney JM. Free radical damage to protein and DNA: Mechanisms involved and relevant observations on brain undergoing oxidative stress. *Ann Neurol* 1992;32:S22-S27.

36. Halliwell B. Reactive oxygen species and the central nervous system. *J Neurochem* 1992;59:1609-1623.

37. Chan PH, Epstein CJ, Li Y, et al. Transgenic mice and knockout mutants in the study of oxidative stress in brain injury. *J Neurotrauma* 1995;12:815-824.

38. Kondo T, Reaume AG, Huang TT, et al. Edema formation exacerbates neurological and histological outcomes after focal cerebral ischemia in CuZn-superoxide dismutase gene knockout mutant mice. *Acta Neurochir (Wien)* 1997;70(Suppl):62-64.

39. Murakami K, Kondo T, Epstein CJ, et al. Overexpression of CuZn-superoxide dismutase reduces hippocampal injury after global ischemia in transgenic mice. *Stroke* 1997;28:1797-1804.

40. Murakami K, Kondo T, Kawase M, et al. Mitochondrial susceptibility to oxidative stress exacerbates cerebral infarction that follows permanent focal cerebral ischemia in mutant mice with manganese superoxide dismutase deficiency. *J Neurosci* 1998;18:205-213.

41. Iadecola C, Zhang F, Casey R, et al. Delayed reduction of ischemic brain injury and neurological deficits in mice lacking the inducible nitric oxide synthase gene. *J Neurosci* 1997;17:9157-9164.

42. Ferriero DM, Holtzman DM, Black SM, et al. Neonatal mice lacking neuronal nitric oxide synthase are less vulnerable to hypoxic-ischemic injury. *Neurobiol Dis* 1996;3:64-71.

43. Hara H, Huang PL, Panahian N, et al. Reduced brain edema and infarction volume in mice lacking the neuronal isoform of nitric oxide synthase after transient MCA occlusion. *J Cereb Blood Flow Metab* 1996;16:605-611.

44. Wang P, Chen H, Qin H, et al. Overexpression of human copper, zinc-superoxide dismutase (SOD1) prevents postischemic injury. *Proc Natl Acad Sci USA* 1998;95:4556-4560.

45. Moskowitz MA, Dalkara T. Nitric oxide and cerebral ischemia. In Siesjö BK, Wieloch T (eds): *Advances in Neurology: Cellular and Molecular Mechanisms of Ischemic Brain Damage.* Philadelphia: Lippincott-Raven Publishers; 1996;365-369.

46. Meldrum BS. The role of nitric oxide in ischemic damage, In Siesjö BK, Wieloch T (eds): *Advances in Neurology: Cellular and Molecular Mechanisms of Ischemic Brain Damage.* Philadelphia: Lippincott-Raven Publishers; 1996;355-363.

47. Ellis HM, Horvitz HR. Genetic control of programmed cell death in the nematode C. elegans. *Cell* 1986;44:817-829.

48. Kerr JFR, Wyllie AH, Currie AR. Apoptosis: A basic biological phenomenon with wide-ranging implications in tissue kinetics. *Brit J Cancer* 1972;26:239-257.

49. Rinner WA, Pifl C, Lassmann H, et al. Induction of apoptosis in vitro and in vivo by the cholinergic neurotoxin ethylcholine aziridinium. *Neuroscience* 1997;79:535-542.

50. Wyllie AH. Glucocorticoid-induced thymocyte apoptosis is associated with endogenous endonuclease activation. *Nature* 1980;284:555-556.

51. Charriaut-Marlangue C, Pollard H, Ben-Ari Y. Is ischemic cell death of the apoptotic type? In Siesjö BK, Wieloch T (eds): *Advances in Neurology: Cellular and Molecular Mechanisms of Ischemic Brain Damage.* Philadelphia: Lippincott-Raven Publishers; 1996;425-431.

52. Uchino H, Elmér E, Uchino K, et al. Cyclosporin A dramatically ameliorates CA1 hippocampal damage following transient forebrain ischemia in the rat. *Acta Physiol Scand* 1995;155:469-471.

53. Li P-A, Hiroyuki U, Elmér E, et al. Amelioration by cyclosporin A of brain damage following 5 or 10 min of ischemia in rats subjected to preischemic hyperglycemia. *Brain Res* 1997;753:133-140.

54. Crompton M, Ellinger H, Costi A. Inhibition by cyclosporin A of a Ca^{2+}-dependent pore in heart mitochondria activated by inorganic phosphate and oxidative stress. *Biochem J* 1988;255:357-360.

55. Bernardi P. The permeability transition pore. Control points of a cyclosporin A-sensitive mitochondrial channel involved in cell death. *Biochim Biophys Acta* 1996;1275:5-9.

56. Duchen MR, McGuinness O, Brown LA, et al. On the involvement of a cyclosporin A sensitive mitochondrial pore in myocardial reperfusion injury. *Cardiovasc Res* 1993;27:1790-1794.

57. Griffiths E, Halestrap A. Mitochondrial non-specific pores remain closed during cardiac ischemia, but open upon reperfusion. *Biochem J* 1995;307:93-98.

58. Bernardi P, Broekemeier KM, Pfeiffer DR. Recent progress on regulation of the mitochondrial permeability transition pore; A cyclosporin-sensitive pore in the inner mitochondrial membrane. *J Bioenerg Biomemb* 1994;26:509-517.

59. Zoratti M, Szabó I. The mitochondrial permeability transition. *Biochim Biophys Acta* 1995;1241:139-176.

60. Wang HG, Reed JC. Mechanisms of Bcl-2 protein function. *Histol Histopathol* 1998;13:521-530.

61. Isenmann S, Stoll G, Schroeter M, et al. Differential regulation of Bax, Bcl-2, and Bcl-X proteins in focal cortical ischemia in the rat. *Brain Pathol* 1998;8:49-62.

62. Susin SA, Zamzami N, Castedo M, et al. Bcl-2 inhibits the mitochondrial release of an apoptogenic protease. *J Exp Med* 1996;184:1331-1341.

63. Yang JC, Cortopassi GA. Induction of the mitochondrial permeability transition causes release of the apoptogenic factor cytochrome c. *Free Radic Biol Med* 1998;24:624-631.

64. Kroemer G, Dallaporta B, Resche-Rigon M. The mitochondrial death/life regulator in apoptosis and necrosis. *Annu Rev Physiol* 1998;60:619-642.

65. Mignotte B, Vayssiere JL. Mitochondria and apoptosis. *Eur J Biochem* 1998;252:1-15.

66. Hirsch T, Susin SA, Marzo I, et al. Mitochondrial permeability transition in apoptosis and necrosis. *Cell Biol Toxicol* 1998;14:141-145.

67. Deshpande JK, Siesjö BK, Wieloch T. Calcium accumulation and neuronal damage in the rat hippocampus following cerebral ischemia. *J Cereb Blood Flow Metab* 1987;7:89-95.

68. Siesjö BK. Mechanisms of ischemic brain damage. *Crit Care Med* 1988;16:954-963.

69. Kuroda S, Siesjö BK. Postischemic administration of FK506 reduces infarct volume following transient focal brain ischemia. *Neurosci Res Comm* 1996;19:83-90.

Chapter 18

Debate: Heparin Should Be Used to Treat Patients Presenting with Acute Stroke or Stroke-in-Evolution
Affirmative Position

Louis R. Caplan, MD

The use of anticoagulants in the treatment of stroke patients continues to be a very controversial issue. Many neurologists use heparin during the acute phase of stroke[1] while others do not use heparin and believe strongly that it should not be used.[2]

My position can be stated as follows:

1) Heparins, low-molecular weight heparins, and heparinoids should not be indiscriminately given to all patients with acute brain ischemia.

2) The efficacy and safety of these agents has not been adequately tested in patients with defined stroke subtypes and occlusive lesions.

3) More trials are needed testing these agents in patients whose stroke subtypes and vascular lesions have been clarified by modern brain imaging and vascular investigations.

4) Knowledge of the causes and pathophysiology of thromboembolism, my own clinical experience, and the experience of others leads me to posit that these agents should be effective in preventing red thrombus development, propagation, and embolization.

From: Choi D, Dacey RG, Hsu CY, Powers WJ. *Cerebrovascular Disease: Momentum at the End of the Second Millennium.* Armonk, NY: Futura Publishing Company, Inc., © 2002.

5) Until more definitive trials are performed, I continue to use and recommend the use of these drugs in patients with:
- large artery occlusions and severe stenosis
- cardiogenic and aortic origin embolism in conditions that have a high risk of acute reembolism
- dural sinus and venous occlusive intracranial disease

The Drugs Used and Their Functions

Standard unfractionated heparin is a biological compound that consists of a heterogeneous mixture of polysaccharides with molecular weights ranging from 3,000 to 30,000.[3] Low-molecular weight heparins are fragments of standard heparin with molecular weights of 4,000 to 6,000.[4,5] Heparinoids are heparin analogues- natural or semisynthetic sulfated glycosaminoglycans that are structurally related to heparin and have similar anticoagulant activity.[5]

Heparins, low-molecular weight heparins, and heparinoids act as anticogulants by binding to plasma antithrombin III. This interaction induces a conformational change in antithrombin III that increases its ability to inactivate coagulation enzymes including thrombin and activated Factor X (Factor Xa).

Low-molecular-weight heparins have more favorable bioavailability and pharmacokinetics than standard heparin. Their plasma half-lives are two to four times that of heparin.[4] Low-molecular weight heparins are thought to cause fewer hemorrhagic complications than standard heparin because they have less pronounced effect on platelet function and vascular permeability.[4] Low-molecular-weight heparins also cause less heparin-related thrombocytopenia, and fewer heparin-related skin necroses and white-clot syndromes. While heparin is monitored closely using prothrombin times and International Normalized Ratios (INRs), low-molecular-weight heparins and heparinoids can be monitored by measuring anti-factor Xa activity. Heparinoids and low-molecular-weight heparins are more convenient to use than standard heparin and now are being used frequently in patients outside of acute hospital settings.

Heparins, low-molecular-weight heparins, and heparinoids are thought to have their major effectiveness in inhibiting the formation of red erythrocyte-fibrin clots. Prothrombin is converted to thrombin. Thrombin in turn catalyzes the final step in the coagulation cascade which is the conversion of the soluble protein fibrinogen into insoluble polymers termed fibrin. Strands of fibrin form a network of fibers that entangle erythrocytes, platelets, and some leukocytes into a firm red clot that often adheres to an endothelial surface.

Red clots tend to form in regions of reduced flow. Activated platelets also promote the formation of red clots. The situations in which red thrombi are thought to form are: 1) stasis in veins in the limbs and pelvis; 2) in large arteries in which there is severe narrowing or occlusion; 3) dilated regions of the heart and aorta in which there is stasis, eg, dilated cardiac atria, ventricular aneurysms, akinetic regions within the ventricles; 4) irregular injured surfaces such as recent myocardial infarctions.

The Data

Unfortunately, there are no hard data from randomized trials that have adequately studied the efficacy and safety of these drugs in patients who have the conditions that are likely to respond to treatment. The available trials lumped patients with brain ischemia together without diagnostic investigations that defined the etiology, stroke subtypes, or vascular lesions among the patients studied. I cannot cite convincing data to support my position but, on the other hand, my opponent in this debate cannot show data that adequately refutes my position. There is simply no hard data available. There is some suggestive data that I believe supports my position that can be gleaned from recent studies in patients with dural sinus and venous thrombosis, and from several studies of treatment of patients with acute ischemic stroke.

Intracranial Dural Sinus and Venous Thrombosis

Beginning in the 1960s a number of single case reports and retrospective reviews suggested that heparin was a safe and effective treatment for patients with intracranial venous thrombosis. In some patients a dramatic improvement occurred a day or so after the start of heparin in patients who had previously been steadily worsening. Some patients worsened when high dose heparin was changed to oral anticoagulants, and then improved after full-dose heparin was reinstituted. Case reports and retrospective reviews showed that patients did not worsen or have new hemorrhages after heparin was given. Bousser et al. noted that, among 82 patients treated with heparin, there were no deaths and 77% of patients had a complete recovery.[6] Among 79 patients given anticoagulants, 94% improved and survived while only about one-half of the 157 patients not given anticoagulants survived.[7]

The only randomized double-blinded prospective trial of heparin use in patients with intracranial venous thrombosis was that of Einhaupl and colleagues.[8] During 1982-1984, these investigators studied 28 patients with angiographically proven sinus venous thrombosis. Ten of the 20 patients that met inclusion criteria were given heparin by intravenous bolus of 3,000 IU and then 25,000-65,000 IU each day by continuous intravenous infusion. The dose was adjusted to double the initial prothrombin time but not to exceed 120 seconds (target 80-100 seconds). The other 10 patients were given placebo. At the start of treatment three patients in the heparin treated group and two in the placebo group had hemorrhages on computed tomography (CT) scans. The authors used the results of a specially designed severity score (1-9 with 9 = death) and the development of intracerebral hemorrhaging (ICH) on treatment as outcome measures. To evaluate the occurrence of brain hemorrhage, each patient had at least two CT scans and a CT was performed when hemorrhage was clinically suspected. The investigators planned to admit 60 patients with an interim analysis after the first 20 patients. The interim analysis was considered so positive for anticoagulation that the study was terminated after the first 20 patients were entered.[8]

The severity scores in the heparin treated group were much improved over the placebo group. Complications in the group treated with heparin included hematuria, a groin hematoma, and a still-birth. One patient in the placebo group died after pulmonary infarction. No patient in the heparin treated group had a new brain hematoma. In the placebo group there were 3 new brain hemorrhages; 2 of the new hematomas were inpatients who did not have hemorrhages at onset. In the 3 patients with brain hemorrhages present before heparin treatment, two had a complete recovery.[8]

Einhaupl and colleagues also retrospectively analyzed their data from 102 patients with angiographically proven intracranial dural sinus and venous occlusions studied between 1977 and 1991.[8,9] Among the 102 patients, 43 had an ICH. Two patients had their first ICH after heparin treatment and one patient who had an ICH before treatment had another on heparin. Altogether six patients had ICH after heparin and 33 not treated with heparin had new hemorrhages. They also analyzed data from 40 patients who had known ICH before heparin treatment (27 patients) and before no heparin treatment (13 patients). Among those treated with heparin, 14/27 had full recovery and 4 died; among those not treated with heparin, only 3/13 recovered fully and 9/13 died. The patients not treated with heparin clearly fared worse and had a higher mortality. I find the data quite convincing that heparin does not worsen or predispose to ICH and heparin leads to a better outcome. The available data supports the proposition that heparin should be given to patients with intracranial dural and venous thrombosis unless there is a strong contraindication.

Acute Ischemic Stroke Due To Large Artery Thromboembolism

In the recently published TOAST trial, the low-molecular-weight heparinoid ORG 10172 was given within 24 hours of the onset of symptoms of an acute ischemic stroke.[10] This heparinoid was then given by continuous intravenous infusion for 7 days with the dose adjusted after 24 hours to maintain the antiXa factor activity at 0.6-0.8 antifactor Xa units/mL. ORG 10172 (Danaparoid) is a mixture of glycosaminoglycans with a mean molecular weight of 5,500 isolated from porcine intestinal mucosa. The antifactor Xa activity of Danaparoid is attributed to its heparin sulfate component, which has a high affinity for antithrombin III.

Although Danaparoid treatment was not effective in terms of the entire group of patients with ischemic stroke, there was some effectiveness in the group of patients that were diagnosed as having large artery atherosclerosis. In the TOAST trial, in patients classified as having large artery atherosclerosis, heparinoid reduced the number of recurrences of stroke during the 7 days of infusion, and the rates of favorable and very favorable outcomes were significantly higher in patients given heparinoid when compared with placebo. Sixty-eight percent of patients with large artery atherosclerosis treated with Danaparoid had favorable outcome versus 54.7% treated with placebo (P = 0.04); 43% of patients with large artery atherosclerosis treated with Danaparoid had very favorable outcomes versus 29.1% treated with placebo (P = 0.02). Recurrent strokes developed in 6% of Danaparoid-treated patients with large artery atherosclerosis versus 11% of those treated with placebo and 2.8% of patients with cardioembolism treated with Danaparoid had recurrent strokes versus 7.3% of patients treated with placebo. Because of the small numbers the figures for recurrent strokes did not meet statistical significance.

Perhaps of even more importance, Danaparoid was effective among the group of patients with large artery atherosclerosis who had severe internal carotid artery stenosis in the neck (> 50% luminal narrowing or occlusion).[11] This was the only subgroup of patients in the TOAST study in which all of the patients had vascular tests that defined the large artery lesions. Table 1 shows the results in these patients. Significantly more patients had favorable and very favorable outcomes among patients treated with heparinoid.

Table 1.

Outcomes in patients with carotid artery stenosis (>50%) or occlusion treated with Danaparoid vs placebo in the TOAST trial[11]; kindly submitted to me by B Bendixen from a slide presented at the 1998 meeting of the American Academy of Neurology

	Danaparoid	Placebo	P value
outcome at 7 days			
favorable	47/90 (52%)	32/91 (35%)	0.025
very favorable	26/90 (29%)	14/91 (15%)	0.032
outcome at 3 months			
favorable	62/91 (68%)	48/92 (52%)	0.035
very favorable	41/91 (45%)	27/92 (29%)	0.033

In a trial performed in Hong Kong, among 312 patients with acute ischemic stroke, low-molecular-weight heparin was more effective than placebo.[12] There was a significant dose-dependent reduction in the risk of death or dependency among the patients treated with low-molecular-weight heparin (chi-square for trend = 8.066, P = 0.005). Although vascular studies were not mandated in this study, the bulk of patients with ischemic stroke in Hong Kong have intracranial artery occlusive disease. Patients with cardiac lesions that required anticoagulation were not entered in this study.

Thus in these two studies, one of the group of patients that would be expected to respond to treatment with heparin compounds, those with large artery occlusive disease, did respond. Although heparin would be predicted to prevent acute recurrence of embolism in patients with cardiac origin embolism, there are cogent reasons why these studies did not show an effect in this group. Patients with high-risk embolic sources thought to require anticoagulation were excluded from the Hong Kong study. Many such patients were probably not admitted to the TOAST study. Also among all patients with cardioembolism, a task force that studied embolism recurrence showed that most recurrences do not occur during the first week after a first embolus.[13] There were results in the TOAST trial among patients with cardioembolism that suggested fewer recurrences developed among patients treated with Danaparoid, but the numbers were too small to be statistically significant.

A recent study of acute anticoagulation with heparin in patients with documented large artery atherostenosis and cardiac origin embolism showed that the treatment could be performed safely with a minimum of hemorrhagic complications.[14]

Conclusions and Recommendations

Brain ischemia is a complex condition caused by a very heterogeneous mix of different cardiac, hematological, and cerebrovascular conditions. No one panacea has or ever will prove effective against all the conditions that cause brain ischemia. Treatment must be tailored to the problem in each individual patient, and will depend to a great extent on four major characteristics: 1) the location, nature, and severity of the causative cardio-cerebrovascular lesion(s), 2) the mechanism of ischemia-hypoperfusion or embolism, 3) the coagulability and other functions of the blood, and 4) the state of the brain- irreversibly infarcted, normal, or stunned (not functioning normally but not yet infarcted- a penumbral state). These four attributes can now be defined quickly and safely using modern diagnostic technology.

I favor therapeutic trials of patients whose stroke subtypes and mechanisms have been defined by modern technology. Further trials should be designed that compare various treatment strategies for specific conditions (such as carotid artery atherostenosis, atrial fibrillation). Trials that study large groups of inadequately evaluated patients with lumped ischemia are a waste of effort, time, and money. When will we learn this important lesson? Until such trials have been completed and the data becomes available, I continue to use heparin in patients with intracranial venous occlusive disease, extracranial and intracranial large artery atherostenosis or recent occlusion, and those patients with high-risk cardiac lesions that have a strong likelihood of acute reembolism. I use two different strategies- diagnose first using modern technology (MR & MRA, CT & CTA, or either brain imaging modality with extracranial and transcranial ultrasound) and then selectively treat the group of patients mentioned. Alternatively when diagnosis is highly likely clinically -treat first before definitive testing and maintain treatment until the diagnosis can be verified or found to be in error.

References

1. Marsh EE, Adams HP, Biller J, et al. Use of antithrombotic drugs in the treatment of acute ischemic stroke: A survey of neurologists in practice in the United States. *Neurology* 1989;39:1631-1634.
2. Scheinberg P. Heparin anticoagulation. *Stroke* 1989;20:173-174.
3. Hirsh J. Heparin. *N Engl J Med* 1991;324:1565-1574.
4. Weitz JI. Low-molecular-weight heparins. *N Engl J Med* 1997;337:688-698.
5. Gordon DL, Linhardt R, Adams HP. Low-molecular-weight heparins and heparinoids and their use in acute or progressing ischemic stroke. *Clin Neuropharm* 1990;13:522-543.

6. Ameri A, Bousser M-G. Cerebral venous thrombosis. *Neurol Clin* 1992;10:87-111.

7. Jacewicz M, Plum F. Aseptic cerebral venous thrombosis. In Einhaupl K, Kempkti O, Baethmann A (eds): *Cerebral Sinus Thrombosis. Experimental and Clinical Aspects.* New York, Plenum, 1990:157-170.

8. Einhaupl KM, Villringer A, Meister W, et al. Heparin treatment in sinus venous thrombosis. *Lancet* 1991;338:597-600.

9. Meister W, Einhaupl K, Villringer A, et al. Treatment of patients with cerebral sinus and vein thrombosis with heparin. In Einhaupl K, Kempski O, Baethmann A (eds): *Cerebral Sinus Thrombosis. Experimental and Clinical Aspects.* New York, Plenum, 1990:225-230.

10. The Publications Committee for the Trial of ORG 10172 in Acute Stroke Treatment (TOAST) Investigators. Low molecular weight heparinoid, ORG 10172 (Danaparoid), and outcome after acute ischemic stroke. A randomized controlled trial. *JAMA* 1998;279:1265-1272.

11. Bendixen BH, Adams HP, Leira EC, et al. Responses to treatment with a low molecular weight heparinoid or placebo among patients with acute ischemic stroke secondary to large artery atherosclerosis. *Neurology* 1998;50:A345.

12. Kay R, Wong KS, Yu YL, et al. Low-molecular-weight heparin for the treatment of acute ischemic stroke. *N Engl J Med* 1995;333:1588-1593.

13. Cerebral embolism task force. Cardiogenic brain embolism. *Arch Neurol* 1986;43:71-84.

14. Camerlingo M, Casto L, Censori B, et al. Immediate anticoagulation with heparin for first-ever ischemic stroke in the carotid artery territories observed within 5 hours of onset. *Arch Neurol* 1994;51:462-467.

Chapter 19

Debate:Anticoagulation in Acute Ischemic Stroke:
Not Indicated

Roger P. Simon, MD and William J. Powers, MD

For many neurologists, anticoagulation remains a mainstay of treatment of acute ischemic stroke.{{sup1}} While data are available supporting its efficacy in reducing deep venous thrombosis accompanying stroke, extension of this benefit to neurological or functional outcome of ischemic stroke has not been conclusively demonstrated.[2,3]

Randomized clinical trials should offer an answer to a clearly defined therapeutic question such as this. In 1986, Duke and colleagues performed such a trial at four hospitals in Canada.[4] Two hundred twenty-five patients with stable, partial stroke occurring in the previous 48 hours were randomly assigned to receive placebo or continuous intravenous heparin sufficient to maintain the APTT at 50-70 seconds for seven days. Computed tomography (CT) scanning at randomization eliminated hemorrhage as a possible confounding variable. The patients were evaluated at 7 days, 3 months, and 1 year after cessation of treatment. Progression within the first 7 days occurred in 19.5% of the placebo group and 17% of the heparin group (n.s.). No differences between the two groups were found with regard to change in neurologic function at 7 days or functional activity at 7 days, 3 months or 1 year following treatment. There was a significantly higher incidence of death in the heparin treated group at 1 year (P < 0.01) due to an

Supported by NSO6833, NS35966

From: Choi D, Dacey RG, Hsu CY, Powers WJ. *Cerebrovascular Disease: Momentum at the End of the Second Millennium.* Armonk, NY: Futura Publishing Company, Inc., © 2002.

excess of deaths that occurred from 3 to 12 months following randomization. These late fatalities appeared unrelated to the treatment. Presumably, this study should have settled the matter of heparin treatment in acute stroke. However, the numbers were relatively small and 95% confidence limits still included a possible modest benefit for heparin at 7 days. The authors pointed out that the patients with partial stroke included those with both large and small artery disease, since the clinical distinction between the two types was difficult to establish at stroke onset. The importance of this etiologic distinction is based on the unproven supposition that the clinical algorithm used to define stroke subtype also define groups which respond differently to treatment.

Three new larger trials have recently provided data in a further attempt to definitively deal with this issue. Two of these trials have capitalized on the recent development of low molecular weight heparins and heparinoids. Like heparin, low molecular weight heparins and heparinoids produce their major anticoagulant effect by binding to antithrombin III. These compounds have reduced activity against thrombin, but retain inhibitory action against factor Xa. Thus, the partial thromboplastin time (which is sensitive to thrombin activity but insensitive to factor X activity) is an inappropriate measure of anticoagulant activity for these newer agents and has been replaced by the anti-factor Xa assay.[5] Low molecular weight heparins have been shown to be more effective in the treatment of deep venous thrombosis than standard heparin, to have a longer half life and not to produce thrombocytopenia.[5,6]

The Low Molecular Weight Heparin for the Treatment of Acute Ischemic Stroke study was performed in Hong Kong.[7] Two doses of the low molecular weight heparin nadroparin calcium were used with a placebo control. No data regarding anti-factor Xa levels were given but published data suggests that the higher doses of 4100 U IV BID would produce peak anti-factor Xa levels of approximately 1 U/mL, while the lower dose of 4100 U QD would produce peak anti-factor Xa levels of 0.4U/mL.[8,9] For comparison, the recommended therapeutic range for heparin in treatment of deep venous thrombosis (that used in the Canadian study) produces anti-factor Xa levels of 0.3 to 0.7 U/mL.[7] The primary outcome measure in the Hong Kong trial was death or dependency six months after randomization. Patients were admitted within 48 hours of the onset of symptoms and treated for 10 days. During the 10-day treatment period, recurrent stroke occurred in 21-1 high-dose patients, 1/101 low-dose patient, and 1/105 placebo patients (n.s.). Major gastrointestinal bleeding, requiring transfusion, occurred in only one patient (in the placebo group). There was no difference among the three groups in the proportion of patients with hemorrhagic transformation. The primary outcome measure of death or dependency at six months showed that there was a significant dose dependent effect in favor of low molecular weight heparin. This effect was not seen at 3 months and was primarily due to deaths in the placebo group during the 3- to 6-month interval. Favorable outcome was most pronounced in the subgroup with lacunar infarcts. The results of this study are similar, but opposite, to the Canadian study with no difference during the early period and an excess of late deaths in one group providing the margin for statistical significance.

A second clinical trial of nadroparin in acute ischemic stroke similar in design to the Hong Kong study recently has been completed. No beneficial effect of low dose or high dose nadroparin was demonstrated. The percent of patients with poor outcome was strikingly similar in all treatment groups: placebo 56.8%, low dose 57.2% and high dose 59.2%.[10]

The second trial is the International Stroke (IST).[11] This was an open label trial of 19,435 patients. The patients were entered within 48 hours after stroke and a negative CT brain scan and were assigned to high-dose (12,500 U BID) or low-does (5,000 U BID) subcutaneous heparin or aspirin (300 mg/day) or a control group or combinations of the above. These doses of heparin can be expected to produce APTT of 50-60 seconds for the high does group and 30-40 seconds for the low dose group with corresponding antifactor Xa levels of 0.2-0.3 U/mL and 0.04-0.05 U/mL, respectively.[12,13] Treatment was for up to 14 days. The primary outcome measures were death during the 2-week treatment period or death or dependency at 6 months. During the first 14-day treatment period, the heparin group had fewer recurrent ischemic strokes (2.9% vs. 3.8%) but an increase in hemorrhagic strokes (1.2% vs. 0.4%) resulting in no difference in death or total nonfatal recurrent strokes. These data suggest that the effect of heparin was primarily to cause hemorrhagic conversion of recurrent strokes without affecting the occurrence. In addition, there was a significant increase in systemic hemorrhage in the heparin group, especially the high-dose group, resulting in an increased number of deaths. At six months, there was no difference in outcome between the patients who received heparin and those who did not. No subgroup, including patients with atrial fibrillation, showed a benefit. Patients with large anterior circulation infarcts fared the worst on heparin. This trial was performed without laboratory monitoring of anticoagulant effect using a lower dose of heparin than is considered adequate for full anticoagulation of deep venous thrombosis. The complicated four-way design and analysis did not allow direct comparison of heparin versus placebo. Nevertheless, several very important facts emerge from this study. Heparin in the higher of the doses used produced an excess of both intracranial and extracranial hemorrhage without benefit for short-term recurrence or long-term outcome. The risk of early recurrence within 14 days, even in patients with atrial fibrillation, was low (approximately 5%) regardless of treatment.

The most recent study is TOAST (Trial of ORG10122 in Acute Stroke Treatment) which utilized danaparoid, a heparinoid.[14] The trial was randomized, double blinded, and placebo controlled.

One-thousand, two hundred and eighty-one patients admitted within 24 hours prior to stroke onset and with a nonhemorrhagic CT scan were randomized to a 7-day course of heparinoid or placebo. Patients were treated for 7 days with the heparinoid dose adjusted to maintain antifactor Xa levels at 0.6 - 0.8 U/mL. The primary endpoint was favorable functional outcome assessed at 3 months. During the 7-day treatment period, recurrent strokes occurred in 7 of 638 patients (1.1%) in the treatment group and 8 of 628 patients (1.3%) in the placebo arm. Serious bleeding occurred in 26 of 328 patients (8%) on active therapy and 7 of 628 patients (1%) randomized to placebo. Intracerebral hemorrhage occurred during the first 7 days in 11 patients in the treatment group and three in the control group. The primary analysis revealed no difference in favorable functional outcome in the treated patients versus control was found at 3 months. This lack of benefit occurred despite of the fact that patients with large strokes (NIH stroke scale < 15) began to be excluded part way through the trial due to an excess of hemorrhages in the early stages of the trial, thus potentially further biasing the results in favor of heparin treatment. As in the IST trial, anticoagulation produced an excess of hemorrhagic side effects without short-term effect on recurrence or long term benefit on outcome. The recurrence rate was low regardless of treatment.

A variety of secondary analyses were also performed in TOAST. At 7 days, a higher percentage of patients treated with heparin had a "very favorable outcome" (33% vs. 27.5%). When the patients were subdivided into stroke type (large vessel atherosclerosis, cardioembolic stroke, lacune, other, and undetermined) there was a favorable outcome in the large vessel atherosclerosis group for patients treated with heparin. However, no reduction in recurrent strokes were found in the large vessel atherosclerosis group during the 7 days of treatment and, within the first week and a half, 14 hemorrhages occurred in the treatment group versus four in the placebo group. All of the subgroup analyses were reported without statistical adjustment to account for the increased chance of finding differences due to the multiple comparisons performed. If the primary analysis of a trial is positive, such secondary analyses can be valuable in demonstrating how generalizable the benefit is and sometimes provide insight into mechanisms. The value of such analyses in a negative trial such as TOAST is problematic. Conclusions regarding statistical significance based on P < 0.05 are rendered invalid by failure to adjust for multiple comparisons. Thus, none of the reported differences in secondary analyses can be considered as evidence for the benefit of anticoagulation, although they may provide hypotheses for future trials.

Unfortunately, although an appropriately designed trial could study the possibility of a treatment effect in the large vessel atherosclerosis group during acute anticoagulant therapy, such a group cannot be defined prospectively. In TOAST, the subdivision of stroke types was done at 3 months when all data from clinical and radiographic studies was available as this was not possible at admission (Adams H.P., personal communication). This is the same problem pointed out by Duke et al. 12 years ago.

Reviewing these four randomized, controlled trials of anticoagulation in acute ischemic stroke with heparin or heparin-like drugs reveals no consistent evidence to support the use of heparin. No trial demonstrated short-term benefit in preventing progression or early recurrence. Long term benefit due to an excess of late deaths was demonstrated in the single trial with a positive result. However, an excess of late deaths in the heparin treated group was also demonstrated in another trial. The Hong Kong trial remains an anomaly because it demonstrated both a benefit of treatment and no excess of intracranial or systemic bleeding with an anticoagulation regimen that was intermediate between two other trials which demonstrated no benefit and increased bleeding (Table 1). Failure to confirm these results in a subsequent trial suggests that the observed difference in outcome was not a result of the anticoagulant treatment. No subgroup showed a consistent benefit across trials or statistically significant benefit in a single trial. These trials confirmed the danger of acute anticoagulation. An excess of systemic hemorrhagic side effects was reported in two of the three trials and an excess of intracranial hemorrhage was reported in two of four trials. Previous data in patients with cerebrovascular disease have indicated that heparin causes symptomatic intracranial hemorrhage in 1%-4% and serious systemic hemorrhage in 2%-3%.[15,16]

The answer to the acute therapy for stroke is found in the aspirin arm of the International Stroke Trial as well as the Chinese Acute Stroke Trial (CAST) which also studied aspirin therapy.[11,17] Aspirin produces a small but real reduction of about 10 deaths or recurrent strokes per 1,000 during the first few weeks. This treatment is without high hemorrhagic risk. As Caplan has noted, the overview of antiplatelet therapy for stroke has shown an improved outcome of 20-25 percent versus placebo.[18]

The efficacy of aspirin treatment in acute ischemic stroke is established. The evidence for the value of heparin and heparin-like drugs

Table 1.

Clinical Trials of Anticoagulation in Acute Ischemic Stroke.

	Canadian	Hong Kong	IST	TOAST
Number	225	2750	19,435	1281
Entry Time/ Treatment Time	<48 hrs/7 days	<48 hrs/ 10 days	<48 hrs/ 14 days	<24 hrs/ 7 days
Active Treatment Dose(s)	IV heparin APTT 60-70 s	IV nadroparin 4100 U BID 4100 U QD	SC heparin 12,500 U BID 5000 U BID	IV danaparoid antifactor Xa 0.6-0.8 U/ml
Anticoagulant Effect-antifactor Xa equvalent	0.3 -0.7 U/mL	1 U/ml (peak) 0.3 -0.4 U/mL (peak)	0.2 -0.3 U/mL 0.04 -.05 U/mL	0.6 -0.8 U/mL
Primary Endpoint	Neurological score/ function/death 7 d/3 mo/1 yr	6 mo death/dependency	6 mo death /dependency	3 mo favorable outcome
Primary Analysis	Negative	Positive	Negative	Negative
Early Recurrence		HD 2% LD 1% PLC 1%	Heparin 4% No heparin 4%	RX 1% PLC 1%
Hemorrhage- Intracranial	No difference	No difference	Significantly increased with heparin	Significantly increased with danaparoid
Hemorrhage- Major Extracranial	No difference	No difference	Significantly increased with heparin	Significantly increased with danaparoid

HD -high dose; LD - low dose; PLC-placebo; RX - treatment

is overwhelmingly negative. The value of heparin in some yet-to-be-defined subgroup of patients from some yet-to-be-defined dose or preparation remains to be proven. A dangerous drug like heparin should not be used unless it efficacy is established.

References

1. Marsh EE 3rd, Adams HP Jr, Biller J, et al. Use of antithrombotic drugs in the treatment of acute ischemic stroke:a survey of neurologists in practice in the United States. *Neurology* 1989;39:1631-1634.

2. Sandercock PAG, van den Belt AGM, Lindley RI, et al. Antithrombotic therapy in acute ischemic stroke; an overview of the completed randomised trials. *J Neurol Neurosurg Psychiatr* 1993;56:17-25.

3. Sherman DG, Dyken ML Jr, Gent M, et al. Antithrombotic therapy for cerebrovascular disorders. An update. *Chest* 1995;108(4 Suppl):444S-456S.

4. Duke RJ, Bloch RF, Turpie AGG, et al. Intravenous heparin for the prevention of stroke progression in acute partial stroke. *Ann Int Med* 1986;105:825-828.

5. Hirsch J, Raschke R, Warkentin TE, et al. Heparin: Mechanism of action, pharmacokinetcs, dosing considerations, monitoring efficacy, and safety. *Chest* 1995;108(4 Suppl):258S-275S.

6. Lensing WA, Prins MH, Davidson BL, et al. Treatment of deep venous thrombosis with low-moloecular weight heparins. *Arch Int Med* 1995;155:601-607.

7. Kay R, Wong KS, Yu YL, et al. Low-molecular weight heparin for the treatment of acute ischemic stroke. *N Engl J Med* 1995;333:1588-1593.

8. Agnelli G, Iorio A, Renga C, et al. Prolonged antithrombin activity of low-molecular weight heparins. Clinical implications for the treatment of thromboembolic diseases. *Circualation* 1995;92:2819-2824.

9. Freedman MD, Leese P, Prasad R, et al. An evaluation of the biological response to Fraxiparine, (a low molecular weight heparin) in the healthy individual. *J Clin Pharm* 1990;30:720-727.

10. Hommel M. Fraxiparine in ischemic stroke study.Cerebrovascular Diseases 1998;8(Suppl 4):64.

11. International Stroke Trial Collaborative Group. The International Stroke Trial(IST): A randomized trial of aspirin, subcutaneous heparin, both, or neither among 19,435 patients with acute ischemic stroke. *Lancet* 1997;349:1569-1581.

12. Turpie AGG, Robinson JG, Doyle DJ, et al. Comparison of high-dose with low-dose subcutaneous heparin to prevent left ventricular mural thrombus in patients with acute transmural anterior myocardial infarction. *N Engl J Med* 1989;320:352-357.

13. Turpie AGG, Gent M, Cote R, et al. A low-molecular-weight heparinoid compared with unfractionated heparin in the prevention of deep vein thrombosis in patients with acute ischemic stroke. *Ann Int Med* 1992;117:353-357.

14. The Publications Committee for the Trial of ORG 10172 in Acute Stroke Treatment (TOAST) Investigators. Low molecular weight heparinoid, ORG

10172 (danaparoid), and outcome after acute ischemic stroke. A random-ized controlled trial. *JAMA* 1998;279:1265-1272.

15. Rothrock JF, Hart RG. Antithrombotic therapy in cerebrovascular disease. *Ann Int Med* 1991;115:885-895.

16. Camerlingo M, Casto L, Censori B, et al. Immediate anticoagulation with heparin for first-ever ischemic stroke in the carotid artery territories ob-served within 5 hours of onset. *Arch Neurol* 1994;51:462-467.

17. CAST (Chinese Acute Stroke Trial) Collaborative Committee. CAST: ran-domized placebo-controlled trial of early aspirin use in 20 000 patients with acute ischemic stroke. *Lancet* 1997;49:1641-1649.

18. Caplan LR. Stroke treatment-promising but still struggling. *JAMA* 1998;279:1304-1306.

Beyond Diffusion: Imaging Measurements of Cerebral Blood Flow and Metabolism

Chapter 20

Overview

Justin A. Zivin, MD, PhD and
Marc Fisher, MD

At the present time, there are divergent opinions concerning the value of diffusion weighted imaging (DWI) and perfusion imaging (PI) magnetic resonance techniques to evaluate acute stroke therapies for clinical trial purposes. In this chapter, we will present both sides of the argument.

Advocate–MF

The availability of two new magnetic resonance imaging (MRI) techniques, DWI and PI, provides novel ways to evaluate stroke patients very rapidly after onset and to potentially monitor the effects of therapeutic interventions. In animal stroke models, it is well documented that DWI and PI can detect the ischemic region within minutes after stroke onset and follow its evolution when serial studies are performed. These two complementary MRI studies provide information about the reduction of blood flow to the ischemic region and where blood flow declines have caused alterations of ion and water homeostasis, leading to the accumulation of cytotoxic edema. Animal studies with these MRI techniques can also be used to evaluate *in-vivo* the effects of thrombolytic and neuroprotective therapies to promote reperfusion and to reduce the extent of the ischemic injury. The *in-vivo* information provided is complementary to the traditional endpoint used in animal stroke studies, reduction of post-mortem infarct volume. Surprising results, such as a delayed reduction of ischemic injury,

From: Choi D, Dacey RG, Hsu CY, Powers WJ. *Cerebrovascular Disease: Momentum at the End of the Second Millennium.* Armonk, NY: Futura Publishing Company, Inc., © 2002.

several hours after initiation of therapy, have been observed with a glycine antagonist by two research groups. This type of treatment effect could not be discerned, if only post-mortem infarct volume measurements were obtained. With thrombolytic therapy in embolic stoke models, the relationship between reperfusion effects on PI and effects on ischemic lesion growth on DWI can be correlated to demonstrate that reperfusion does in deed affect the development of ischemic lesions *in-vivo*. DWI and PI studies are now used in many centers along with post-mortem infarct size reduction and behavioral evaluations during the preclinical assessment of purported acute stroke therapies to determine if application in patients is appropriate.

Human applications of DWI and PI are accelerating with the increasing availability of MRI units capable of performing ultrafast imaging that is necessary for the routine acquisition of high quality images. With PI, the ischemic region can be identified and in the majority of stroke patients the size of the hypoperfused region is larger than the size of the DWI abnormality when the studies are obtained within 6 hours of onset. This region of so-called "diffusion-perfusion mismatch" may in part identify that portion of the ischemic territory most likely to respond to therapeutic intervention, because it is a region where cerebral blood flow is impaired, but diffusion abnormalities have not yet occurred. As treatment trials using DWI and PI are performed this hypothesis can be tested. It is clear from several studies that without therapeutic intervention, the size of the ischemic region on DWI will increase in most stroke patients and that this evolution of ischemic lesion volumes occurs up to and beyond 24 hours after stroke onset. Currently, DWI and PI provide the earliest imaging capability to determine the location, and information about the age of acute focal ischemic lesions. This capability to rapidly localize where a stroke is evolving is important when stroke subtyping for clinical trials is considered. For example, if a drug with no effect on white matter ischemia is being developed, then patients with lacunar stroke should not be randomized for inclusion in the trial. Clinically, distinguishing lacunar from cortical strokes may be difficult in some cases. This distinction can be easily made in most cases with DWI/PI. Patients with brainstem and cerebellar strokes are not included in some acute stroke trials, because of difficulties with adapting clinical outcome measures to posterior circulation strokes. The ability of DWI/PI to rapidly localize could be used to exclude posterior circulation stroke or to include them, if an imaging outcome will be used primarily to assess therapeutic response (as will be described). Concerns have arisen that using DWI/PI as the only early imaging study will not provide the means to accurately identify hemorrhagic stroke. The paramagnetic effects of fresh blood within intracerebral hemorrhages should theoretically induce susceptibility effects and allow for the relatively easy identification of hemorrhages. Preliminary studies have supported this hypothesis, but larger studies with direct comparisons of hemorrhage identification by MRI and CT are needed. In studies of most neuroprotectants, the precise identification of hemorrhage may not be critical. Conversely, in thrombolytic trials where hemorrhage identification is critical, computed tomography (CT) could be included in the early imaging protocol until the presumed diagnostic accuracy of MRI is confirmed.

An important but unresolved question remains: what is the utility of DWI/PI in clinical, acute stroke trials? The information provided by DWI/PI in animal stroke models has encouraged clinical stroke trialists to consider using these MRI modalities for stroke drug assessment in patients. Currently, the results of only one moderately sized trial, that with Citicoline has been presented at meetings. This study had a 24-hour enrollment window and was stopped early before the prospectively defined sample size was obtained. The preliminary results are encouraging in that beneficial effects on MRI parameters reflected clinical benefit. This treatment effect occurred only in patients treated within 12 hours of stroke onset. This is an outcome with biologic plausibility because later treatment is less likely to affect lesion evolution, the main MRI endpoint of the trial. The endpoint used in this trial, the effect of treatment on ischemic lesion evolution between the baseline, pretreatment ischemic lesion volume on DWI and late lesion volume 3 months later on T2 imaging is currently the approach suggested by myself and colleagues to measure therapeutic response. This endpoint was chosen because of substantial information from natural history studies that suggests that early ischemic lesions depicted by DWI are likely to enlarge considerably in most cases when compared to T2 ischemic lesion volumes at 1-3 months after stroke onset. As mentioned previously, the majority, but not all patients will have a smaller DWI lesion volume than PI determined hypoperfused volume during the first few hours after stroke onset. This group represents approximately 70% of stroke patients studied within 6 hours of onset and likely represents the best target for acute stroke patients, while patients with equal DWI and hypoperfused volumes or larger DWI than hypoperfused volumes may have less chance to respond to therapy. This hypothesis will have to be tested in future clinical stroke trials with adequate numbers of patients enrolled.

What is the current status of DWI/PI based acute stroke trials? There are at least four phase II or phase III acute stroke trials that include these MRI techniques in the trial, including both neuroprotective and thrombolytic agents. Other trials are being planned. The trials currently being performed and planned should help considerably to determine the usefulness of DWI/PI in acute stroke drug development. Currently, we can only hypothesize that they should be helpful to determine if a drug affecting ischemic lesion evolution or promoting reperfusion will then affect clinical outcome. The predominant proof of this concept will come from a phase III trial with an adequate sample size that demonstrates a significant effect towards improving clinical outcome on an accepted rating scale that is correlated with a significant effect on lesion evolution by early DWI and late T2 imaging. Such an outcome should clearly relate clinical benefit to an affect on the ultimate size of the ischemic lesion. Another potential role for DWI/PI studies is in phase III clinical trials.

For example, if an intervention designed to reduce infarct size by preclinical assessment has no effect at all on ischemic lesion evolution determined by early and late MRI studies, then it is very unlikely that it would achieve significant improvement effects on clinical outcome scales. Current information suggests that appropriately targeted stroke populations with less than 100 patients per treatment group will be needed to perform an adequately powered phase II study. A number that is considerably smaller than the 300-400 patients per group widely used in trials with strictly a clinical outcome measure that are designed to have enough power to detect a drug treatment effect. Conversely, a significant treatment effect on ischemic lesion evolution determined by MRI studies should provide some added confidence to the costly and time consuming performance of a large phase III trial. MRI-based acute stroke drug development could provide a means to evaluate potential therapies in a more cost-effective and expeditious manner, if current ongoing studies clarify the utility of imaging supported stroke drug development. The ongoing MRI-based trials will conclude during the next 1-2 years and hopefully confirm or refute the hypotheses generated about the utility of DWI-PI in acute stroke drug development. Additionally, as in traditional clinical outcome-based stroke trials, much unanticipated information will likely be derived from these trials that will help to refine and perhaps expand their role in the future when we begin to move into the era of multitherapy trials. Hopefully, MRI and other imaging technologies, better therapeutic interventions and carefully designed and implemented acute stroke trials will improve our capability to develop effective acute stroke therapies.

Skeptic – JAZ

Although DWI/PI is a potentially exciting advance in MRI technology, a good deal of work will be required to prove its value for clinical trials purposes. The histological or biochemical basis of image abnormalities is not yet known in any detail, so it is unclear what is actually detected by the abnormal signals. Lacking a theoretical understanding, it is essential to develop empiric methods for utilizing this tool. The only way that it will be possible to prove the utility of such empiric observations is to conduct detailed clinical trials of the technique. This has not yet been accomplished. As a result, it is too early to say whether DWI/PI will be useful in clinical trials.

Ultimately, the regulatory agencies that are responsible for approving drugs will require evidence that a new form of treatment improves neurologic function. This is a standard that is also widely accepted within the medical community. This is a behavioral measure, and until it is shown that DWI/PI is a reliable surrogate, it will not be usable as a primary outcome variable for a pivotal phase III trial.

At this time, it remains uncertain whether DWI/PI will even be useful as a marker for phase II protocol development purposes. It is unknown whether the variance of the image volumes is less than that for clinical rating scales. In fact, it is probable that DWI/PI is less efficient than clinical rating scales for defining neurological deficits. It is well established that there is a relatively poor correlation between lesion volumes, as defined by CT or histological studies, and neurological deficits after a stroke. The reason is that a small lesion in a critical place causes more functional loss than a large region of tissue destruction in a relatively silent brain region. There is no reason to expect that MRI methods will be superior to these other types of images.

The coefficient of variation of the abnormal images may be smaller than that of clinical rating scales, but that remains to be established. Therefore, assertions that fewer patients will be required to establish a trend in a phase II study are not warranted at the present time.

A realistic goal for the developers of DWI/PI technology may be to develop new types of inclusion or exclusion criteria that can be established rapidly, before treatment is initiated. For example, it might be possible for DWI/PI to define the age of a lesion. If the technique is sufficiently accurate shortly after ischemia onset, it might be valuable for distinguishing new from old abnormalities. Also, if a distinctive signal pattern can be found that indicates that a stroke is very severe or likely to resolve without treatment, it might be helpful for selecting a patient cohort that can benefit from therapy. Examples of such anomalies that are detectable with CT technology are intracerebral hemorrhages and the "dense middle cerebral artery sign" which is associated with the presence of a large clot in that artery. Both indicate lesions that cannot be effectively managed with thrombolytic drugs. The sensitivity of MRI for detection of hemorrhage or clot is not known.

The usefulness of DWI/PI as a method for identifying abnormal blood flow shortly after the onset of ischemia is unproven, although advocates cite this as a major advance. This capability is not unique to the DWI/PI. A number of technologies can do so, such as single photon emission CT (SPECT), positron-emission tomography (PET), and xenon inhalation cerebral blood flow measurement methods. In some instances, these older methods can provide a quantitative survey of regional blood flow whereas DWI/PI , as it is currently used, provides only qualitative information. The older cerebral blood flow measurement devices lack meaningful clinical applicability, and, in the absence of compelling evidence to the contrary, it is unlikely that the DWI/PI blood flow detection capability will provide information that is important for making clinical decisions. Furthermore, none of these methods has been proven to reliably define salvageable ischemic brain tissue and that is also true for DWI – PI mismatch.

Aside from the theoretical issues, there are a number of practical problems that will discourage adoption of DWI/PI methods. These are mainly related to the need to administer drugs rapidly to stroke victims. Although the scans can be performed relatively rapidly, making sure that the patients are protected from materials that can be dangerous in high magnetic fields, and the delays associated with the rather cumbersome process of maneuvering patients into and out of the machines is an impediment. Acute stroke victims are usually elderly and may be gravely ill with concomitant problems at the time of their initial presentation. Placing such people in the relatively inaccessible interior of the MRI scanner can interfere with urgent patient care. Also, it has not been proven that any sizeable number of patients can be recruited and scanned within the three-hour limit required for effective thrombolytic therapy.

Some clinical trials of acute stroke therapies have included DWI/PI studies in at least part of the patient population. If these investigations prove that the technique is clinically useful and better than less expensive strategies, resistance to its adoption should end. However, the advocates bear the burden of proof in demonstrating the importance of the techniques. Testimonials without solid evidence will not suffice.

Chapter 21

Measuring Oxygen Saturation Using Magnetic Resonance Imaging

E. Mark Haacke, PhD, Weili Lin, MD,
Benjamin Lee, MD, Daniel Kido, MD,
Chung Y. Hsu, MD, and
William J. Powers, MD

Introduction

Neuroimaging has become a major component of assessing tissue damage noninvasively following ischemic insults. Currently, a variety of imaging modalities exist to study this problem and each offers some unique capability to examine specific pathophysiological conditions associated with stroke including tissue perfusion, morphology, and metabolism with some overlap between modalities. In the case of computed tomography (CT), images with high sensitivity and specificity in detecting acute hemorrhage can be obtained. Unfortunately, CT offers limited soft tissue contrast and fails to reveal the true extent of the stroke in the early time period. However, the easy accessibility, short data acquisition times, and the distinct ability in revealing acute hemorrhage have made CT the primary imaging tool for stroke management. The ability to visualize acute hemorrhage is of critical importance in determining the treatment that the patient ultimately receives.

Positron-emission tomography (PET) or single proton emission CT (SPECT) have low spatial resolution and yield limited anatomical

From: Choi D, Dacey RG, Hsu CY, Powers WJ. *Cerebrovascular Disease: Momentum at the End of the Second Millennium.* Armonk, NY: Futura Publishing Company, Inc., © 2002.

information. Nevertheless, both are routinely utilized to provide information associated with cerebral hemodynamics such as cerebral blood volume (CBV), cerebral blood flow (CBF). PET provides quantitative measurements of oxygen metabolism as well. Extensive research on animals has demonstrated that the alterations of cerebral hemodynamics and oxygen metabolism are both dynamic and complex in nature particularly during the acute state after ischemic insult. The knowledge of this information could reveal the status of the affected tissue.[1-5] Using PET, many investigators have observed that the oxygen extraction fraction (OEF) is first increased during ischemia in an attempt to maintain the cerebral mateabolic rate for oxygen (CMRO$_2$), in response to the reduction of CBF followed by a decline in both OEF and CMRO$_2$ concurrent with a low CBF. These dynamic changes of oxygen metabolism and cerebral hemodynamics further suggest that the regions with increased OEF represent the penumbra whereas the regions with subsequent reduction of OEF and CMRO$_2$ reflect tissue with irreversible damage.

Despite the recognition of the importance of cerebral hemodynamics and oxygen metabolism, none of this information is usually taken into account in the determination of the patients' treatment nor used for patient management. This could simply be explained by the fact that PET is an inconvenient and expensive procedure that is not widely available. These limitations make it difficult to establish the relationship between changes in cerebral hemodynamics and oxygen metabolism with the patient outcomes.

Magnetic resonance imaging (MRI) has made significant advances in evaluating stroke. Today, diffusion weighted images (DWI) are being used clinically to help diagnose acute ischemia.[6] In addition, MRI is able to noninvasively study the major vessels and show any major stenoses or blockages of blood flow. Efforts have also been made to measure CBF,[7] blood volume,[8-12] and oxygen saturation of the major vessels[13] and brain parenchyma.[14] The focus of this chapter will be on oxygen saturation measurements and visualizing changes in tissue associated with changes in local venous blood volume and/or oxygen saturation. In this chapter, clinical applications of a new, high resolution, BOLD (blood oxygen level dependent) venographic imaging approach will be presented.

Magnetic Resonance Concepts

MR imaging provides high soft tissue contrast which depends on a number of different tissue properties. These properties are referred to as spin density (ρ), the T1 or longitudinal relaxation time, and the

T2 or transverse relaxation time. Gradient echo sequences can be used to probe two other quantities of interest: the T2* relaxation time and the phase (θ). For blood, both these quantities depend on the local oxygen saturation through its effect on the local magnetic field.[15-17] Changes in the blood's phase or T2* can lead to signal loss, and are referred to as intravascular effects. As the magnetic field inside the blood vessel changes, so does the field outside it. This leads to a further loss of signal referred to as the extravascular effect.

Intravascular T2*

Deoxyhemoglobin (Hb) is paramagnetic in nature. For this reason, the magnetic field changes (increases) as the amount of Hb in the blood changes. If Y is used to refer to the fractional amount of oxyhemoglobin (HbO$_2$) present in the blood, then 1-Y represents the fractional amount of Hb. In MRI, the signal is proportional to exp(-TE/T2*) where TE is the echo time and T2* the transverse relaxation time. Finding the signal loss from blood in humans at 1.5T requires finding T2* as a function of Y. Using R2*=1/T2* and R_{20}=1/T_{20}*, it is known that

$$R_2^* (Y) = R_{20}^* + 14(1-Y)/sec \qquad [1]$$

where $R_{20}^* = 5$/sec and $0.7 \leq Y \leq 1.0$. The numerical values come from measurements in the human aorta and vena cava.[18] It is difficult to perform these measurements on smaller vessels when fast flow is present, but it is important to at least characterize T2*(Y) when attempting to estimate signal changes. If T2*(Y) can be accurately measured, then the oxygen saturation Y can be extracted from the data.

Intravascular Phase (θ)

Another route to assess Y is to find the local magnetic field $\Delta B(Y)$ within a vessel.[13] For a vessel parallel to the main field B_0, the dependence on Y is given by

$$\Delta B(Y) = 4\pi\chi_{do}B_0 \text{ Hct } (1-Y)/3 \qquad [2]$$

The phase as a function of echo time and Y is given by

$$\theta = -\gamma \Delta B(Y) T_E \qquad [3]$$

With a hematocrit (Hct) of 0.4, χ_{do} = 0.18 ppm, and γ = 2.67×10^8 rad/sec/T, the phase is approximately

$$\theta = -40\pi(1-Y)T_E \qquad [4]$$

Using specially designed sequences, θ can be found for a given vessel. It has been shown for pial vessels in the brain that Y=0.544 +/− 0.029.[13]

Intravoxel Effects

As discussed earlier, the phase of the blood changes with Y. This will cause signal loss when a blood vessel occupies only a fraction of a voxel. This partial volume effect arises because the MR signal is vectorial in nature. The sum of brain parenchymal signal with blood signal has a complicated oscillatory dependence on Y and an amplitude dependence on λv, the fractional venous blood volume. If the blood volume fraction is small compared to that from brain parenchyma, then this partial volume effect plays less of a role compared to the signal loss from extravascular effects.

Despite this complicated behavior, there is one aspect of this effect that can be used to visualize small venous vessels in the brain.[19] If a high resolution scan is run so that the phase of the veins is roughly π, then, apart from T2* effects, the signal from the brain will be roughly 1- λv and that from the venous blood will be $-\lambda v$ yielding a reduced total signal of 1-2 λv. High resolution here implies that the vessel occupies a large fraction of the pixel and therefore λv may approach 0.5. This suggests that the veins can cause a dramatic signal loss under the right circumstances. The resulting images are referred to as High Resolution, BOLD, Venographic (HRBV) images.

Extravascular Signal Loss

Even if there is no signal from blood, the local magnetic field caused by the Hb will produce a signal dephasing in the brain parenchyma outside the vessels.[17] For a random system of vessels,[20] this term depends directly on λv and 1-Y via

$$R_2^* = R_{20}^* + 40\pi \lambda v (1-Y) \qquad [5]$$

By performing experiments which change only Y or λv, the change in R_2^* can be measured and the remaining unknown found from

$$\Delta R2^* = 40\pi \ \Delta \ (\lambda\nu(1\text{-}Y)) \qquad\qquad [6]$$

If blood signal is suppressed, this will be the only source of signal loss.

Materials and Methods

Human Studies

The cancellation of veins with background tissue is best accomplished with a long echo time (40 ms), three-dimensional, fully velocity compensated gradient echo sequence at 1.5 T (VISION whole body imager, Siemens Medical Systems, Erlangen, Germany). High-resolution scans are most revealing. Given the fact that pial veins are roughly 0.5 to 1mm in diameter, we chose to fix the resolution at 0.5 mm × 1.0 mm in plane and 2 mm through plane. Any smaller voxel size causes a significant loss in signal-to-noise. A slab of 9.6 cm is usually excited and a flip angle of 20° is used. With TR = 60 ms, the total imaging time is about 10 minutes for 48 slices. (Reducing the coverage to 6.4 cm with 32 slices reduces the scan time to less than 7 min.) The matrix size is 192 phase encoding steps by 512 read points using a rectangular field of view of 192 mm x 256 mm. These HRBV scans were run both on volunteers (Institutional Review Board-approved consent forms were signed by all volunteers) and on patients with venous lesions. Processing to enhance venous vessels is performed as discussed in Reichenbach et al.[19]

Animal Studies

To evaluate tissue signal changes as a function of oxygen saturation, rat brains were studied under a variety of physiological conditions. Male Long-Evans rats weighing 275-350 g were used. General anesthesia was induced with a single intraperitoneal injection of pentobarbital (30 mg/kg). Both the right femoral artery and vein were cannulated with PE-50 polyethylene catheters (Becton-Dickinson, Sparks, MD) to obtain arterial samples (Hct assays, blood gas analysis) and to deliver drugs. Tracheotomy and tracheal cannulation were performed to provide ventilation (Harvard Apparatus Inc., South Natick, MA) after the animals were transferred to the MR scanner. An intravenous neuromuscular blocking agent was administered (pancuronium hydrochloride, 0.1 mg/kg/hour), and appropriate mechanical ventilation was provided.

The right jugular vein was also exposed midway between the clavicle and the mandible and cannulated with a heparinized PE-50 catheter so that jugular blood samples could be collected. All jugular venous samples were collected anaerobically via the combined effects of capillary action and gravity drainage into heparinized glass tubes

(Chiron Diagnostics Co., Norwood, MA). We have extensive experience in collecting jugular blood samples and have demonstrated that a good correlation of oxygen saturation can be obtained between blood samples collected from the jugular vein and the superior sagittal sinus suggesting that the oxygen saturation obtained in the jugular vein can be used as a good indicator for the cerebral venous oxygen saturation.[12] All blood samples were analyzed less than 3 minutes after collection with a blood gas analyzer (Ciba-Corning Diagnostics, Medfield, MA) in order to maintain strict anaerobic conditions during the sampling process and minimize time dependent alterations of pH and blood gas tension. For each blood sample, parameters measured included pH, pCO_2, and pO_2.

All animal images were acquired on the same 1.5 T whole body VISION system with a gradient strength of 25 mT/m and a ramp time of 0.6 msec to the maximum gradient. A small, custom made, receive only radiofrequency coil and a 2D gradient echo FLASH sequence was used to acquire all images. First order velocity compensation was used along both the slice select and frequency encoding directions. The imaging parameters were: TR = 83 msec; TE = 40 msec; slice thickness = 2 mm; field-of-view = 60 x 60 mm^2; flip angle = 40°; and matrix size = 80*128. Twenty scans (each taking 2 minutes to collect) were acquired continuously with rats in the baseline state, and 50 scans were then acquired after a specific animal manipulation (which lasted 5 minutes) including hypoxemic hypoxia and hemodilution. The average differences in signal intensity from these images were used to calculate $\Delta R2^*$ in the brain parenchyma.

Results and Discussion

The effects of venous blood signal cancellation in a normal patient and in two patients with venous abnormalities will be presented. Although these results are not quantitative, they do reveal any abnormal major and micro-vascular changes in tissue. The dependence of brain signal on both λv and Y is demonstrated under controlled conditions in an animal model. These results are indicative of what will be required technically to accomplish quantitative measurements of oxygen saturation in humans.

Human Studies

A representative HRBV image from a patient with no known history of cerebral vascular disease is shown in Figure 1 to demonstrate the normal pattern of cerebral venous structures. This image was obtained by post-processing the individual slices after which a

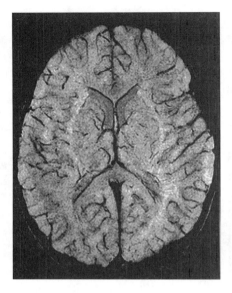

Figure 1. A high resolution, venographic image showing the major veins in a 1 cm slice of the brain in the region of the ventricles. Both the central and peripheral draining veins are shown.

minimum intensity projection over five adjacent slices was performed. All venous structures are shown as low signal intensity in the processed image.

An example of the clinical utility of this technique is illustrated by the following example. A patient presented with multiple hemangiomas. Little information was present on the T1-weighted spin echo image but a low resolution T2*-weighted echo planar scan (Figure 2A) did show two hemangiomas. However, the HRBV scan (Figure 2B) showed, in addition, multiple lesions.

Another study of a patient with a complex venous malformation reveals how even changes in the microvasculature can be seen with the HRBV approach (Figure 3). The major affected vessels are shown in the post-contrast T1-weighted scan (Figure 3A). Multiple additional abnormal vessels are shown around the major vessels. The large dark regions (the vessels) in the venography study are surrounded by a reduction of tissue signal. These obvious signal losses may be caused from an increase in venous blood volume (ie, $\lambda\nu$ increases) or a decrease in Y (ie, an increase in deoxyhemoglobin, 1-Y).

Animal Studies

Hemodilution

Theory indicates that R2* and, hence, signal loss, will depend on the product of Hct, $\lambda\nu$ and (1-Y). The change in R2* should be directly proportional to ΔHct if both $\lambda\nu$ and 1-Y remain constant. In order to

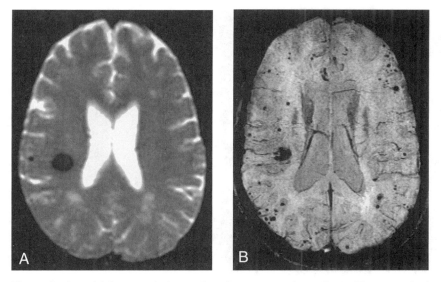

Figure 2. A rapid, low resolution, echo-planar scan of a patient with suspected hemangiomas (**A**). Two lesions in the right hemisphere are clearly visible. A minimum intensity projection of 5 slices from the HRBV study demonstrates many additional hemangiomas (**B**).

validate the signal dependence on Hct, normovolemic hemodilution was achieved by withdrawing either 3 cc (mild group) or 6 cc (moderate group) of blood from the arterial catheter at a constant rate of 1.5 - 2.0 cc/min. Concurrently, a sterile 5% solution of serum albumin in isotonic sodium chloride was infused intravenously as surrogate plasma at 3 cc/min. The addition of albumin to the saline serves to maintain the oncotic pressure of the hemodiluted blood and circulating volume and, therefore, prevents hypotension. $\Delta R2^*$ as a function of time prior to and after HD is shown in Figure 4, for both groups. The mild HD group shows a smaller $R2^*$ reduction when compared to the moderate HD group in good agreement with the current understanding of the BOLD effect. Furthermore, when quantitation of the BOLD effect is desired, the results shown here underscore the importance of the need to take the variation of Hct into account.

Hypoxemic Hypoxia

In contrast to hemodilution, the dependence of $\Delta R2^*$ on signal loss can also be shown by changing Y via an alteration of blood oxygenation. When Hct and $\lambda\nu$ remain constant, the change in signal is anticipated to be linearly dependent on the change in Y. In order to test this hypothesis, graded hypoxemic hypoxia was induced by an alteration

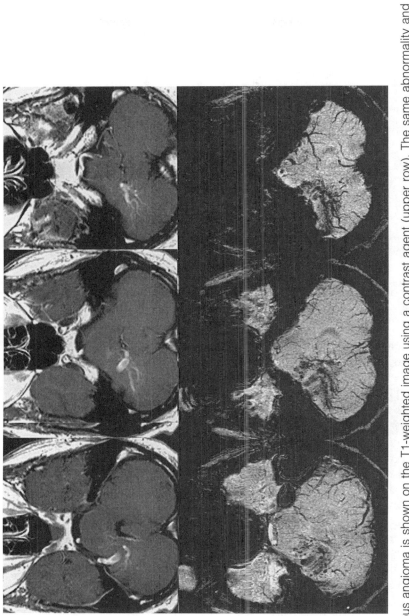

Figure 3. A venous angioma is shown on the T1-weighted image using a contrast agent (upper row). The same abnormality and numerous additional vessels were shown without contrast agent on the HRBV images (bottom row).

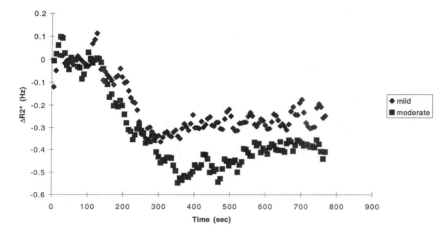

Figure 4. The changes of R2* (ΔR2*) in the brain parenchyma in response to graded acute hemodilution are shown. A reduction of R2* is observed immediately after hemodilution suggesting a positive BOLD effect and an increase in MR signal intensity. The degree of change in R2* depends on the degree of hematocrit reduction. The moderate group (solid boxes) shows larger R2* changes when compared with the mild group (solid diamonds). This is consistent with the current understanding of the BOLD mechanisms.

of the ratio of nitrogen to oxygen in the inspired gas mixture. Both arterial and jugular venous blood samples were collected before and after each episode. An effective change of Yb (Yb=αYa+(1-α)Yb and α=0.75)[21] in the brain parenchyma was calculated by a linear weighted sum of the changes of both arterial and venous blood oxygen saturation[12] while taking into account the volume distribution of cerebral arterial (1-α) and venous blood volume (α). Subsequently, ΔR2* measurements in the brain parenchyma (in response to the induced hypoxemic hypoxia) were correlated against the changes of Y. The results are shown in Figure 5. Notice a general linear relationship exists when changes of arterial and venous oxygen saturation were correlated with ΔR2*, respectively, but neither one exhibits a strong correlation. In contrast, a stronger correlation was obtained when ΔR2* was correlated with the effective oxygen saturation changes of both arterial and venous blood. These findings are perhaps not surprising since both arterial and venous blood become desaturated in responding to hypoxemic hypoxia and it follows that the signal changes are best represented by the combined effects of both pools of blood.

Conclusions

The ability to visualize the effects of oxygen saturation levels in venous blood in MR images and to quantify oxygen saturation in the

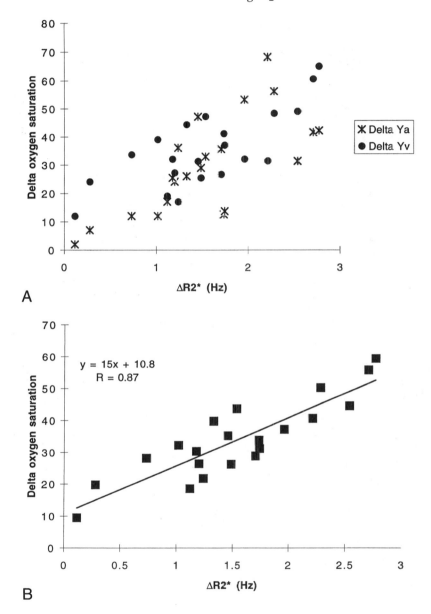

Figure 5. The changes of R2* in the brain parenchyma in response to hypox-emic hypoxia are correlated to the changes of oxygen saturation measured from the arterial and jugular venous blood samples, respectively. Correlating R2* changes with oxygen saturation changes obtained from either arterial or jugular venous blood samples alone, a linear relationship is obtained but neither of them are strong (**A**). However, a stronger linear relationship is obtained when R2* changes are correlated with the weighted sum of both arterial and jugular venous blood oxygen saturation changes (**B**).

brain have become possible through utilization of the BOLD phenomena. This approach opens a new avenue for utilizing MR to investigate oxygen metabolism changes in response to the pathophysiological alterations associated with cerebrovascular disease. In this paper, we have demonstrated that the cerebral venous structures can be visualized with HRBV, an imaging method based on BOLD effects. Specifically, we have shown that vascular lesions can be visualized using HRBV. In both clinical cases, the true extent of abnormal venous structures can only be observed in HRBV images.

Even though the anatomical aspects of the venous vessels and their patterns in association with cerebral venous disease were the main focus of this paper, the fact that the underlying mechanisms of HRBV imaging depend on both cerebral blood oxygen saturation and echo time makes it possible to utilize this method to assess information associated with local oxygen extraction fraction. In other words, the absence of regional cerebral venous structures in HRBV does not necessarily translate to the absence of vessels but rather, the images can be used as an indication of a reduction of oxygen extraction fraction locally. This is because the reduction of OEF would increase the oxygen saturation in the vessels and, therefore, require a much longer TE to develop the desired signal cancellation, between the vessels and the adjacent brain parenchyma (see, for example, Eq. (4)). This property could potentially be applicable in the study of stroke patients. For example, we might hypothesize that when an increase of conspicuity of venous structures is observed in association with a peri-infarcted region, this could suggest that the adjacent brain tissues are still metabolically active (ie, no decrease in OEF occurs). This implies a low cerebral blood oxygen saturation, hence, making the vessels visible using HRBV. In contrast, when the venous structures are absent in a peri-infarcted region, it could be indicative of tissue infarction since a low oxygen extraction is anticipated, resulting in an increase in cerebral venous blood oxygen saturation. Further clinical studies utilizing this BOLD contrast mechanism are needed to expand our understanding of the pathophysiological conditions associated with cerebrovascular disease as we enter the 21st century.

References

1. Heiss WD, Graf R, Lottgen J, et al. Repeat positron emission tomographic studies in transient middle cerebral artery occlusion in cats: Residual perfusion and efficacy of postischemic reperfusion. *JCBFM* 1997;17:388-400.
2. Marchal G, Beaudouin V, Rioux P, et al. Prolonged persistence of substantial volumes of potentially viable brain tissue after stroke: A correlation PET-CT study with voxel-based data analysis. *Stroke* 1992;27:599-606.

3. Touzani O, Young AR, Derlon JM, et al. Sequential studies of severely hypometabolic tissue volumes after permanent middle cerebral artery occlusion: A positron emission tomographic investigation in anesthetized baboons. *Stroke* 1995;26:2112-2119.

4. Weiss WD, Graf R, Fujita T, et al. Early detection of irreversibly damaged ischemic tissue by flumazenil positron emission tomography in cats. *Stroke* 1997;28:2045-2052.

5. Furlan M, Marchal G, Viader F, et al. Spontaneous neurological recovery after stroke and the fate of the ischemic penumbra. *Ann Neurol* 1996;40:216-226.

6. Warach S, Li W, Rontahl M, et al. Clinical outcome in ischemic stroke predicted by early diffusion weighted and perfusion magnetic resonance imaging: A preliminary analysis. *JBCFM* 1996;16:53-59.

7. Rosen BR, Belliveau JW, Vevea JM, et al. Perfusion imaging with NMR contrast agents. *Magn Reson Med* 1990;14:249-265.

8. Rosen BR, Belliveau JW, Aronen HJ, et al. Susceptibility contrast imaging of cerebral blood volume: Human experience. *Magn Reson Med* 1991;22:293-299.

9. Schwarzbauer C, Syha J, Haase A. Quantification of regional blood volumes using rapid T1 mapping. *Magn Reson Med* 1993;29:709-712.

10. Moseley ME, Chew WM, White DL, et al. Hypercarbia-induced changes in cerebral blood volume in the cat: A ^1H MRI and intravascular contrast agent study. *Magn Reson Med* 1992;23:21-30.

11. Kuppusamy K, Lin W, Cizek G, et al. In Vivo regional cerebral blood volume: Quantitative assessment with 3D T1- weighted pre- and post contrast MR imaging. *Radiology* 1996;201:106-112.

12. Lin W, Paczynski RP, Kuppusamy K, et al. Quantitative Measurements of Regional Cerebral Blood Volume Using MRI in Rats: Effects of Arterial Carbon Dioxide Tension and Mannitol. *Magn Reson Med* 1997;38:420-428.

13. Haacke EM, Lai S, Reichenbach JR, et al. In vivo measurement of blood oxygen saturation using magnetic resonance imaging. *Human Brain Mapping* 1997;5:341-346.

14. Lin W, Paczynski RP, Celik A, et al. Experimental hypoxemic hypoxia: Changes in R2* of brain parenchyma accurately reflect the combined effects of changes in arterial and cerebral venous oxygen saturation. *Magn Reson Med* 1998;39:474-481.

15. Ogawa S, Lee TM. Magnetic resonance imaging of blood vessels at high field: In vivo and in vitro measurements and image simulation. *Magn Reson Med* 1990;16:9-18.

16. Ogawa S, Lee TM, Kay AR, et al. Brain magnetic resonance imaging with contrast dependent on blood oxygenation. *Proc Natl Acad Sci USA* 1990;87:9868-9872.

17. Ogawa S, Menon RS, Tank DW, et al. Functional brain mapping by blood oxygenation level-dependent contrast magnetic resonance imaging. *Biophysical J* 1993;64:803-812.

18. Li D, Wang Y, Waight DJ. Blood oxygen saturation assessment in vivo using T2* estimation. *MRM* 1998;39:685-690.

19. Reichenbach JR, Venkatesan R, Schillinger DJ, et al. Small vessels in the human brain: MR venography with deoxyhemoglobin as an intrinsic contrast agent. *Radiology* 1997;204:272-277.

20. Yablonskiy DA, Haacke EM. Theory of NMR signal behavior in magnetically inhomogeneous tissue: The static dephasing regime. *Magn Reson Med* 1994;32:746-763.

21. Pollard V, Prough DS, DeMelo AE, et al. The influence of carbon dioxide and body position on near-infrared spectroscopic assessment of cerebral hemoglobin oxygen saturation. *Anesthes & Analg* 1996;82:278-287.

Chapter 22

Quantitative Measurement of Regional Blood Flow by Magnetic Resonance with Arterial Spin Tagging

Alan C. McLaughlin, PhD, Frank Q. Ye, PhD, Venkata S. Mattay, MD, Joseph A. Frank, MD, and Daniel R. Weinberger, MD

Introduction

Arterial spin tagging approaches[1,2] are similar to steady-state $H_2{}^{15}O$ positron-emission tomography (PET) approaches[3] for imaging cerebral blood flow, but use a tracer (magnetically "tagged" arterial water) that can be detected using magnetic resonance imaging (MRI). This chapter briefly summarizes how arterial spin tagging approaches can be used to provide quantitative cerebral blood flow images, and presents two applications. The first application involves focal decreases in cerebral blood flow in infarcted areas, while the second application involves focal increases in cerebral blood flow in "activated" areas of the brain. Finally, the potential of spin tagging approaches for studying cerebrovascular disease is discussed.

Theory

In "steady-state" arterial spin tagging approaches, arterial water is continuously tagged (by inversion of water protons) as it passes

From: Choi D, Dacey RG, Hsu CY, Powers WJ. *Cerebrovascular Disease: Momentum at the End of the Second Millennium.* Armonk, NY: Futura Publishing Company, Inc., © 2002.

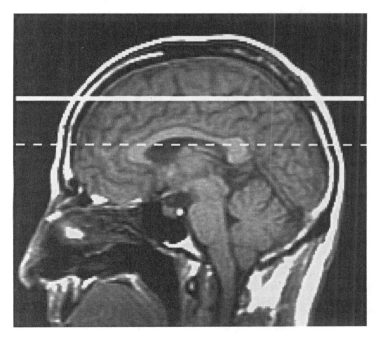

Figure 1. Sagittal image of a human head, showing the approximate location of the imaging slice (solid line) and the inversion plane (dashed line) for a typical steady-state arterial spin tagging experiment.

through a "tagging plane" (see Figure 1). After the tag is turned on, the amplitude of MRI signals in the brain reach a new steady-state, in which inflow of tagged water into the brain is counter-balanced by outflow of tagged water from the brain and magnetic "relaxation" of tagged water in the brain. Cerebral blood flow, Q, can be calculated using the following equation[2,4]

$$\frac{\Delta M}{M_{SS}} = \frac{2 \alpha Q/\lambda}{1/T_1} \tag{1}$$

where ΔM is the steady-state change in the MRI signal from intracellular brain water when arterial spins are perturbed, M_{ss} is the steady-state MRI signal from intracellular brain water, α is the degree of arterial water proton inversion ($\alpha = 1$ for complete inversion), {{lambda}} is the brain/blood partition coefficient for water, and $1/T_1$ is the observed longitudinal relaxation rate of brain water protons.

One disadvantage of arterial spin tagging approaches is that magnetic relaxation of arterial blood will reduce the extent of tagging in capillary blood by a factor exp $(-\tau_a/T_{1a})$, where τ_a is the arterial transit time, ie, the time required for tagged blood to move from the tagging plane to the capillary exchange sites in the imaging slice, and T_{1a} is

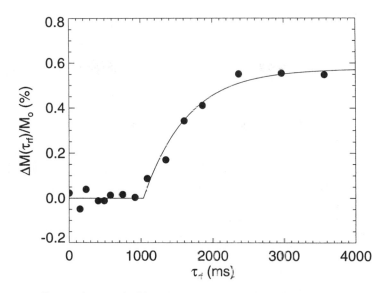

Figure 2. Dependence of ΔM on the length of the tagging period. ΔM values were averaged for a large grey matter ROI, and data were acquired in the presence of bipolar crusher gradients. The solid curve is the best fit of the data to a theoretical expression. (Modified with permission from Ye et al.[5])

the longitudinal relaxation time of arterial water protons. Cerebral blood flow values can be corrected for longitudinal relaxation during arterial transit if τ_a is known. One way to estimate τ_a is to measure the delay in the observed wash-in curve of tagged water into the brain. Figure 2 illustrates a wash-in curve measured for a grey matter region of interest (ROI). The arterial transit time can be obtained from the fit of the delayed wash-in curve to a simple theoretical model.[5] For the data shown in Figure 2, the average arterial transit time for grey matter ($\tau_{a,grey}$) was ~1.0 s.

Figure 3 shows a ΔM image, and a cerebral blood flow image calculated from the ΔM image using equation (1) and the calculated value of $\tau_{a,grey}$. One problem with this approach is that deviations in τ_a from $\tau_{a,grey}$ could add significant error to the calculated cerebral blood flow values. Alsop and Detre[6] recently proposed that the sensitivity of calculated cerebral blood flow values to variations in τ_a could be substantially reduced if acquisition of the MR images were delayed. Alsop and Detre[6] used a two-compartment model (arterial bed and brain tissue) to interpret the delayed acquisition data. Other groups have utilized crusher gradients to reduce contributions from tagged water in the arterial bed, and used a one-compartment model (brain tissue) to interpret the data.[7,8] Both the one-compartment and the two-compartment delayed acquisition approaches can be used to estimate cerebral blood flow values using approximate estimates of the arterial transit time. One estimate of the arterial transit time can be obtained using the mean value of $\tau_{a,grey}$ calculated for a control group of subjects.[5] While this estimate of τ_a may be useful for "normal" brain tissue, it may not be useful for brain regions where perfusion is severely compromised.

A number of groups have used "pulsed" arterial spin tagging approaches, eg, EPISTAR,[9] FAIR,[10,11] and QUIPSS II,[12] instead of steady-state arterial spin tagging approaches. Although pulsed and steady-state spin tagging approaches are similar, there are some subtle differences. For example, although steady-state approaches generally have slightly higher sensitivity than pulsed approaches, pulsed approaches are easier to use experimentally, especially at high magnetic field strengths (ie, 3 or 4 Tesla).

Survey of Experimental Results

The accuracy of cerebral blood flow values calculated using arterial spin tagging approaches can be tested by comparison with cerebral blood flow values determined using $H_2^{15}O$ PET. Average cerebral blood flow values determined using single-compartment delayed-acquisition spin tagging approaches were 10% higher than average cerebral blood flow values determined in the same slice using $H_2^{15}O$ PET approaches.[13] These results suggest that one-compartment delayed-acquisition spin tagging approaches can provide accurate estimates of cerebral blood flow.

One application of spin tagging approaches is to study focal decreases in cerebral blood flow. Figure 4 shows a quantitative cerebral blood flow image taken from a 29-year-old female with a chronic infarction. The cerebral blood flow was substantially reduced in the infarcted area, which is shown as a dark area in the T_1-weighted anatomical image.

Another application of spin tagging approaches is to study focal increases in cerebral blood flow during cerebral activation. Figure 5 shows quantitative cerebral blood flow images obtained from the same axial slice during rest (top, right) and during right-hand finger-tapping at 2Hz (top, left). The difference image (bottom, left) shows the effect of finger tapping on cerebral blood flow. The data in the difference image were processed using standard statistical methods to obtain the "activation" image shown in the bottom right of Figure 5. Areas having statistically significant increase in cerebral blood flow during finger tapping are shown in black, superimposed on an anatomical image.

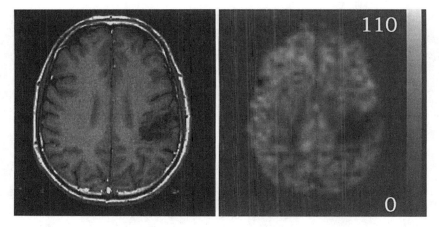

Figure 4. (left) T_1-weighted anatomical image, and (right) cerebral blood flow image from a 55-year-old male with a chronic infarction.

The data shown in Figure 5 demonstrate cerebral blood flow increases in the primary sensorimotor cortex, as expected from previous PET studies.[14] Similar results were observed for all subjects involved in the study.[7] For example, activation was observed in the primary sensorimotor cortex for all subjects, while activation was observed in the supplementary motor area for five of seven subjects. The mean increase in cerebral blood flow in activated primary sensorimotor cortex regions (averaged over all activated regions in all subjects) was 39 ± 6 cc/100g/min (63% ± 22%). If the difference in point spread functions is taken into account these increases are consistent with increases in cerebral blood flow observed using PET approaches.[7]

Cognitive tasks that involve working memory components would be expected to produce focal increases in cerebral blood flow in several cortical areas, especially prefrontal cortex.[15-17] Figure 6 shows a cerebral blood flow activation map obtained for a simple "two-back" working memory task, showing activation in the prefrontal cortex. Similar results were observed for all subjects involved in the study.[8] For example, all subjects showed statistically significant increases in cerebral blood flow in prefrontal cortex, although the pattern of activation varied widely from subject to subject. The mean increase in cerebral blood flow in activated prefrontal cortex (averaged over all activated regions in all subjects) was 22 ± 5 cc/100g/min (23% ± 7%).

All of the cerebral blood flow images discussed above were obtained using two-dimensional approaches. Figure 7 shows a three-dimensional cerebral blood flow activation image taken during finger tapping.[18] Statistically significant increases in cerebral blood flow were observed in the primary sensorimotor cortex.

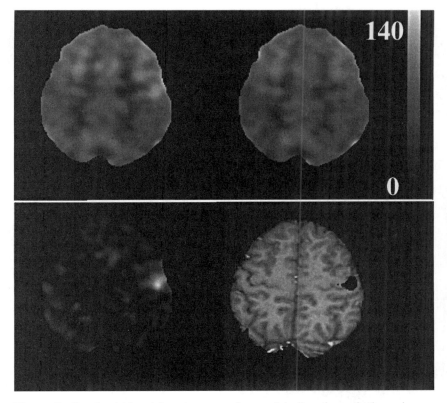

Figure 5. Cerebral blood flow images of an axial slice through the primary sensorimotor cortex during rest (top right), and finger tapping conditions (top left). A difference image (bottom left) shows the effect of finger tapping on cerebral blood flow, and a cerebral blood flow "activation image" (bottom right) shows regions that had statistically significant differences in cerebral blood flow during finger tapping (dark areas). The scale is in cc/100g/min. (Modified with permission from Ye et al.[7])

Potential Applications to Cerebrovascular Disease

Quantitative arterial spin tagging approaches will be useful in studying the pathophysiology of ischemic cerebrovascular disease. For example, Schmitz et al.[19] used spin tagging approaches to investigate relative perfusion changes during somatosensory stimulation at different times after transient global ischemia in the rat. They concluded that full recovery of brain function was substantially delayed compared to recovery of ionic homeostasis and recovery of CBF/CMRO$_2$ coupling. In a clinical study, Detre et al.[21] used spin tagging approaches

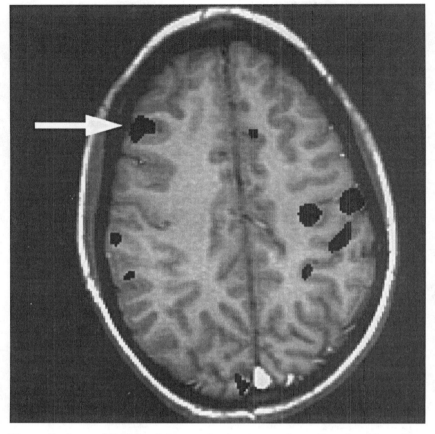

Figure 6. A cerebral blood flow activation image for a "two-back" working memory task. Regions marked in black (superimposed on an anatomical image) had statistically significant differences in cerebral blood flow during the task. The arrows point to activated regions in the prefrontal cortex. (Modified with permission from Ye et al.[8])

to investigate the response of cerebral perfusion to "augmentation" testing before and after therepeutic intervention. They observed that patients with symptomatic middle cerebral artery stenosis had a substantial increase in "cerebrovascular reserve" after anticoagulation treatment.

Quantitative arterial spin tagging approaches may not be useful in clinical management of individual patients with acute stroke. One reason is that the long arterial transit times in infarcted areas may make quantitation of cerebral blood flow difficult. Another reason is that cerebral blood flow measurements alone may not be able to predict which areas of the ischemic penumbra will eventually recover.[20]

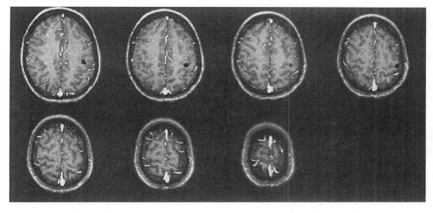

Figure 7. Three-dimensional cerebral blood flow activation image for a finger tapping task. Regions marked in black (superimposed on an anatomical image) had statistically significant increases in cerebral blood flow during finger tapping.

Comparison with Other MRI Approaches

Other MRI techniques that provide important information on cerebral perfusion are "bolus tracking" approaches with paramagnetic contrast agents[21] and functional MRI (fMRI) approaches with BOLD contrast.[22-24] Both techniques are complementary to arterial spin tagging approaches. For example, bolus tracking techniques can provide quantitative maps of mean transit times, and fMRI techniques are more sensitive than arterial spin tagging techniques in following cerebral activation. However, neither bolus tracking techniques or fMRI techniques can provide absolute blood flow measurements.[25]

Spin tagging approaches may also prove useful, in conjunction with ^{17}O MRI techniques, for obtaining quantitative images of cerebral oxygen consumption ($CMRO_2$). ^{17}O MRI approaches[26] are similar to ^{15}O PET approaches,[3] except they use a stable isotope of oxygen that can be detected by MRI. In particular, both approaches require an independent measure of cerebral blood flow in order to calculate $CMRO_2$. Previous ^{17}O MRI studies with animals used concurrent ^{19}F MRI detection of inhaled CHF_3 to determine CBF, but this approach may not be feasible with humans.[27] However, concurrent spin tagging/ ^{17}O techniques could provide simultaneous CBF and $CMRO_2$ images in humans, and give detailed information on the metabolic consequences of cerebrovascular lesions.[19]

Conclusions

Arterial spin tagging approaches can provide quantitative images of cerebral blood flow in humans, and can be used to follow resting cerebral blood flow and focal increases or decreases in cerebral blood flow. Arterial spin tagging approaches will have important applications in studying cerebrovascular disease, but may not have immediate applications in clinical management of individual patients.

References

1. Detre JA, Leigh JS, Williams DS, et al. Perfusion imaging. *Magn Reson Med* 1992;23:37-45.
2. Williams DS, Detre JA, Leigh JS, et al. Magnetic resonance imaging of perfusion using spin inversion of arterial water. *Proc Nat Acad Sci USA* 1992;89: 212-216.
3. Frackowiak RSJ, Lenzi G-L, Jones T, et al. Quantitative measurement of regional cerebral blood flow and oxygen metabolism in man using ^{15}O and positron emission tomography: Theory, procedure, and normal values. *J Comput Assist Tomogr* 1980;4:727-736.
4. McLaughlin AC, Ye FQ, Pekar JJ, et al. Effect of magnetization transfer on the measurement of cerebral blood flow using steady-state arterial spin tagging approaches: A theoretical investigation. *Magn Reson Med* 1997;37: 501-510.
5. Ye FQ, Mattay VS, Jezzard P, et al. Correction for vascular artifacts in cerebral blood flow values measured by using arterial spin tagging techniques. *Magn Reson Med* 1997;37:226-235.
6. Alsop DC, Detre JA. Reduced transit time sensitivity in noninvasive magnetic resonance imaging of human cerebral blood flow. *J Cereb Blood Flow Metab* 1996;16:1236-1249.
7. Ye FQ, Smith AM, Yang Y, et al. Quantitation of regional cerebral blood flow increases during motor activation: A steady-state arterial spin tagging study. *NeuroImage* 1997;6:104-112.
8. Ye FQ, Smith AM, Mattay VS, et al. Quantitation of regionial cerebral blood flow increases in the prefrontal cortex during a working memory task: A steady-state arterial spin tagging study. *NeuroImage* 1998;8(1):44-49.
9. Edelman RR, Siewart B, Darby DG, et al. Qualitative mapping of cerebral blood flow and functional localization with echo-planar imaging and signal targeting with alternating radio frequency. *Radiology* 1994;192:513-520.
10. Kim S-G. Quantification of relative cerebral blood flow changes by flow-sensitive alternating inversion recovery (FAIR) technique: Application to functional mapping. *Magn Res Med* 1995;34 293-301
11. Kwong KK, Chesler DA, Weisskoff RM, et al. MR perfusion studies with T1-weighted echo planar imaging. *Magn Reson Med* 1995;34:878-887.
12. Wong EC, Buxton RB, Frank LR. Quantitative imaging of perfusion using a single subtraction (QUIPSS and QUIPSS II). *Magn Reson Med* 1998;39: 702-708.
13. Ye FQ, Berman KF, Ellmore T, et al. H_2^{15}O validation of arterial spin tagging measurements of cerebral blood flow in humans. *Abstr Int Soc Magn Reson Med* 1997;5:87.
14. Roland PE, Larsen B, Lassen NA, et al. Supplementary motor area and other cortical areas in organization of voluntary movements in man. *J Neurophysiol* 1980;43:118-136.

15. Paulesu E, Frith CD, Frackowiak RSJ. The neural correlates of the verbal component of working memory. *Nature* 1993;362:343-345.

16. Jonides J, Smith EE, Koeppe RA, et al. Spatial working memory in humans as revealed by PET. *Nature* 1993;363:623-625.

17. Berman KF, Ostrem J, Randolph C, et al. Physiological activation of a cortical network during performance of the Wisconsin card sorting task: A positron emission tomography study. *Neuropsychologia* 1995;33:1027-1046.

18. Ye FQ, Smith AM, Yang Y, et al. 3D imaging of cerebral blood flow changes during motor activation. *Abstr Int Soc Magn Reson Med* 1998;6:1467.

19. Schmitz B, Hoehn-Berlage M, Kerskens CM, et al. Recovery of the rodent brain after cardiac arrest: A functional MRI study. *Magn Reson Med* 1998;39:783-788.

20. Furlan M, Marchal G, Viader F, et al. Spontaneous neurological recovery after stroke and the fate of the ischemic penumbra. *Ann Neurol* 1996;40:216-226.

21. Ostergaard L, Sorenson AG, Kwong KK, et al. High-resolution measurement of cerebral blood flow using intravascular tracer bolus passage. Part II: Experimental comparison and preliminary results. *Magn Reson Med* 1996;36:726-736.

22. Kwong KK, Belliveau JW, Chesler DA, et al. Dynamic magnetic resonance imaging of human brain activity during primary sensory stimulation. *Proc Nat Acad Sci USA* 1992;89:5675-5679.

23. Ogawa S, Tank, DW, Menon R, et al. Intrinsic signal changes accompanying sensory stimulation: Functional brain mapping with magnetic resonance imaging. *Proc Nat Acad Sci USA* 1992;89:5951-5955.

24. Bandettini P, Wong EC, Hinks R, et al. Time course EPI of human brain function during task activation. *Magn Reson Med* 1992;25:390-397.

25. McLaughlin AC, Ye FQ, Berman KF, et al. Use of diffusible and non-diffusible tracers in studies of brain perfusion. In Moonen CTW, Bandettini PA, (eds): *Functional MRI.* Heidleberg: Springer Verlag;1998.

26. Pekar JJ, Sinnwell T, Ligeti L, et al. Simultaneous measurement of cerebral oxygen consumption and blood flow using ^{17}O and ^{19}F magnetic resonance imaging. *J Cereb Blood Flow Metab* 1995;15:312-320.

27. Fagan SC, Rahill AA, Balakrishnan G, et al. Neurotoxicity and physiologic effects of trifluoromethane in man. *J Toxicol Environ Health* 1994;45:221-229.

Section VI.

Delayed Neuronal Death

Chapter 23

The GluR2 Hypothesis of Ischemia-Induced Damage: Implications for Neuroprotection and Rescue

Domenico E. Pellegrini-Giampietro, MD, PhD, Keiji Oguro, MD, PhD, Thoralf Opitz, PhD, Agata Calderone, MD, Michael V.L. Bennett, PhD, and R. Suzanne Zukin, PhD

Cerebral Ischemia: Clinical Features and Neuropathology

Stroke is a dehabilitating disorder and major cause of death in the world. Approximately 150,000 people suffer from stroke each year in the United States alone. Major forms of acute brain damage include focal ischemia (localized brain hypoxia associated with reduced blood flow to a restricted region within the brain) and global ischemia (transient reduction in blood flow to both cerebral hemispheres). Focal ischemia, observed in patients who suffer subarachnoid hemorrhage, embolic obstruction or traumatic brain injury,[1,2] or induced experimentally in animals by surgical occlusion (transient or permanent) of the

This work was supported in part by a grant from the Italian Government (MURST/ PNR Neurobiology) to Dr. Pellegrini-Giampietro and by National Institutes of Health Grants nos. NS 20752 to Dr. Zukin and NS 07412 to Dr. Bennett. Dr. Bennett is the Sylvia and Robert Olnick Professor of Neuroscience.

From: Choi D, Dacey RG, Hsu CY, Powers WJ. *Cerebrovascular Disease: Momentum at the End of the Second Millennium.* Armonk, NY: Futura Publishing Company, Inc., © 2002.

middle cerebral artery[3] leads to rapid onset, relatively nonspecific neurodegeneration. Histopathological hallmarks of focal ischemia include pan-necrosis involving neurons, glia and endothelial cells in the core[4] and more restricted cell loss in the ischemic "penumbra," a zone of moderately ischemic tissue that surrounds the core.[5,6]

In contrast, severe, transient global ischemia, observed in patients successfully resuscitated from cardiac arrest[7] or induced experimentally in animals,{{sup3}} leads to delayed, highly selective neuronal cell death. Pyramidal neurons of the hippocampal CA1 and CA4 are particularly vulnerable.[8] Histologically detectable neurodegeneration of CA1 pyramidal neurons is not apparent until 48 to 72 hours after circulation has been restored. Longer ischemic episodes (20 to 30 minutes) lead to delayed cell death in hippocampus, subiculum; neocortical layers III, V and VI; and small- to medium-sized striatal neurons, first evident in the striatum at 24 hours.[8] The most common cause of global ischemia is cardiac arrest following myocardial infarction, open heart surgery or ventricular fibrillation, asphyxia and near drowning. Despite its status as a major, world-wide cause of death and disability, molecular mechanisms underlying ischemia-induced damage are not well understood. This chapter reviews recent studies that shed light on molecular mechanisms associated with ischemia-induced cell death. The present chapter is an adaptation of the earlier review published by the same authors.[9]

Pathogenesis: Excitotoxicity and the GluR2 Hypothesis

Neuronal injury resulting from glutamate receptor-mediated excitotoxicity has been implicated in a wide spectrum of neurological disease states, including cerebral ischemia, hypoglycemia, trauma, epilepsy and some types of neurodegenerative or psychiatric diseases. The existence of diseases in the central nervous system (CNS) in which excitotoxicity is involved may have important clinical consequences, such as the possibility of more effective therapeutic intervention. The hypothesis that ischemia might have an excitotoxic pathophysiological component is supported by a number of findings reported in the course of the past two decades.[10-12] These include neuropathological changes resembling the pattern of neurodegeneration induced by excitotoxic agents; accumulation of extracellular glutamate due to both increased release or decreased uptake; alteration in the number or subunit composition of glutamate receptors; abnormal and sustained increase in cytosolic free Ca^{2+}; dependence on excitatory afferents; and delayed onset of neuronal damage.

Probably, however, the most compelling piece of evidence implicating glutamate toxicity in cerebral ischemia is the finding that glutamate receptor antagonists are neuroprotective in a variety of experimental models. Moreover, NMDA antagonists are currently in early-phase clinical trials for stroke injury. Glutamate-induced rise in intracellular Ca^{2+} is thought to play a critical role in this neurodegeneration. Possible causes of a rise in intracellular Ca^{2+} include activation of Ca^{2+} permeable ionotropic glutamate receptors, activation of metabotropic glutamate receptors positively linked to inositol phosphates, activation of voltage-sensitive Ca^{2+} channels, and/or deactivation or extrusion and/or sequestration systems.[13-16] This rise in intracellular Ca^{2+} may lead to the onset of cell death by a number of mechanisms including activation of proteases, phospholipases and endonucleases, generation of free radicals that destroy cellular membranes by lipid peroxidation[1,16-18] and induction of apoptosis.[17,19]

Until recently, the NMDA receptor was the only glutamate receptor known to be permeable to Ca^{2+}. It is now well established that AMPA receptors lacking the GluR2 subunit are permeable to a number of divalent cations including Ca^{2+} and potentially provide an important source of Ca^{2+} overload. The *GluR2 hypothesis* predicts that specific neurological insults lead to a decrease in GluR2 expression and increase in formation of Ca^{2+} -permeable AMPA receptors, and thereby, enhanced pathogenicity of endogenous glutamate. This article reviews recent experimental evidence that Ca^{2+} -permeable AMPA receptors contribute to the delayed and cell- specific neurodegeneration associated with transient forebrain ischemia.

Ca^{2+} - Permeability of AMPA Receptors is Controlled by the GluR2 Subunit

AMPA-type glutamate receptors mediate fast excitatory synaptic transmission in the vertebrate central nervous system[20] and are encoded by four genes, GluR1-4 (or GluR-A-D) subunits.[21] GluR subunits appear to be expressed by virtually all neurons in the brain, although each cell may differ in the number and type of subunits expressed. Individual neurons predominantly form heteromeric AMPA receptors made up of at least two different subunits, but they may also form homomers.[22,23]

The GluR2 subunit governs the Ca^{2+} -permeability of AMPA receptors. AMPA receptors assembled from GluR1, GluR3 and/or GluR4 subunits are permeable to Ca^{2+} and have doubly rectifying current/voltage relations.[24-26] GluR2, expressed with other GluR subunits, forms channels that are Ca^{2+} -impermeable and electrically linear or outwardly rectifying. The dominance of the GluR2 subunit in determining permeability to Ca^{2+} and other divalent ions is attributed to the presence of a positively charged arginine (R) in place of a glutamine (Q) residue within the TM2 domain.[26,27] Rectification of receptors lacking GluR2 arises from fast voltage- dependent channel block by intracellular polyamines.[28,29] Some positively charged polyamine spider toxins like argiotoxin[30] and Joro spider toxin[31] block Ca^{2+} -permeable AMPA receptors selectively (presumably they fail to block GluR2 containing receptors because they are repelled by the positively charged arginine residue in the GluR2 subunit) and therefore serve as pharmacological probes to detect the presence or absence of GluR2 in recombinant (as well as in native) receptor assemblies. The functionally critical arginine within TM2 is not encoded by the GluR2 gene, but rather arises within the pre-mRNA by editing of a codon for the neutral glutamine residue.[32,33] RNA editing at the "Q/R" site of AMPA receptors is specific to GluR2 and is extremely efficient. In neonatal and adult rat brain, virtually 100% of GluR2 mRNA undergoes editing; in embryonic brain, only a small percentage of GluR2 subunits (about 1%) are unedited.[26]

The Ca^{2+} -permeability of native AMPA receptors varies widely. Since editing of GluR2 mRNA at the Q/R site is virtually complete under physiological conditions, Ca^{2+} -permeable AMPA receptors occur in neurons only as a consequence of low expression of GluR2 mRNA. Studies involving patch-clamp recording and RT-PCR (reverse transcriptase-polymerase chain reaction) demonstrate that AMPA receptor permeability to Ca^{2+} varies inversely with abundance of GluR2 mRNA in a wide range of cell types. Excitatory principal neurons such as hippocampal[34,35] and neocortical[36] pyramidal cells and dentate gyrus granule cells[35] exhibit low AMPA receptor Ca^{2+} - permeability and more abundant GluR2 mRNA. Hippocampal[34,37] and neocortical[37] GABAergic interneurons and dentate gyrus basket cells[36] display higher AMPA receptor Ca^{2+} - permeability and less abundant GluR2 mRNA. Bergmann glia cells of the cerebellum exhibit high AMPA receptor Ca^{2+} -permeability and undetectable GluR2.[35]

Hippocampal GABA-ergic interneurons (which are known to lack GluR2) are viable and relatively resistant to postischemic delayed neurodegeneration.[38] In addition, transgenic mice with targeted disruption of the GluR2 gene survive and their principal neurons (that express GluR2 in wild-type animals) are functional.[39] Possible explanations for the survival of these neurons may include an increase in compensatory mechanisms for Ca^{2+} buffering and extrusion (as, for example, expression of Ca^{2+} binding proteins)[40] or reduced AMPA currents due to expression of receptors with faster and more profound desensitization.[35,41] Hence, the GluR2 hypothesis will apply primarily to principal neurons that normally express Ca^{2+} -impermeable AMPA receptors and that are not required to cope with Ca^{2+} influx via AMPA receptors.

In these cells, acute changes in permeability of AMPA receptors to Ca^{2+} could account for cell death. High rate of Ca^{2+} influx through AMPA receptors in cultured rat cerebellar Purkinje cells[42] and in a subpopulation of neocortical neurons[43-45] leads to enhanced vulnerability to kainate toxicity.

Ca^{2+}-Permeable AMPA Receptors in Ischemia-Induced Neuronal Cell Death

Transient, severe global ischemia observed in patients during cardiorespiratory arrest,[7] cardiac surgery[46-48] or experimentally in animals, induces selective and delayed neuronal death.[8,49] Although during the ischemic insult all forebrain areas experience oxygen and glucose deprivation, only selected neuronal populations degenerate and die.[50] Pyramidal neurons in the CA1 region of the hippocampus are particularly vulnerable. Histological evidence of degeneration, exhibiting characteristics of apoptosis, is not observed until 2 to 3 days after induction of ischemia in rats.[8,49,51,52]

Considerable evidence implicates Ca^{2+}-permeable AMPA receptors in delayed neuronal cell death after ischemia. The initial observation came from studies in which AMPA receptor antagonists were administered to rats at times after induction of global ischemia. NBQX (2,3-dihydroxy-6-nitro-7-sulfamoylbenzo(f)-quinoxaline) administered as late as 16 hours after the induction of global ischemia afforded neuroprotection (ie, prevented ischemia-induced neurodegeneration[53-57]). In contrast, MK-801, a selective N-methyl-D-aspartate (NMDA) receptor antagonist, is not neuroprotective.[54,57,93] These findings are consistent with a model in which activation of AMPA receptor is necessary, and possibly sufficient, for the delayed neurodegeneration.

Ischemia-Induced Down Regulation of GluR2 Expression

GluR2 mRNA expression is dramatically reduced in CA1 pyramidal cells of the hippocampus following transient forebrain ischemia (Figure 1).[58-62] The decrease in GluR2 mRNA occurs as early as 12 hours following the ischemic insult and decreases to 30% of control levels within 24 hours.

GluR2 mRNA down regulation directly precedes neural damage, and does not occur in the CA3 or dentate gyrus regions which are resistant to ischemia-induced damage. GluR3 mRNA levels also decrease, but to a lesser degree (50% of control values), and GluR1 and NR1 levels remain constant.

A   **B**

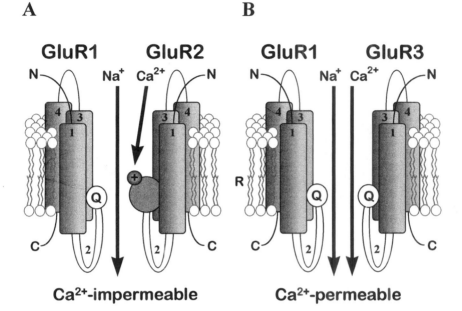

Figure 1. Ca^2+ permeability of AMPA receptors depends on subunit composition. **A.** The GluR2 subunit, expressed with GluR1 and/or GluR3, forms AMPA channels that are Ca^2+ -impermeable. GluR2 limits Ca^2+ gating due to the presence of an edited positively charged arginine (R) in place of a glutamine (Q) residue at the Q/R site. **B.** AMPA channels assembled from GluR1 and/or GluR3 subunits are permeable to Ca^2+.

Down regulation of GluR2 mRNA expression if translated into reduced GluR2 subunit expression would lead to increased formation of Ca^{2+} -permeable AMPA receptors and enhanced pathogenicity of endogenous glutamate (the *GluR2 hypothesis*). We examined possible changes in AMPA receptor subunit expression through Western blot analysis with AMPA receptor subunit-specific antibodies.[63] Important technical advances included not only the development of subunit specific antibodies, but also the development of antibodies directed to specific sequences within both the N-terminal and C-terminal domains of the individual subunits.[64,65] Recent studies provide evidence that the C –terminal domain of GluR1 and possibly other AMPA receptor subunits undergo proteolysis following a global ischemic insult.[66]

Global ischemia was induced in gerbils by the 2-vessel occlusion method. Neuronal cell loss was monitored histologically. At times after ischemia, tissue from the hippocampal CA1, CA3 and dentate gyrus were removed by micro-dissection, protein extracts prepared and subjected to SDS-PAGE and Western blot analysis. Nitrocellulose membranes were probed with polyclonal and monoclonal antibodies that recognized peptide sequences in either the N-terminal or C-terminal domains of the GluR1 and GluR2 subunits of the AMPA receptor. Using enhanced chemiluminescence detection and computer-aided densitometry, the relative amount of GluR2 protein could be determined with either GluR1 or actin as a standard. Global ischemia led to a 60% reduction in GluR2 protein expression at 72 hours after reperfusion. GluR1 subunit expression was reduced by 20%. The reduction in GluR2 protein expression was first detected at 60 hours after ischemia. No changes in GluR1 or GluR2 subunit expression were detected in the CA3 or dentate gyrus. Thus, protein expression changes specific to vulnerable CA1 neurons. The decrease of GluR2 could be detected with antibodies raised against both the C- and the N-terminal sequence of the protein, suggesting that limited proteolysis of the C-terminus is not the reason for measuring lower amounts of GluR2. Thus, the ratio of GluR2:GluR1, which may predict Ca^{2+}-permeability of AMPA receptors, decreased after ischemia. These findings provide further support for the *GluR2 hypothesis*.

Ischemia-Induced Changes in Glutamate Receptor Function

Global ischemia induces a number of functional changes in the hippocampal CA1 indicative of increased expression of Ca^{2+}-permeable AMPA receptors. AMPA –receptor mediated excitatory postsynaptic currents (EPSCs) at the CA1/Schaffer collateral synapse are prolonged after ischemia and exhibit increased sensitivity to Joro spider toxin and 1-naphthyl acetyl spermine (Figure 2)[67] channel blockers selective for Ca^{2+}-permeable AMPA receptors.[32,31]

These findings are consistent with a mechanism whereby postischemic CA1 neurons generate slow EPSCs mediated by newly expressed Ca^{2+}-permeable AMPA receptors.[68] Many postischemic CA1 pyramidal neurons are irreversibly depolarized by prolonged low frequency stimulation of the Schaffer collateral/commisural input.[18] Moreover, postischemic neurons fail to exhibit long-term potentiation following tetanic stimulation.[69] Hippocampal neurons in culture subjected to sublethal oxygen-glucose deprivation exhibit increased AMPA- or kainate- induced Ca^{2+} accumulation, increased sensitivity of AMPA receptors to Joro spider toxin, and increased vulnerability to AMPA receptor-mediated excitotoxity, suggesting increased formation of GluR2-lacking, Ca^{2+}-permeable AMPA receptors.[69]

To determine whether down regulation of GluR2 expression translates into enhanced AMPA receptor-mediated Ca^{2+} entry in CA1 neurons, we used a combination of electrophysiological intracellular re-

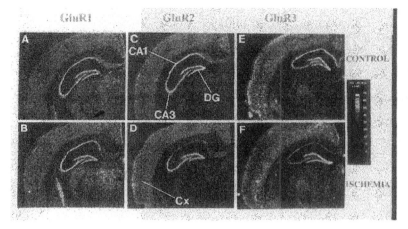

Figure 2. Pseudo-color display of density of autoradiograms of GluR1, GluR2 and GluR3 mRNA localization in coronal sections of control and postischemic rat brain at the level of the hippocampus.**A.** GluR1 expression in control (sham-operated) brain; **B.** GluR1 expression in ischemic rats 24 hrs after 10 min of global ischemia; **C.** GluR2 expression in control; **D.** GluR2 expression 24 hours postischemia, showing dramatic and selective reduction in CA1 labeling; **E.** GluR3 expression in control brain; **F.** GluR3 expression 24 hours postischemia, showing that reduction in CA1 is not marked as in **D** and extends through CA3. DG: dentate gyrus, Cx: neocortex.

cording and optical imaging with Ca^{2+} indicator dye fura-2.[62] In hippocampal slices from gerbils 48 hours after ischemia, AMPA elicits only a small rise in $[Ca^{2+}]_1$, which is not significantly different from Ca^{2+} rises in control neurons. At 72 hours after the ischemic insult individual CA1 neurons that retain the ability to fire action potentials exhibit a greatly enhanced AMPA-elicited rise in $[Ca^{2+}]_1$ (Figure 3). Basal $[Ca^{2+}]_1$ does not differ in control and postischemic pyramidal cells. These findings indicate that AMPA receptor functional responses are altered following global inschemia and provide direct evidence for Ca^{2+} -influx directly through AMPA receptors in vulnerable CA1 postischemic neurons at times preceding obvious cell loss.

Recent evidence implicates Zn^{2+} entry as a critical component of neuronal death after transient global ischemia in rates.[70] As a result of ischemia, Zn^{2+} translocated from presynaptic terminals accumulates in degenerating neurons in the hippocampal CA1.[70] This accumulation precedes the onset of neurodegeneration and is prevented by intraventricular administration of the Zn^{2+} chelator Ca-EDTA just prior to induction of ischemia.

Ca-EDTA administration 1 hour after reperfusion is not neuroprotective, indicating that Zn^{2+} entry during or immediately after ischemia is toxic. Moreover, ischemia induces mRNA expression of the trans-

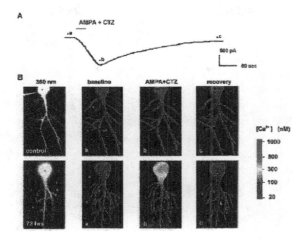

Figure 3. AMPA-elicited inward current and rise in intracellular free Ca^{2+} concentration in a CA1 pyramidal neuron after ischemia. **A.** Inward current elicited by AMPA (30 μM with 10 μM cyclothiazide (CTZ) in a CA1 pyramidal neuron in a hippocampal slice from an animal 72 hours after ischemia. AMPA and CTZ were both applied for 30 seconds (bar). Then the AMPA was washed out with saline containing the NMDA, Ca^{2+} and Na^+ channel blockers. After 5 min, CNQX (20 μM) was added to the other blockers to cause more rapid recovery. In the control neuron illustrated in **B**, the AMPA-elicited inward current in the presence of 30 μM CTZ was of somewhat lower amplitude but similar in time course. **B.** Optical imaging [350 nm excitation images] of individual CA1 pyramidal neurons injected with fura-2 in hippocampal slices from a control animal *(upper row)* and an experimental animal 72 hours after ischemia (*lower row*, same cell as in **A**). **a**, image taken before bath application of agonist (time indicated in current trace above); **b**, image taken at peak inward current after application of AMPA (30 μM with 10 μM CTZ); **c**, image taken after recovery to near baseline current. Highlight represents Ca^{2+} concentration determined from the ratio of fluorescence obtained at two excitation wavelengths (350 nm and 380 nm); calibration at right. AMPA elicited little change in intracellular free Ca^{2+} in the control neuron. In contrast, AMPA elicited a rise in Ca^{2+} in the soma of the postischemic neuron and a smaller increase in its proximal dendrites.

porter gene ZNT-1 in CA1 neurons that are destined to die, presumably in response to the Zn^{2+} accumulation, since Zn^{2-} induces expression of the gene in cultured neurons.[71] Although one can interpret the induction as a homeostatic response, it does not prevent cell death. Since GluR2-lacking AMPA receptors are permeable to Zn^{2+},[72] delayed entry of Zn^{2+} may contribute to degeneration. If so, Ca-EDTA treatment delayed by several days after the ischemic insult would also be neuroprotective.

Finally, evidence in support of a role for Ca^{2+}-permeable AMPA receptors in ischemia-induced damage comes from studies involving dissociated primary cultures of cortical neurons.[73] This study reveals that activation of Ca^{2+} -permeable AMPA receptors, in addition to activation of NMDA channels, leads to the generation of oxygen radicals, a well-established cause of cell damage. Together these studies provide compelling evidence that "switching off" of GluR2 expression in CA1 after transient global ischemia leads to formation of new AMPA receptors lacking the GluR2 subunit. This change in receptor composition increases AMPA receptor-mediated entry of Ca^{2+} (or possibly Zn^{2+}) in response to endogenous glutamate and causes, or contributes to, delayed post-ischemic neurodegeneration (the "*GluR2 hypothesis*").[74,75] Since editing of GluR2 mRNA at the Q/R site is unaltered after global ischemia,[69,76-78] the change in AMPA receptor properties is likely to arise as a direct consequence of altered gene expression, rather than of a change in editing efficiency at the Q/R site.

Neuroprotection Strategies

Although the molecular mechanisms by which global ischemia alters GluR2 expression are as yet unknown, it is possible to design strategies for neuroprotection. Three possible approaches are 1) suppression of down regulation of GluR2 expression; 2) direct block of GluR2-lacking, Ca^{2+} -permeable AMPA receptors by selective polyamines and toxins; and 3) block of subsequent apoptosis. It is important to consider the therapeutic window for each treatment modality and to distinguish between protection prior to the ischemic episode and rescue following the ischemic episode of neurons otherwise destined to die. In principle, rescue can be carried out at any stage of the cascade, which leads to cell death.

A number of neuroprotective strategies and drug treatments in animal models of global ischemia prevent down regulation of GluR2 expression in CA1. Pre-conditioning with a sublethal ischemic insult or administration of agonists of adenosine A1 receptors and activators of ATP-sensitive K+ channels just prior to induction of ischemia block the down regulation of GluR2 mRNA expression and prevent cell death.[61] Aurintricarboxylic acid, a nonspecific endonuclease inhibitor that can prevent apoptosis, is neuroprotective when given intraventricularly prior to ischemia and blocks down regulation of GluR2 (Figure 1.)[79] However, ATA administered 6 hours after ischemia is not neuroprotective, and does not prevent the down regulation of GluR2. These observations suggest that ATA does not act by directly blocking apoptosis (or other programmed cell death) in CA1 neurons (which processes are likely to be initiated after formation of Ca^{2+} -permeable AMPA receptors), but rather acts directly to block down regulation of GluR2 gene expression. In contrast, the AMPA/kainate receptor antagonist NBQX is neuroprotective,[53-57] but does not block down regulation of GluR2,[59] suggesting that NBQX affords neuroprotection by a direct block of GluR2-lacking, Ca^{2+}-permeable AMPA receptors.

There is some disagreement as to the duration of protection by NBQX. Some authors report that although neurons in animals treated with NBQX within 24 hours survive for seven days, many of these cells die after several weeks.[80] The delayed mortality could be a result of lack of recovery of GluR2 expression.

Global ischemia induces changes in gene expression in the vulnerable CA1, including expression of immediate early genes,[81,82] enzymes,[83] stress proteins[84,82] and neurotrophic factors.[85,86] All of these are possible candidates for the down regulation of GluR2 expression after an insult. The observation that some mRNAs (and proteins) are up-regulated in the CA1 following ischemia suggests that the down regulation of GluR2 is likely to be a result of a specific regulatory mechanism rather than of nonspecific decrease in transcription, RNA processing or RNA stability.

Genetic Approaches to the Role of GluR2 in Neuronal Cell Deat

Gene inactivation (knock-out) and antisense (knock-down) approaches have proven useful in determining the function of a particular protein under physiological and pathological conditions. Altogether four animal models have been developed using genetic techniques: 1) the Q/R editing deficient mouse (lacking intron 11 of the GluR2 gene); 2) the GluR2 knock-out mouse; 3) the GluR2-flip over expressing mouse; and 4) the gerbil acutely treated with GluR2 antisense oligonucleotides (knock-down). This section briefly reviews the consequences of these genetic manipulations on brain development and susceptibility to excitotoxic cell death.

Heterozygous transgenic mice engineered for a Q/R editing deficient GluR2 allele express AMPA receptors with increased Ca^{2+}-permeability, particularly in hippocampal and neocortical principal neurons.[87] The primary consequence is the onset of spontaneous and recurrent seizures.[87] The mice develop recurrent seizures and die within the first three weeks of life, with cell loss in the hippocampus. In these animals, unedited GluR2 may contribute to the formation of a greater number of Ca^{2+}-permeable AMPA receptors than in the GluR2 knock-out mice (see below).

Transgenic mice with targeted disruption of the GluR2 gene ("GluR2 knock-out mice") differ considerably from GluR2 Q/R editing deficient mice; the knock-out mice are viable and fertile. The knockout mice exhibit a nine-fold increase in kainate-elicited Ca^{2+} -influx into individual CA1 pyramidal neurons and increased inward rectification of kainate-elicited responses and of the AMPA receptor mediated component of EPSCs.[39] The passive membrane properties at the resting potential are unchanged, except that input resistance is increased, perhaps due to reduced cell size. EPSCs are little changed in amplitude and the decay rate is unchanged (unlike the EPSCs in postischemic gerbil).[18] The AMPA receptor mediated component of the EPSCs is reduced relative to the NMDA receptor mediated component, possibly due to reduction in AMPA receptor density as a result of inefficient receptor assembly. Long-term potentiation (LTP) in GluR2 knock-out animals is increased and has a substantial NMDA receptor independent component. These strongly suggest that LTP can be mediated by Ca^{2+} influx through Ca^{2+} -permeable AMPA receptors.[88] The GluR2 knockout animals exhibit significant behavioral changes. Ca^{2+} -permeable AMPA receptors, which are expressed at higher levels in the postnatal animal than in the adult, may be involved in synaptic plasticity during brain development, and failure to decrease Ca^{2+} -permeability of AMPA receptors at later stages may lead to aberrant development.

Viability of the GluR2 knock-out mice in contrast to that of the GluR2 editing deficient mice may be the result of a number of mechanisms. There may be 1) compensatory increases in Ca^{2+} buffering and extrusion (as, for example, enhanced expression of Ca^{2+} -binding proteins),[41,89] 2) reduced AMPA receptor currents, due to slower receptor assembly or reduced expression of GluR1 and GluR3, and/or 3) expression of receptors with altered properties, such as enhanced desensitization.[35,41]

Modifications other than down regulation of GluR2 expression can increase excitotoxicity. The presence of the GluR2-flip splice-variant subunit in heteromeric AMPA receptors leads to a larger current flow through these channels.[35, 90] Transgenic mice that over-express GluR2-flip show enhanced susceptibility to excitotoxic glutamate-mediated damage after permanent middle cerebral artery occlusion, and glutamate excitotoxicity is increased relative to that of wild-type in neurons cultured from the transgenic mice.[91] Excitotoxicity may be caused by increased Ca^{2+} influx through voltage-gated Ca^{2+} channels and through NMDA receptor channels[1,10,12] following increased depolarization mediated by AMPA receptors containing primarily the flip isoform of GluR2.[35,90] GluR2 knock-down as a technique offers the advantage of examining the effects of GluR2 suppression in an animal that has developed under normal conditions. Injection of antisense oligonucleotides directly into the brain of gerbils and rats has been used to demonstrate a probable causal relationship between down regulation of GluR2 expression and delayed neuronal cell death.[92] This study demonstrates that knock-down of GluR2 by intraventricular injection of specific anti-sense oligonucleotides leads to death of CA1 and CA3 neurons. Scrambled antisense administered under the same conditions is without effect. Since the induced neurotoxicity is blocked by 1-naphthyl acetyl spermine, the cause of death is likely to be Ca^{2+} influx through GluR2-lacking AMPA receptors. Furthermore, antisense administered to animals subjected to a brief ischemic episode (which, by itself, causes no neuronal damage) leads to greater cell death than is observed for antisense administration to control animals.[93]

Given the prominent role of GluR2 in normal physiology, brain development, and excitotoxicity, an important future direction would be to apply spatial and temporal restrictions to the regulation of GluR2 expressions as, for example, by conditional knock-out or knock-in approaches. Such studies would be expected to aid in our understanding of the role of the GluR2 subunit during synaptogenesis and formation of neuronal circuitry and in the neurodegeneration associated with stroke.

Conclusions

A series of events, studied in neuronal primary cultures as well as in experimental models *in vivo*, are thought to be involved in the process linking brain ischemia to neuronal death. Some of them have been shown to be susceptible to modulation by pharmacological agents. These pathogenic mechanisms include glutamate release and glutamate receptor activation, expression of inducible early genes (c-fos, c-jun), downregulation of GluR2 mRNA and protein, increased Ca^{2+} permeability of AMPA receptors, impairment of intracellular Ca^{2+} homeostasis, free radical formation, and induction of apoptosis. Effective therapeutic measures to limit neurological damage once stroke has occurred have been elusive so far. A better understanding of the pathophysiologic mechanisms of stroke is an important factor, together with the realization of the need for rapid diagnosis and initiation of therapy following the acute event that makes this goal more attainable in the near future.

References

1. Choi DW. Cerebral hypoxia: Some new approaches and unanswered questions. *J Neurosci* 1990;10:2493-2501.
2. Siesjo BK. Pathophysiology and treatment of focal cerebral ishcemia ischemia. Part II: Mechanisms of damage and treatment. *J Neurosurg* 1992;77:337-354.

3. Ginsberg MD, Busto R. Rodent models of cerebral ischemia. *Stroke* 1989;20: 1627-1642.

4. Pulsinelli W. Pathophysiology of acute ischaemic stroke. *Lancet* 1992;339: 533-536.

5. Astrup J, Siesjo BK, Symon L. Thresholds in cerebral ischemia; the ischemic penumbra. *Stroke* 1981;12:723-725.

6. Ginsberg MD, Pulsinelli WA. The ischemia penumbra, injury thresholds, and the therapeutic window for acute stroke. *Ann Neurol* 1994;36:553-554.

7. Petito CK, Feldmann E, Pulsinelli WA, et al. Delayed hippocampal damage in humans following cardiorespiratory arrest. *Neurology* 1987;37:1281-1286.

8. Pulsinelli WA, Brierley JB, Plum F. Temporal profile of neuronal damage in model of transient forebrain ischemia. *Ann Neurol* 1982;11:491-498.

9. Oguro K, Grooms S, Calderone A, et al. Molecular mechanisms of delayed neurodegeneration in ischemia and status epilepticus. *In Pharmacology of Cerebral Ischemia*, Kreiglstein J (ed): 1999 Marburg.

10. Meldrum B, Garthwaite J. Excitatory amino acid neurotoxicity and neurodegenerative disease. *Trends Pharmacol Sci* 1990;11:379-387.

11. Olney JW. Excitotoxic amino acids and neuropsychiatric disorders. *Ann Rev Pharmacol Toxicol* 1990;30:47-71.

12. Lipton SA, Rosenberg PA. Excitatory amino acids as a final common pathway for neurological disorders. *New Engl J Med* 1994;330:613-622.

13. Tsubokawa H, Oguro K, Robinson HP, et al. Intracellular inositol 1,3,4,5-tetrakisphosphate enhances the calcium current in hippocampal CA1 neurones of the gerbil after ischaemia. *J Physiol (Lond)* 1996;497:67-78.

14. Tsubokawa H, Oguro K, Robinson HP, et al. Inositol 1,3,4,5-tetrakisphosphate as a mediator of neuronal death in ischemic hippocampus. *Neuroscience* 1994;59:291-297.

15. Oguro K, Nakamura M, Masuzawa T. Histochemical study of Ca(2+)-ATPase activity in ischemic CA1 pyramidal neurons in the gerbil hippocampus. *Acta Neuropathol* 1995;90:448-453.

16. Siesjo BK, Bengtsson F. Calcium fluxes, calcium antagonists, and calcium-related pathology in brain ischemia, hypoglycemia, and spreading depression: A unifying hypothesis. *J Cereb Blood Flow Metab* 1989;9:127-140.

17. Choi DW. Calcium: Still center-stage in hypoxic-ischemic neuronal death. *Trends Neurosci* 1995;18:58-60.

18. Tsubokawa H, Oguro K, Robinson HP, et al. Abnormal Ca2+ homeostasis before cell death revealed by whole cell recording of ischemic CA1 hippocampal neurons. *Neuroscience* 1992;49: 807-817.

19. Takei N, Endo Y. Ca2+ ionophore-induced apoptosis on cultured embryonic rat cortical neurons. *Brain Res* 1994;652:65-70.

20. Nicoll RA, Malenka RC, Kauer JA. Functional comparison of neurotransmitter receptor subtypes in mammalian central nervous system. *Physiol Rev* 1990;70:513-565.

21. Seeburg PH. The TINS/TiPS Lecture. The molecular biology of mammalian glutamate receptor channels. *Trends Neurosci* 1993;16:359-365.

22. Martin LJ, Blackstone CD, Levey Al, et al. AMPA glutamate receptor subunits are differentially distributed in rat brain. *Neuroscience* 1993;53(2): 327-358.

23. Wenthold RJ, Petralia RS, Blahos J II, et al. Evidence for multiple AMPA receptor complexes in hippocampal CA1/CA2 neurons. *J Neurosci* 1996;6:1982-1989.

24. Hollmann M, Hartley M, Heinemann S. Ca2+ permeability of KA-AMPA--gated glutamate receptor channels depends on subunit composition. *Science* 1991;252: 851-853.

25. Verdoorn TA, Burnashev N, Monyer H, et al. Structural determinants of ion flow through recombinant glutamate receptor channels. *Science* 1991;252:1715-1718.

26. Burnashev N, Monyer H, Seeburg PH, et al. Divalent ion permeability of AMPA receptor channels is dominated by the edited form of a single subunit. *Neuron* 1992;8:189-198.

27. Hume RI, Dingledine R, Heinemann SF. Identification of a site in glutamate receptor subunits that controls calcium permeability. *Science* 1991;253: 1028-1031.

28. Kamboj SK, Swanson GT, Cull-Candy SG. Intracellular spermine confers rectification on rate calcium-permeable AMPA and kainate receptors. *J Physiol (Lond)* 1995;486 (Pt 2):297-303.

29. Koh DS, Burnashev N, Jonas P. Block of native Ca(2+)-permeable AMPA receptors in rat brain by intracellular polyamines generates double rectification. *J Physiol (Lond)* 1995;486 (Pt2):305-312.

30. Herlitze S, Raditsch M, Rupperberg JP, et al. Argiotoxin detects molecular differences in AMPA receptor channels. *Neuron* 1993;381:793-796.

31. Blaschke M, Keller BU, Rivosecchi R, et al. A single amino acid determines the subunit-specific spider toxin block of alpha-amino-3-hydroxy-5-methyl-isoxazole-4-propionate/kainate receptor channels. *Proc Natl Acad Sci USA* 1993;90:6528-6532.

32. Sommer B, Kohler M, Sprengel R, et al. RNA editing in brain controls a determinant of ion flow in glutamate- gated channels. *Cell* 1991;67:11-19.

33. Higuchi M, Single FN, Kohler M, et al. RNA editing of AMPA receptor subunit GluR-B: A base-paired intron-exon structure determines position and efficiency. *Cell* 1993;75:1361-1370.

34. Bochet P, Audinat E, Lambolez B, et al. Subunit composition at the single-cell level explains functional properties of a glutamate-gated channel. *Neuron* 1994;12(2):383-388.

35. Geiger JRP, Melcher T, Koh D-S, et al. Relative abundance of subunit mRNAs determination gating and Ca2+ permeability of AMPA receptors in principal neurons and interneurons in rat CNS. *Neuron* 1995;15:193-204.

36. Jonas P, Racca C, Sakmann B, et al. Differences in Ca2+ permeability of AMPA-type glutamate receptor channels in neocortical neurons caused by differential GluR-B subunit expression. *Neuron* 1994;12:1281-1289.

37. Racca C, Catania MV, Monyer H, et al. Expression of AMPA-glutamate receptor B subunit in rat hippocampal GABAergic neurons. *Eur J Neurosci* 1996;8(8):1580-1590.

38. Johansen FF. Interneurons in rat hippocampus after cerebral ischemia. Morphometric, functional, and therapeutic investigations. *Acta Neurol Scand Suppl* 1993;150:1-32.

39. Jia Z, Agopyan N, Miu P, et al. Enhanced LTP in mice deficient in the AMPA receptor GluR2. *Neuron* 1996;17: 945-956.

40. Ribak CE, Nitsch R, Seress L. Proportion of parvalbumin-positive basket cells in the GABAergic innervation of pyramidal and granule cells of the rate hippocampal formation. *J Comp Neurol* 1990;300(4):449-461.

41. Lambolez B, Ropert N, Perrais D, et al. Correlation between kinetics and RNA splicing of alph-amino-3-hydroxy-5-methylisoxazole-4-propionicacid receptors in neocortical neurons. *Proc Natl Acad Sci USA* 1996;93(5):1797-1802.

42. Brorson JR, Manzolillo PA, Miller RJ. Ca2+ entry via AMPA/KA receptors and excitotoxicity in cultured cerebellar Purkinje cells. *J Neurosci* 1994;14(1):187-197.

43. Turetsky DM, Canzoniero LM, Sensi SL, et al. Cortical neurones exhibiting kainate-activated Co^{2+} uptake are selectively vulnerable to AMPA/kainate receptor-mediated toxicity. *Neurobiol Dis* 1994;1(3):101-110.

44. Weiss JH, Turetsky D, Wilke G, et al. AMPA/kainate receptor-mediated damage to ADPH-diaphorase-containing neurons is Ca2+ dependent. *Neurosci Lett* 1994;67(1-2):93-96.

45. Lu YM, Yin HZ, Chiang J, et al. Ca(2+)-permeable AMPA/kainate and NMDA channels: High rate of Ca2+ influx underlies potent induction of injury. *J Neurosci* 1996;16(17):5457-5465.

46. Brillman J. Central nervous system complications in coronary artery bypass graft surgery. *Neurol Clin* 1993;11: 475-495.

47. Roach GW, Kanchuger M, Mangano CM, et al. Adverse cerebral outcomes after coronary bypass surgery. Multicenter Study of Perioperative Ischemia Research Group and the ischemia Research and Education Foundation Investigators [see comments]. *N Engl J Med* 1996;335:1857-1863.

48. Swain JA. Cardiac surgery and the brain [editorial; comment]. *N Engl J Med* 1993;329:1119-1120.

49. Kirino T. Delayed neuronal death in the gerbil hippocampus following ischemia. *Brain Res* 1982;239:57-69.

50. Schmidt-Kastner R, Freund TF. Selective vulnerability of the hippocampus in brain ischemia. *Neuroscience* 1991;40:599-636.

51. Chen J, Zhu RL, Nakayama M, et al. Expression of the apoptosis-effector gene, Bax, is up-regulated in vulnerable hippocampal CA1 neurons following global ischemia. *J Neurochem* 1996;67:64-71.

52. Rosenbaum DM, D'Amore J, Llena J, et al. Pretreatment with intraventricular aurintricarboxylic acid decreases infarct size by inhibiting apoptosis following transient global ischemia in gerbils. *Ann Neurol* 1998;43:654-660.

53. Buchan AM, Li H, Cho S, et al. Blockade of the AMPA receptor prevents CA1 hippocampal injury following severe but transient forebrain ischemia in adult rats. *Neurosci Lett* 1991;132:255-258.

54. Pulsinelli W, Sarokin A, Buchan A. Antagonism of the NMDA and non-NMDA receptors in global versus focal brain ischemia. *Prog Brain Res* 1993;96:125-135.

55. Pulsinelli WA. The therapeutic window in ischemic brain injury [editorial]. *Curr Opin Neurol* 1995;8:3-5.

56. Sheardown MJ, Nielsen EO, Hansen AJ, et al. 2,3-Dihydroxy-6-nitro-7-sulfamoyl-benzo(F)quinoxaline: A neuroprotectant for cerebral ischemia. *Science* 1990;247:571-574.

57. Sheardown MJ, Suzdak PD, Nordholm L. AMPA, but not NMDA, receptor antagonism is neuroprotective in gerbil global ischemia, even when delayed 24 h. *Eur J Pharmacol* 1993;236:347-353.

58. Pellegrini-Giampietro DE, Zukin RS, Bennett MVL, et al. Switch in glutamate receptor subunit gene expression following global ischemia in rats. *Proc Natl Acad Sci USA* 1992;89:10499-10503.

59. Pellegrini-Giampietro DE, Pulsinelli WA, Zukin RS. NMDA and non-NMDA receptor gene expression following global brain ischemia in rats: Effect of NMDA and non-NMDA receptor antagonists. *J Neurochem* 1994;62:1067-1073.

60. Pollard H, Heron A, Moreau J, et al. Alterations of the GluR-B AMPA receptor subunit flip/flop expression in kainate-induced epilepsy and ischemia. *Neuroscience* 1993;57:545-554.

61. Heurteaux C, Lauritzen I, Widmann C, et al. Essential role of adenosine, adenosine A1 receptors, and ATP-sensitive K+ channels in cerebral ischemic preconditioning. *Proc Natl Acad Sci USA* 1995;92:4666-4670.

62. Gorter JA, Petrozzino JJ, Aronica EM, et al. Global ischemia induces downregulation of GluR2 mRNA and increases AMPA receptor mediated Ca2+ influx in hippocampal CA1 of gerbil. *J Neurosci* 1997;17:6179-6188.

63. Opitz T, Grooms SY, Zukin RS, et al. Global ischemia decreases GluR2 protein level in the hippocampal CA1 prior to cell death. *Soc Neurosci Abstr* 1998;24:231.20.

64. Petralia RS, Wang YX, Mayat E, et al. Glutamate receptor subunit 2-selective antibody shows a differential distribution of calcium-impermeable AMPA receptors among populations of neurons. *J Comp Neurol* 1997;385(3):456-476.

65. Vissavajjhala P, Janssen WG, Hu Y, et al. Synaptic distribution of the AMPA-GluR2 subunit and its colocalization with calcium-binding proteins in rat cerebral cortex: An immunohistochemical study using a GluR2-specific monoclonal antibody. *Exp Neurol* 1996;142(2):296-312.

66. Bi X, Chen J, Dang S, et al. Characterization of calpain-mediated proteolysis of GluR1 subunits of alpha-amino-3-hydroxy-5-methylisoxazole-4-propionate receptors in rat brain. *J Neurochem* 1997;68:1484-1494.

67. Tsubokawa H, Oguro K, Masuzawa T, et al. Effects of a spider toxin and its analogue on glutamate-activated currents in the hippocampal CA1 neuron after ischemia. *J Neurophysiol* 1995;74:218-225.

68. Kirino T, Robinson HP, Miwa A, et al. Disturbance of membrane function preceding ischemic delayed neuronal death in the gerbil hippocampus. *J Cereb Blood Flow Metab* 1992;12:408-417.

69. Ying HS, Weishaupt JH, Grabb M, et al. Sublethal oxygen-glucose deprivation alters hippocampal neuronal AMPA receptor expression and vulnerability to kainate-induced death. *J Neurosci* 1997;17:9536-9544.

70. Koh JY, Suh SW, Gwag BJ, et al. The role of zinc in selective neuronal death after transient global cerebral ischemia. *Science* 1996;272:1013-1016.

71. Tsuda M, Imaizumi K, Katayama T, et al. Expression of zinc transporter gene, ZnT-1, is induced after transient forebrain ischemia in the gerbil. *J Neurosci* 1997;17:6678-6684.

72. Sensi SL, Canzoniero LM, Yu SP, et al. Measurement of intracellular free zinc in living cortical neurons: Routes of entry. *J Neurosci* 1997;17:9554-9564.

73. Carriedo SG, Yin HZ, Sensi SL, et al. Rapid entry through Ca^{2+} permeable AMPA/kainate channels triggers marked intracellular Ca^{2+} rises and consequent oxygen radical production. *J Neurosci* 1998;18:7727-7738.

74. Bennett MVL, Pellegrini-Giampietro DE, Gorter JA, et al. The GluR2 hypothesis: Ca(++)-permeable AMPA receptors in delayed neurodegeneration. *Cold Spring Harb Symp Quant Biol* 1996;61:373-384.

75. Pellegrini-Giampietro DE, Bennett MVL, Zukin RS. The GluR2 (GluR-B) hypothesis: Ca(2+)-permeable AMPA receptors in neurological disorders. *Trends Neurosci* 1997;20:464-470.

76. Kamphuis W, de Leeuw FE, Lopes da Silva FH. Ischemia does not alter the editing status at the Q/R site of glutamate receptor-A, -B, -5 and –6 subunit mRNA. *Neuroreport* 1995;6:1133-1136.

77. Paschen W, Schmitt J, Uto A. RNA editing of glutamate receptor subunits GluR2, GluR5 and GluR6 in transient cerebral ischemia in the rat. *J Cereb Blood Flow Metab* 1996;16: 548-556.

78. Rump A, Sommer C, Gass P, et al. Editing of GluR2 RNA in the gerbil hippocampus after global cerebral ischemia. *J Cereb Blood Flow Metab* 1996;16:1362-1365.

79. Aronica EM, Gorter JA, Grooms S, et al. Aurintricarboxylic acid prevents GluR2 mRNA down-regulation and delayed neuro-degeneration in hippocampal CA1 neurons of gerbil after global ischemia. *Proc Natl Acad Sci USA* 1998;95:7115-7120.

80. Nurse S. Corbett DJ. Neuroprotection after several days of mild, drug-induced hypothermia. *J Cereb Blood Flow Metab* 1996;16:474-480.

81. Kamme F, Campbell K, Wieloch T. Biphasic expression of the fos and jun families of transcription factors following transient forebrain ischemia in the rat. Effect of hypothermia. *Eur J Neurosci* 1995;7:2007-2016.

82. Nowak TS Jr, Osborne OC, Suga S. Stress protein and proto-oncogene expression as indicators of neuronal pathophysiology after ischemia. *Prog Brain Res* 1993;96:195-208.

83. Kindy MS, Hu Y, Dempsey RJ. Blockade of ornithine decarboxylase enzyme protects against ischemic brain damage. J Cereb Blood Flow Metab 1994;14:1040-1045.

84. Aoki M, Abe K, Kawagoe J, et al. Acceleration of HSP70 and HSC70 heat shock gene expression following transient ischemia in the preconditioned gerbil hippocampus. *J Cereb Blood Flow Metab* 1993;13:781-788.

85. Kokaia Z, Metsis M, Kokaia M, et al. Brain insults in rats induce increased expression of the BDNF gene through differential use of multiple promoters. *Eur J Neurosci* 1994;6:587-596.

86. Takeda A, Onodera H, Sugimoto A, et al. Coordinated expression of messenger RNAs for nerve growth factor, brain-derived neurotrophic factor and neurotrophin-3 in the rat hippocampus following transient forebrain ischemia. *Neuroscience* 1993;55:23-31.

87. Brusa R, Zimmermann F, Koh DS, et al. Early-onset epilepsy and postnatal lethality associated with an editing –deficient GluR-B allele in mice. *Science* 1995;270:1677-1680.

88. Gu JG, Albuquerque C, Lee CJ, et al. Synaptic strengthening through activation of Ca2+ -permeable AMPA receptors. *Nature* 1996;381:793-796.

89. Kondo M, Sumino R, Okado H. Combinations of AMPA receptor subunit expression in individual cortical neurons correlate with expression of specific calcium-binding proteins. 1997;17(5):1570-1581.

90. Mosbacher J, Schoepfer R, Monyer H, et al. A molecular determinant for submillisecond desensitization in glutamate receptors. *Science* 1994;266: 1059-1061.

91. Le D, Das S, Wang YF, et al. Enhanced neuronal death from focal ischemia in AMPA-receptor transgenic mice. *Mol Brain Res* 1997;52:235-241.

92. Oguro K, Oguro N, Koijima T, et al. Knock-down of AMPA receptor GluR2 expression leads to hippocampal neuronal death and increases damage by sublethal ischemia. *Society for Neurosci* (Abstract) 1998;24:231.

93. Buchan A, Li H, Pulsinelli WA. The N-methyl-D-aspartate antagonist, MK-801, fails to protect against neuronal damage caused by transient, severe forebrain ischemia in adults rats. *J Neurosci* 1991;11:1049-1056.

Chapter 24

Fluorescent Indicator Measurements of Ca^{2+} Homeostasis in Postischemic CA1 Hippocampal Neurons

John A. Connor, PhD, Anders C. Greenwood, PhD, Seddigheh Razani-Boroujerdi, PhD, Jeffrey J. Petrozzino, PhD, and Rick C. S. Lin, PhD

Introduction

There are large differences in the severity and the time course of postischemic cell loss in different brain regions. Some areas show widespread, immediate death, eg, striatum. Others, notably area CA1 of the dorsoseptal hippocampus, show very little immediate damage, but nearly total cell loss over several days following a transient ischemic insult. The general description of delayed neuronal death in rodents has been worked out most carefully in two global ischemia models: the 4-vessel occlusion model in the rat,[1] and common carotid artery occlusion in gerbil.[2-4] Delayed neuronal death, prominent in the CA1 hippocampus, has been subsequently described in monkeys,[5] and in humans a similar distribution pattern of neuronal loss is found in individuals who were revived after cardiac arrest.[6,7]

The causes of this delayed death are poorly understood, but the extended time-course involved make it potentially amenable to treat-

Supported by NS35644 from NIH-NINDS

From: Choi D, Dacey RG, Hsu CY, Powers WJ. *Cerebrovascular Disease: Momentum at the End of the Second Millennium.* Armonk, NY: Futura Publishing Company, Inc., © 2002.

ment, given an understanding of these causes. Although abnormally large influxes of Ca^{2+} in the postischemic period, or breakdown of Ca^{2+} regulation are often cited as contributing, or proximal causes of neuronal death,[8-11] a direct examination of the Ca^{2+} physiology of the neurons destined to die has been lacking. Although there is virtually no question at this date that there is a large, long lasting Ca^{2+} increase in neurons during and immediately after ischemic insult,[12,13] the condition of Ca^{2+} homeostasis during the following 1-3 days, when there are many intact and functional CA1 neurons has remained unclear. We have addressed the issue using CA1 pyramidal neurons, given ischemic insults, *in vivo*, and then examined in the slice preparation. We have found that the vulnerable CA1 neurons examined 1-3 days after the ischemic insult, show greatly decreased Ca^{2+} signaling during electrical activity, normal to subnormal basal Ca^{2+} levels, and a near normal ability to recover from Ca^{2+} loads. Morphologically, the dendrites of these same neurons display extensive beading of MAP-2 immuostaining, a marker associated with neuronal damage.[14,15] The results suggest the importance of further research into the possible neuroprotective and/or deleterious roles of reduced Ca signalling after transient ischemia.

Methods

Adult male Mongolian gerbils were anesthetized with 1.5% to 2% halothane, kept at 37° – 38° C rectal temperature with a heating pad and lamp, and subjected to 5 minutes of carotid occlusion with aneurysm clamps.[16] Two strategies were used to evaluate changes in calcium handling in neurons following ischemia. In the first, a unilateral carotid occlusion was used. In susceptible animals this procedure leads to near total pyramidal neuron death in CA1 on the ipsilateral side and spares neurons on the nonischemic (contralateral) side.[17] Use of ipsilateral and contralateral slices made it possible to compare control and ischemia-treated CA1 neurons taken from the same animal, controlling for surgical manipulations and other variables. These experiments were particularly advantageous for studies of the time course of calcium changes. Because of differences in collateral circulation between gerbils, the procedure has a success rate of about 50%–60 % in male gerbils.[17] To determine the effectiveness of the 5 minute unilateral occlusions in producing ischemic conditions in the ipsilateral hemisphere, we examined the slices used in imaging experiments for the appearance of dendritic beading in MAP-2 immunostaining[14,15] or in biocytin fills. Only slices showing extensive dendritic beading were included in the post-ischemic populations. Dendritic beading was not present in the contralateral hemisphere.

The second strategy used 5-minute occlusion of both carotids with controls being provided by data from age-matched, unoperated gerbils. To determine the effectiveness of this operation in our hands, a population of 10 gerbils were sacrificed 10 days after the bilateral occlusion and their hippocampi examined using cresyl violet staining. Consistent with earlier studies in gerbils[2-4,18,19] we observed pyramidal cell loss, exceeding 90%, in area CA1 of both hemispheres in eight of the ten brains, with the remaining two showing near total loss in only one hemisphere

Gerbils from the control population and 1–3 days after ischemia were anesthetized by ketamine/xylazine injection (40/5 mg/Kg), decapitated, and coronal hemispheric slices (400 μm thick) cut using a vibrotome. Slices were incubated for at least 1.5 hours at 25° C in the following solution (mM: 126 NaCl, 3 KCl, 1.25 NaH$_2$PO$_4$, 1 MgSO$_4$, 26 NaHCO$_3$, 2 CaCl$_2$, and 10 dextrose), gassed with a mixture of 95% O$_2$ / 5% CO$_2$. Experiments were run at both 23°-25° C and at 32° C. The progressive loss of Ca-signaling after ischemia was present at both measurement temperatures. Microelectrodes were tip-filled with 10 mM fura-2 in 0.5 mM KAcetate and sometimes 2% biocytin. They were then back-filled with 3 M KCl / 1 M KAcetate. To limit impalement quality as a confounding variable, we selected cells with input resistance > 50 MW and steady resting membrane potentials more negative than −60 mV. Holding current was adjusted to maintain the potential between −65 and −75 mV. After experiments in which biocytin was co-injected along with fura-2, slices were fixed in 3.5% paraformaldehyde in 0.1 M phosphate buffer for 3–6 hours, cryoprotected by addition of 20% sucrose for 3–6 hours and resection at 40-60 μm with a freezing microtome. Sections were processed with the ABC method (Vector kit) for photomicroscopy.

Ester loading of cells with fura-2 followed the basic procedure of Regehr & Tank.[20] A large bore micropipette filled with fura-2/AM:DMSO (10 μM:.3%) was positioned in the alveolus and pressure pulses (1 Hz, 0.5 duty cycle) applied for 15 or more minutes. Basal dendrites of CA1 neurons steadily accumulated fura-2, which diffused to cell bodies and apical dendrites. This positioning of the pipette allowed measurements to be made in the cell body layer, distant from the loading site. Calcium measurements were made by ratio imaging of fura-2,[21] using 350/380 nm excitation, an upright microscope and a cooled frame-transfer CCD-camera system.[22] In Figure 1 Ca²⁺ profiles have been plotted using the National Institute of Health Image program.

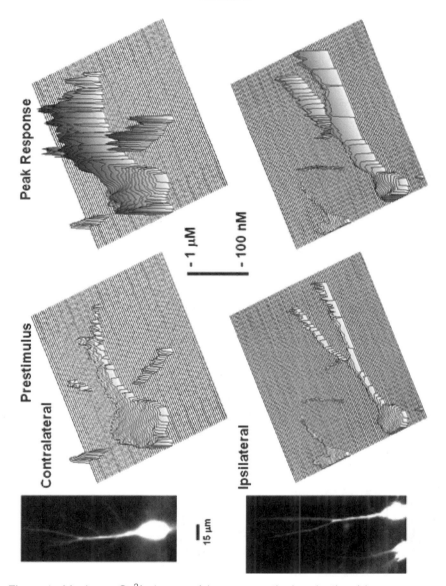

Figure 1. Maximum Ca^{2+} changes (shown as vertical projections) in a neuron from the contralateral hemisphere (upper panels) of an animal given a 5-minute unilateral occlusion compared with a neuron in the ipsilateral hemisphere (lower panels). Stimulus current was 0.6 nA/1 seconds in both neurons. Leftmost panels show fluorescence images of the neurons which had been microinjected with fura-2 (380 nm excitation). Projection images are rotated 90° CW from the fluorescence images. In the postischemic slice two neurons (lower left corner of fluorescence panel) were injected and the electrode withdrawn before the third (responding neuron, right) was penetrated.

Results

Intracellular Ca changes were measured with microelectrode injected fura-2 and non-invasively loaded fura-2/AM. Cells selected for inclusion in the microelectrode based part of this study had steady resting potentials > −60 mV and membrane resistance (Rm) > 70 MOhm. While neurons were often encountered in postischemic (and control) preparations that had lower, often oscillatory membrane potential with spontaneous firing, these were rejected as possibly being near death from either the ischemia or the electrode penetration. Given that 90%–95% of the CA1 neurons are going to die anyway, we selected the more normally behaving population to gain insight into early pathophysiology. Figure 1 shows Ca^{2+} increases driven by depolarizing current injections (0.6 nA, 1 sec) in two neurons from the same animal, one from the normal side of the brain (upper panels) and one from the ischemic side (lower panels). The postischemic neuron typifies the attenuated, depolarization driven Ca^{2+} increases in postischemic neurons (uni- or bilateral occlusion) compared to activity driven increases in control neurons. Resting Ca^{2+} levels tended to be somewhat lower (not higher) in the postischemic neurons than in controls (see Table 1, not absence of a significant difference). In probing for changes in Ca^{2+} homeostasis, Ca^{2+} transients were elicited by injecting depolarizing current through the recording microelectrode. This response avoids complications of stimulation through presynaptic fibers (orthodromic) which might be subject to systematic changes after ischemia such as the number of viable inputs, synaptic efficacy, or differences in stimulus electrode placement in different experiments. Ca^{2+} changes that occur in this protocol are due to activation of voltage gated Ca channels in the postsynaptic neuron. Ca^{2+} release from internal stores does not produce an appreciable signal under these conditions.[23,24]

Table 1.

Parameter	Control	Post-ischemia 3 days
sAHP*	9.3 ± 0.7 mV (n = 7)	6.5 ± 1.0 mV (n = 7)
Rest Potential	-65.2 ± 1.7 mV (n = 13)	-67.9 ± 2.9 mV (n = 7)
Dend. Ca2+ (rest)**	84 ± 10 nM (n = 12)	70 ± 13 nM (n = 11)***

* P = 0.04 (Student's *t*-test, unpaired) n = 7 control; n = 7 day 3
** P = 0.41 (Not Significant, Student's *t*-test, unpaired)
*** More resting Ca²+ measurements are available than others because cells are lost during execution of experiments.

Figure 2 shows Ca^{2+} increases during spike trains in two populations of neurons, from unoperated controls and from animals 2 days after <u>bilateral</u> occlusion of the carotid arteries. Stimulus current levels were adjusted between 0.5 and 0.6 nA to fire 15–18 spikes in the 1-second period in control cells (n = 6) and 16–20 spikes in the postischemic cells (n = 6). The initial 300 ms of spike firing is shown in the right hand traces. For each cell, the time course of the Ca^{2+} change was determined in the most responsive region of primary dendrite. As can be seen, the Ca^{2+} increase elicited by the spike trains was much smaller in the postischemic neurons as compared with the controls, 8-fold smaller peak on average, even though the postischemic neurons fired more spikes. Correspondingly smaller Ca^{2+} signals were seen in all parts of the dendritic tree and in the soma. Results from the unilateral and bilateral occlusion protocols are therefore in good agreement.

The reduction of depolarization induced Ca^{2+} signals after ischemia was found for even large, long lasting depolarizations (4 seconds, 3 nA depolarizing current). Figure 3 compares data gathered from populations of neurons 1, 2, and 3 days following unilateral carotid

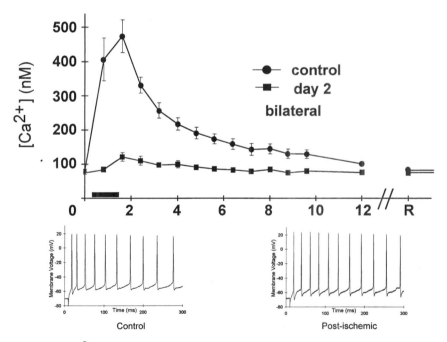

Figure 2. Ca^{2+} increases during spike trains in two populations of neurons, from unoperated controls and from animals 2 days after <u>bilateral</u> occlusion of the carotid arteries (n = 6 in each group, mean ± SEM). Samples of spike trains are given in the lower part of the figure.

occlusion with control data taken from neurons on the unoccluded side (n = 6 neurons in each group). Figure 3A shows the time course of Ca^{2+} increases in the apical dendrite elicited by extended depolarizations. Regions of maximum Ca^{2+} change in the primary dendrite of

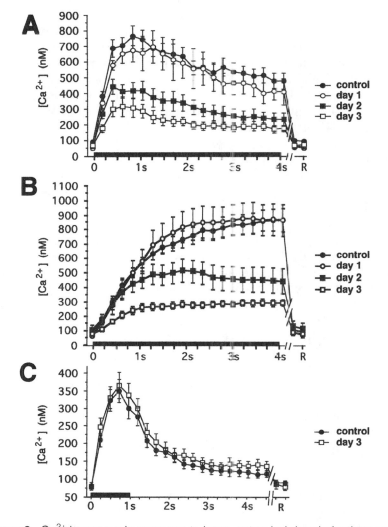

Figure 3. Ca^{2+} increases in response to large, extended depolarizations measured at apical dendrite location **(A)** and soma **(B)**. Neurons sampled from non-ischemic hemisphere (control) and ischemic hemisphere (unilateral occlusions) 1, 2, and 3 days after operation. Data from controls and 1 day postischemia are not significantly different but thereafter the Ca^{2+} response is attenuated. **C.** Recovery time course for matched dendritic Ca^{2+} loads in controls and day 3 postischemics from the same group of cells as A & B. Horizontal black bars indicate stimulus duration. n = 6, all groups.

each neuron were selected for the plots. Ca^{2+} levels actually increased only during the initial 1 second of the stimulus when most of the spike firing occurred. During the remaining period of the stimulus the cells remained depolarized to -20 mV but firing had stopped. Increasing the amplitude of the stimulus current did not significantly increase the amplitude of the Ca^{2+} change because delayed rectification prevented the voltage from moving appreciably beyond -20 mV. Thus the records show that the maximal changes observed in the primary dendrites of the neurons undergo a pronounced fall-off with time after ischemia. Somatic Ca^{2+} levels increased more slowly than levels in the dendrites (Figure 3B), but peak levels followed the same falloff with time between the ischemic insult and the day at which measurements were made. The peak Ca^{2+} increase was not significantly different in the control neurons and at 1 day postischemic.

Figure 3C compares time courses of post stimulus Ca^{2+} recovery. Here, the stimulus amplitude was adjusted so that the maximum Ca^{2+} change in controls and ischemics was approximately the same ($< 20\%$ difference between all maxima). Since the peak Ca^{2+} changes were suppressed in the postischemic neurons, this equalization required a small amplitude stimulus in the controls and a much larger amplitude in the ischemics. Ca^{2+} levels were followed during the 1 second stimulus and for 3 seconds of the recovery, and finally at 30 and 60 seconds. The recovery time courses appear to be identical.

As a confirmation of the unilateral results of Figure 3A, we also examined neurons after bilateral ischemia; 6 CA1 neurons from 4 unoperated gerbils and 6 neurons from 5 gerbils 2 days after bilateral ischemia. At 2 days, the peak value of the mean dendritic Ca^{2+} transient elicited by a 2-second 2 nA current pulse was 57% of the control value ($P < 0.05$, data not shown). With either occlusion operation the greatest contrast in Ca signaling between controls and ischemics was observed using action potential trains as the stimulus rather than maintained depolarization.

Although unlikely, it is possible that the criteria used for microelectrode injection of fura-2 and recordings may lead to selection of a small population of healthy neurons in ischemic slices, and reject the 90%-95% of neurons that are destined to die following this insult. This possibility was addressed by performing a series of experiments in which CA1 neurons were noninvasively loaded with membrane-permeant fura-2/AM to measure Ca^{2+} changes. In contrast to microelectrode filling, this method allows measurements in a number of neighboring cells in the slice, and avoids the selection problem that arises with microelectrode penetration. Figure 4 shows a typical fluorescence image from a control slice (left panel). The somata of three or more neurons could usually be resolved in a slice, but

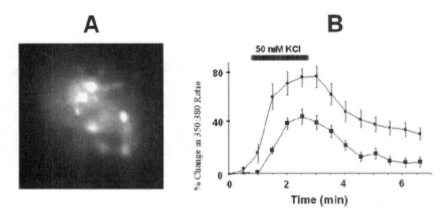

Figure 4. A. Fluorescence image (380 nm excitation) of neuronal somata loaded noninvasively with fura -2 by infusion of membrane permeable fura-2AM into the alveolar region of the slice. The infusion site is not in the field of view. Calibration bar 50 μm. **B.** Ca^{2+} signals in somata of neurons responding to 2 minutes superfusion of high K saline. Open squares: Control population, n = 21. Filled circles: 2 days after bilateral schemia.

dendrites rarely stood out from the background. In each experiment, 50 mM KCl was bath-applied and the fura-2 ratio change in the best resolved somata (somata fluorescence > 6X background) were measured at 30-second intervals. Figure 4 (right panel) compares time courses of the averaged ratio signals from 21 cells from controls and 16 cells on day 2 after bilateral ischemia (7 control animals and 6 postischemic animals). The postischemic ratio signal was markedly reduced (P < 0.05), confirming the results from fura-2 injections despite the different protocol. Ratio signals were not converted to $[Ca^{2+}]$ because of limitations of the fura-2/AM method. First, nonspecific loading produces background from out-of-focus cells, which may include damaged high-Ca^{2+} cells near the slice surface. Second, the fluorescent signal includes a nonquantifiable component from the unconverted ester form of fura-2/AM, which does not bind Ca^{2+}. These two limitations of the method would tend to lessen the observed difference between Ca^{2+} transients in postischemics and controls, which was nonetheless significant (Figure 4).

If the reduced Ca^{2+} changes shown above are due to decreased activity driven influx, as opposed to increased intracellular buffering, then there should also be electrically measurable changes. CA1 neurons are normally capable of generating a modified action potential in the presence of Na channel block, the Ca-spike.[25,26] Figure 5A compares firing patterns before and after the addition of the Na channel blocker, tetrodotoxin (TTX , 2 μM) to the superfusion solution. No K channel blockers were used. In all the control neurons examined (n = 8), there

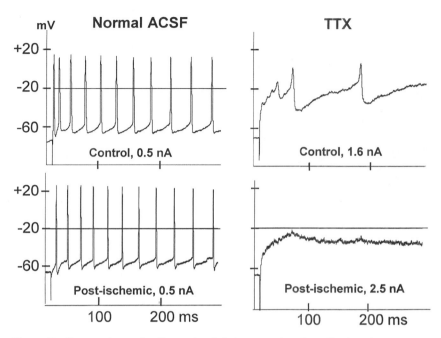

Figure 5. Comparison of action potentials in normal and postischemic neurons. In normal saline, there are subtle differences in spike train characteristics between control and postischemic neurons (see text) but both classes fire robust spike trains (left-hand panels). In the presence of TTX (1 μM) normal neurons fire a Ca-spike (upper right panel), but in the postischemic population (day 2, bilateral occlusion). There was no Ca-spike (lower right panel). Normal ACSF and TTX data taken from the same neuron.

was a prominent action potential remaining in TTX (36.14 ± 4.4 mV amplitude and 13.4 ± 3.8 msec duration, mean ± SEM). The higher threshold for the Ca-spike required a larger stimulus current than was required than for the Na spikes (upper traces, Figure 5A). In all seven of the seven neurons from four gerbils studied 2 days after bilateral ischemia, we could not elicit recognizable spike activity in TTX, despite increasing the stimulus current to very large values (eg, Figure 5A, lower right trace).

The finding of Figure 5A supports the idea that the spike/depolarization-mediated Ca^{2+} transients were reduced after ischemia by a direct effect on VGCCs. First, it is implausible that enhanced K+ currents could prevent normal VGCCs from generating Ca^{2+} spikes, given the large depolarizations achieved and the fact that the repetitive firing pattern in normal saline, more spikes in postischemic neurons than in controls, suggested normal or subnormal K currents. Second, Ca^{2+} spikes would be minimally affected by putative changes in postischemic Ca^{2+} buffering or sequestration that might be invoked to explain the reduced fura-2 signals. The possibility of increased buffering is also unlikely given the normal recovery shown in Figure 2B.

There were also other changes in Ca²⁺-related electrophysiology of post-ischemic CA1 cells. First, the slow afterhyperpolarization (sAHP) that follows depolarization were markedly reduced. The sAHP is attributed to the Ca-dependent K⁺ current, I_{AHP}, while adaptation derives from a mixture of K+ currents, with and without, Ca-dependence.[27] Table 1 summarizes data showing the reduction in sAHP on days 2 and 3 after unilateral ischemia. Second, spike train adaptation, that progressively lowers the firing rate during extended depolarization was greatly reduced after ischemia. Figure 6A shows reduced spike-frequency adaptation on day 3 after unilateral ischemia compared to controls. The population data of Figure 6B were generated by measuring the first 5 interspike intervals in trains elicited by 0.5 nA of injected current. Intervals 2–5 were expressed as percentages of the first spike interval for each cell before the group mean for each interval was calculated and plotted, the day-2 cells showing much less adaptation

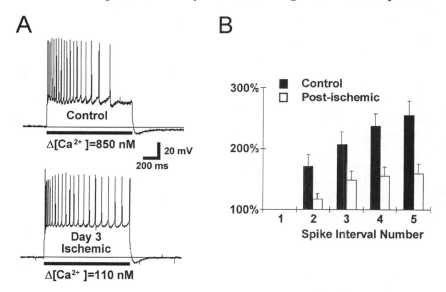

Figure 6. A. Action potential trains generated by depolarizing current, 1 second duration, in control neuron (upper trace) and neuron in affected hemisphere 3 days after unilateral occlusion. Postischemic neuron shows less adaptation in firing rate, but also a much smaller Ca²⁺ increase measured at the end of the depolarization. **B.** Population comparison of the adaptation in firing rate in controls and postischemic neurons. Increase in interspike interval is expressed as a percentage of the interval between spikes 1 and 2. Stimulus current was adjusted to give approximately the same initial firing rate for all cells. Values lay between 4.5–5.5 nA.

(P < 0.05). Because adaptation was reduced, the post-ischemic cells fired more spikes for a given current and were more excitable in this sense. However, these more numerous spikes in post-ischemic cells produced much smaller Ca^{2+} increases. Third, there was marked reduction in the broadening of successive spikes during the trains evoked on day 2 after bilateral ischemia, relative to controls (data not shown).

Discussion

Our measurements of intracellular Ca^{2+} homeostasis in living CA1 cells prepared 1–3 days after brief ischemia, *in vivo*, give no support to the prevailing idea of *chronic* postischemic Ca^{2+} overload during this extended period. There were no qualitative differences in results between unilateral and bilateral occlusions, and the unilateral protocol provided a valuable control for experimental manipulations. Our results are consistent with the view that accumulation of intracellular Ca^{2+} does not appreciably precede cell death in CA1 cells that are dying days after the initial Ca overload that occurs during brief ischemia.[28] Also consistent with this view was the observation of prolonged normal resting levels of Ca^{2+} before delayed excitotoxic death in neuronal/glial co-cultures,[29] despite the common observation of elevated Ca^{2+} levels leading more immediately to neuronal death in vitro.[30,31] Thus, different approaches have provided some precedent for our findings here. We do not question at all that large acute overloads of Ca^{2+} occur during the ischemic episode and perhaps for a short period thereafter.[12,13] The time course and extent of these <u>acute</u> overloads in response to *in vitro* models of ischemia[32] or to prolonged glutamate exposure *in vitro*[33-36] has also been extensively studied.

A downregulation of Ca^{2+} influx might be a defense mechanism against subsequent insults that would normally generate Ca^{2+} overloads, which if expressed too fully, might result in degeneration, given the following things known about Ca^{2+} dependent physiology in neurons. First, VGCC-mediated Ca^{2+} influxes have been shown to play a key role in loading intracellular IP3-sensitive Ca^{2+} stores in whole-cell patched, CA1 cells.[24,37] These IP3-sensitive stores include the rough endoplasmic reticulum and nuclear envelope.[38-40] Second, the chronic, near-complete impairment of protein synthesis observed after ischemia[41] may be maintained by depressed cytoplasmic and nuclear Ca^{2+} levels, which could dysregulate mRNA transcription[11,42] and reduce traffic through nuclear pores.[40,43-45]

Finally, there is evidence that reduced Ca^{2+} influx can lead to apoptotic mechanisms,[46-48] which may contribute to post-ischemic cell death in a manner complicated by the dependence of apoptosis on protein synthesis.[49,50]

References

1. Pulsinelli WA, Brierley JB, Plum F. Temporal profile of neuronal damage in a model of transient forebrain ischemia. *Ann Neurol* 1982;11:491-498.

2. Kirino T. Delayed neuronal death in the gerbil hippocampus following ischemia. *Brain Res* 1982;239:57-69.

3. Kirino T, Sano K. Selective vulnerability in the gerbil hippocampus following transient ischemia. *Acta Neuropathol* 1984;62: 201-208.

4. Crain BJ, Westerkam WD, Harrison AH, et al. Selective neuronal death after transient forebrain ischemia in the Mongolian gerbil: A silver impregnation study. *Neurosci* 1988;27:387-402.

5. Bodsch W, Barbier A, et al. Recovery of monkey brain after prolonged ischemia. II. Protein synthesis and morphological alterations. *J Cereb Blood Flow Metab* 1986;6:22-33.

6. Petito CK, Feldmann E, Pulsinelli WA, et al. Delayed hippocampal damage in human following cardiac arrest. *Neurology* 1987;37:1281-1286.

7. Horn M, Schlote W. Delayed neuronal death and delayed neuronal recovery in the human brain following global ischemia. *Acta Neuropathol* 1992;85: 79-87.

8. Siesjo BK, Bengtsson F. Calcium fluxes, calcium antagonists, and calcium-related pathology in brain ischemia, hypoglycemia, and spreading depression: A unifying hypothesis. *J Cerebral Blood Flow Metabol* 1989;9:1271-40.

9. Kirino T, Robinson HPC, Miwa A, et al. Disturbance of membrane function preceding ischemic delayed neuronal death in the gerbil hippocampus. *J Cerebral Blood Flow Metabol* 1992;12:408-417.

10. Tsubokawa H, Oguro K, Robinson HPC, et al. Abnormal Ca2+ homeostasis before cell death revealed by whole cell recording of ischemic CA1 hippocampal neurons. *Neurosci* 1992;49:807-817.

11. Ghosh A, Greenberg ME. Calcium signalling in neurons: Molecular mechanisms and cellular consequences. *Science* 1995;268:239-246.

12. Silver IA, Erecinska M. Intracellular and extracellular changes of [Ca2+] in hypoxia and ischemia in rat brain in vivo. *J Gen Pysiol* 1990;95:827-836.

13. Silver IA, Erecinska M. Ion homeostasis in rat brain in vivo: Intra- and extracellular [Ca2+] and [H+] in the hippocampus during recovery from short-term, transient ischemia. *J Cerebral Blood Flow Metabol* 1992;12:759-772.

14. Matesic DF, Lin RCS. Microtubule-associated protein 2 as an early indicator of ischemia-induced neurodegeneration in the gerbil forebrain. *J Neurochem* 1994;63:1012-1020.

15. Hori H, Carpenter DO. Functional and morphological changes induced by transient in vivo ischemia. *Experimental Neurology* 1994;129:279-289.

16. Lin CS, Polsk K, Nadler JV, et al. Selective neocortical and thalamic cell death in the gerbil after transient ischemia. *Neurosci* 1990;35:289-299.

17. Gill R, Foster AC, Woodruff GN. Systemic administration of MK-801 protects against ischemia-induced hippocampal neurodegeneration in the gerbil. *J Neurosci* 1987;7:3343-3349.

18. Bonnekoh P, Barbier A, Oschlies U, et al. Selective vulnerability in the gerbil hippocampus: Morphological changes after 5-min ischemia and long survival times. *Acta Neuropathol* 1990;80:18-25.

19. Gorter JA, Petrozzio JJ, Aronica EM, et al. Global ischemia induces down-regulation of Glur2 mRNA and increases AMPA receptor-mediated Ca2+ influx in hippocampal CA1 neurons of gerbil. *J Neurosci* 1997;17(16): 6179-6188.

20. Regehr WG, Tank DW. Selective fura-2 loading of presynaptic terminals and nerve cell processes by local perfusion in mammalian brain slice. *J Neuros Meth* 1991;37:111-119.

21. Grynkiewicz G, Poenie M, Tsien RY. A new generation of Ca2+ indicators with greatly improved fluorescent properties. *J Biological Chem* 1985;260: 3440-3450.

22. Petrozzino JJ, Pozzo Miller LD, Connor JA. Micromolar Ca2+ transients in dendritic spines of hippocampal pyramidal neurons in brain slice. *Neuron* 1995;14:1223-1231.

23. Markram H, Helm PJ, Sakmann B. Dendritic calcium transients evoked by single back-propagating action potentials in rat neocortical pyramidal neurons. *J Physiol Lond* 1995;485:1-20.

24. Garaschuk O, Yaai Y, Konnerth A. Release and sequestration of calcium by ryanodine-sensitive stores in rat hippocampal neurones. *J Physiol (Lond)* 1997;502:13-30.

25. Schwartzkroin PA, Slawsky M. Probable calcium spikes in hippocampal neurons. *Brain Res* 1997;135:157-161.

26. Wong RK, Prince DA, Basbaum AI. Intradendritic recordings from hippocampal neurons. *Proc Natl Acad Sci USA* 1979;76: 986-990.

27. Hotson JR, Prince DA. A calcium activated hyperpolarization follows repetitive firing in hippocampal neurons. *J Neurophysiol* 1980;43:409-419.

28. Bonnekoh P, Kurolwa T, Klolber O, et al. Time profile of calcium accumulation in hippocampus, striatum and frontoparietal cortex after transient forebrain ischemia in the gerbil. *Acta Neuropathol* 1992;84:400-406.

29. Dubinsky JM. Intracellular calcium levels during the period of delayed excitotoxicity. *J Neurosci* 1993;13:623-631. 30. Choi DW. Calcium and excitotoxic neuronal injury. *Ann N Y Acad Sci* 1994;747:162-171.

31. Dubinsky JM. Examination of the role of calcium in neuronal death. *Ann N Y Acad Sci* 1993;679:34-42.

32. Lobner, Lipton P. Intracellular calcium levels and calcium fluxes in the CA1 region of the rat hippocampal slice during in vitro ischemia: Relationship to electrophysiological cell damage. *J Neurosci* 1993;13:4861-4871.

33. Connor JA, Wadman WJ, Hockberger PE, et al. Sustained dendritic gradients of Ca2+ induced by excitatory amino acids in CA1 hippocampal neurons. *Science* 1988;240:649-653.

34. Randall RD, Thayer SA. Glutamate-induced calcium transient triggers delayed calcium overload and neurotoxicity in rat hippocampal neurons. *J Neurosci* 1992;12:1882-1895.

35. Wadman WJ, Connor JA. Persisting modification of dendritic calcium influx by excitatory amino acid stimulation in isolated CA1 neurons. *Neurosci* 1992;48:293-305.

36. Weiss S, Hochman D, MacVicar BA. Repeated NMDA receptor activation induces distinct intracellular calcium changes in subpopulations of striatal neurons in vitro. *Brain Res* 1993;627:63-71.

37. Jaffe DB, Brown TH. Metabotropic glutamate receptor activation induces calcium waves within hippocampal dendrites. *J Neurophysiol* 1994;72:471-474.

38. Malviya AN, Rogue P, Vincendon G. Stereospecific inositol 1,4,5-[32P]trisphosphate binding to isolated rat liver nuclei: Evidence for inositol trisphosphate receptor-mediated calcium release from the nucleus. *Proc Natl Acad Sci USA* 1990;87:9270-9274.

39. Parys JB, Sernett SW, DeLisle S, et al. Isolation, characterization, and localization of the inositol 1,4,5- trisphosphate receptor protein in Xenopus laevis oocytes. *J Biol Chem* 1992;267:18776-18782.

40. Stehno-Bittel L, Luckhoff A, Clapham DE. Calcium release from the nucleus by InsP3 receptor channels. *Neuron* 1995;14:163-167.

41. Thilmann R, Xie Y, Kleihues P, et al. Persistent inhibition of protein synthesis precedes delayed neuronal death in postischemic gerbil hippocampus. *Acta Neuropathol (Berl)* 1986;71:88-93.

42. Hardingham GE, Chawla S, Johnson CM, et al. Distinct functions of nuclear and cytoplasmic calcium in the control of gene expression. *Nature* 1997;385:260-265.

43. Greber UF, Gerace L. Depletion of calcium from the lumen of endoplasmic reticulum reversibly inhibits passive diffusion and signal-mediated transport into the nucleus. *J Cell Biol* 1995;128:5-14.

44. Perez-Terzic C, Pyle J, Jaconi M, et al. Conformational states of the nuclear pore complex induced by depletion of nuclear Ca2+ stores. *Science* 1996;273:1875-1877.

45. Stehno-Bittel L, Perez-Terzic C, Clapham DE. Diffusion across the nuclear envelope inhibited by depletion of the nuclear Ca2+ store. *Science* 1995;270:1835-1838.

46. Franklin JL, Johnson EM Jr. Suppression of programmed neuronal death by sustained elevation of cytoplasmic calcium. *Trends Neurosci* 1992;15:501-508.

47. Gallo V, Kingsbury A, Balazs R, et al. The role of depolarization in the survival and differentiation of cerebellar granule cells in culture. *J Neurosci* 1987;7:2203-2213.

48. Koh JY, Cotman CW. Programmed cell death: Its possible contribution to neurotoxicity mediated by calcium channel antagonists. *Brain Res* 1992;587:233-240.

49. Chalmers-Redman RM, Fraser AD, Ju WY, et al. Mechanisms of nerve cell death: Apoptosis or necrosis after cerebral ischaemia. *Int Rev Neurobiol* 1997;40:1-25.

50. Choi DW. Calcium: Still center-stage in hypoxic-ischemic neuronal death. *Trends Neurosci* 1995;18:58-60.

Chapter 25

Delayed Neuronal Death—A Perspective and Synthesis

Myron D. Ginsberg, MD

Introduction

Delayed neuronal death is usefully viewed as one region along a continuum of cell death which ranges from the very slow to the very rapid. This chapter attempts to construct a framework for conceptualizing key phenomena relevant to delayed neuronal death, as well as to summarize certain issues raised in discussion of the antecedent papers of this section. Studies of our group are cited to illustrate key points.

The Pace of Neuronal Death May be Both Accelerated and Decelerated

Recent experimental studies have clearly established that the pace of neuronal death following an ischemic insult is susceptible to either acceleration or deceleration, depending upon the precise context of the ischemic insult. Known accelerators of ischemic death include hyperthermia,[1] which may have a broad time window;[2,3] multiple ischemic insults repeated at short time intervals;[4] and compound insults such as ischemia plus trauma, or hypoxia plus ischemia. Decelerators of the rate of ischemic cell change include hypothermia;[5,6] adrenalectomy,[7] probably acting via induced hypothermia; and tolerance-inducing preconditioning paradigms.[8,9] Certain drugs may also delay the pace of

Our studies are supported by program-project grant NS 05820.

From: Choi D, Dacey RG, Hsu CY, Powers WJ. *Cerebrovascular Disease: Momentum at the End of the Second Millennium.* Armonk, NY: Futura Publishing Company, Inc., © 2002.

ischemic change, in some instances due to hypothermia.[10] In general, factors which accelerate the pace of ischemic neuronal death also appear to exacerbate the extent of injury while, conversely, factors which decelerate the pace of ischemic injury typically lead to less extensive changes. Furthermore, milder ischemic insults appear to be more susceptible to the influence of modulatory factors than severe insults.

Highly Determined Neuronal Death: 2-Hour Focal Cerebral Ischemia

At one extreme, certain ischemic insults are strongly deterministic, assuring that cell death swiftly ensues. An apposite example is cerebral infarction following sufficiently long periods of focal ischemia. In transient middle cerebral artery occlusion (MCAo), events transpiring during the first 2–3 hours of occlusion hours may be entirely sufficient to determine the subsequent pattern and extent of infarctive histopathology. This was demonstrated in our recent investigations of a highly reproducible model of 2-hour MCAo by intraluminal suture, studied by correlative autoradiographic and histopathologic image analysis.[11,12] By pixel comapping, we showed that approximately 90% of the eventual infarct is already predicted by local blood flow below mid-penumbral values (0.3 mL/g/min) measured at the end of 2 hours of MCAo (Figure 1). Furthermore, the development of infarctive histopathology is precisely reflected in a depression of local cerebral glucose utilization (lCMRgl) measured at just 1 hour of recirculation (Figure 1). These two measurements in conjunction very precisely predict those pixels destined to infarct.[12]

These observations, however, must be qualified by pointing out that they apply only to a prediction of *pan-necrosis*. Selective injury to neurons with preservation of the neurophil at the periphery of brain infarct,[13] referred to as "incomplete infarction,"[14] also occurs to a variable degree, depending upon the model.[15] The latter neuropathological changes are known to be ameliorated by hyperglycemia[16,17] and to be accentuated by periinfarct depolarizations.[18,19] Even in the context of pan-necrosis, however, postischemic factors may also play a role. For example, the incomplete return of postischemic cortical recirculation may encourage the development of maximal infarcts following only two hours of MCAo.[11]

Less Highly Determined Neuronal Death: 30-Minute Focal Cerebral Ischemia

In contrast to the above scenario, shortening the duration of MCAo tends to render the process of neuronal death much less highly deter-

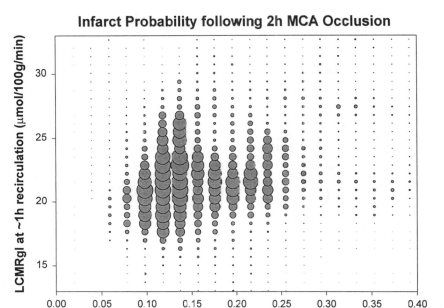

Figure 1. Pixel-based analysis of the probability of histopathological infarction resulting from 2 hours of MCA occlusion, as a function of local cerebral blood flow (LCBF) measured autoradiographically at the end of the occlusion period, and as a function of local glucose utilization (LCMRgl) measured autoradiographically at approximately 1 hour of postischemic recirculation. Data are replotted from the study of Zhao et al[2] and were derived by comapping of LCBF, LCMRgl, and infarct frequency maps into the same computer-template. Bubble sizes are proportional to numbers of affected pixels. This analysis clearly shows that LCBF values below approximately 0.30 mL/g/min, measured at 2h MCA occlusion, strongly predict infarctive pathology. Regions destined to infarct already show depressed LCMRgl values at 1 hour of recirculation.

mined. Under such conditions, *delayed* cell death may then emerge. Du et al.[20] contrasted the sequelae of 90- and 30-minute periods of MCAo plus bilateral carotid artery occlusions. As expected, the 90-minute insult led to fully developed morphological evidence of infarction within 24 hours, whereas no infarction was evident at 24 hours following the 30-minute insult. However, rats with the 30-minute insult began to show infarction at 3 days, and by 2 weeks they had infarcts as large as those induced by the 90-minute insult. The participation of apoptotic mechanisms was suggested by prominent TUNEL staining and internucleosomal DNA fragmentation, and by reduction of infarct size with cycloheximide treatment.[20] This work clearly illustrates that the severity of an insult may not only modulate the pace of neuronal death but also its *mechanism*, and it suggests that necrosis and apoptosis may not be mutually exclusive injury processes in the ischemic context.

Normal Neurons, Lateral CA1 Hippocampus

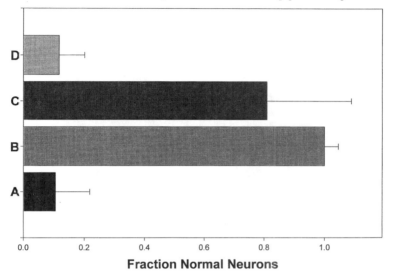

Fraction Normal Neurons

Figure 2. Normal pyramidal-neuron counts (expressed as a fraction of total neurons) in the lateral subsector of hippocampal CA1 in rats subjected to 10 minutes of global forebrain ischemia by two-vessel occlusion plus hypotension. Values are means ± SD, replotted from the data of reference.[6] Normothermic-ischemic rats (brain temperature 37°C) surviving for 2 months show greatly reduced numbers of normal neurons **A.** Rats with *intraischemic* brain cooling to 30°C and 2-month survival show high-grade permanent neurorotection **B.** By contrast, rats with normothermic periods of brain ischemia followed by *postischemic* brain hypothermia (30°C x 3 hours) appear to be neuroprotected when examined histologically following only 3-day survival (**C**); but in similar animals surviving for 2 months (**D**), this protection is no longer evident. Thus, postischemic hypothermia of this magnitude and duration merely *delays*, but does not prevent, neuronal death.

Global Ischemia: Modulation of the Pace of Cell Death by Hypothermia

Instructive clues as to the mechanisms of delayed neuronal death are to be found in studies comparing the influence of intra- versus postischemic brain hypothermia on the histological outcome of a 10-minute global ischemic insult.[5,6] While brain temperature reductions to 30°C *during* the insult conferred permanent protection (at 2 months) in the hippocampal CA1 sector and striatum, *postischemic* cooling (30°C × 3 hours, begun at 5 minutes of recirculation) appeared to protect at 3 days, but this effect was progressively lost at 7 days and 2 months (Figure 2).[6] The clear implication of these results is that both intra- and postischemic events determine the pace of neuronal death. Postischemic contributory factors might include the secondary release of excitotoxic neurotransmitters, impaired neurotransmitter re-uptake mechanisms, or the delayed infiltration of cells such as microglia, which might in turn initiate cytotoxic processes related to cytckine release, oxygen radical production, or secondary neurotransmitter effects.[21] The precise contributions of these putative factors remain to be determined.

The permanent protection associated with intraischemic hypothermia, contrasting with the only temporary protection afforded by postischemic cooling, might suggest that fundamentally different mechanisms are at play in the two contexts. This view is challenged, however, by the observations of Corbetts's group[22] that lengthening the duration of postischemic hypothermia (eg, up to 24 hours) appears to provide long-lasting protection (at 1 year) in CA1 neurons. These readily manipulable experimental settings provide a fertile milieu for the study of the biochemical and molecular processes underlying neuroprotection.

Does a Delay in the Pace of Neuronal Death Imply an Expanded Therapeutic Window of Opportunity?

It is possible that the experimental induction of delay in the pace of neuronal death (as with postischemic hypothermia) might broaden the therapeutic window for other interventions. This was tested by the delayed administration of the NMDA antagonist MK-801 on days 3, 5, and 7 following a 10-minute global ischemic insult in rats in which early postischemic hypothermia (30°C × 3 hours) had been used.[23] Postischemic hypothermia with delayed MK-801 therapy approximately doubled the number of normal-appearing neurons in hippocampal CA1 sector at 2 months when compared to the group with postischemic hypothermia alone, but considerable inter-animal variability precluded demonstration of a statistically significant inter-group difference in this respect.[23] Corroborative behavioral data have also been published in this model.[24] This question is deserving of further exploration, as its clinical implications are far-reaching.

Multiple Ischemic Insults as a Modulator of the Pace and Extent of Injury

The paradigm of multiple global ischemic insults (5-minutes × 3, separated by 1 hour), when compared to a single 15-minute insult, yields data showing that both the pace of neuronal death and its eventual extent may be thereby accentuated, although not necessarily *pari passu*.[4] For example, in the striatum, multiple insults led to the earlier emergence of neuronal death (at 2 vs. 24 hours) but did not affect the final number of ischemic cells. By contrast, in the thalamus, the single-insult paradigm produced virtually no ischemic neuronal death, whereas the multiple insults did.[4] Neurochemically, multiple insults gave rise to a delayed and sustained increase in a composite index of excitatory / inhibitory neurotransmitter imbalance—the "excitotoxic index."[4,25] This was not present following single insults.

It is obvious that the exacerbatory/acceleratory influence of multiple ischemic insults and the protective/deceleratory influence of ischemic preconditioning paradigms[8,9] are anti-parallel processes which may therefore possibly partake, to some degree, of shared molecular and biochemical mechanisms. This is yet another area requiring renewed study.

An Example of Very Delayed Cell Death after Normothermic Global Ischemia

Even relatively brief normothermic global ischemic insults may be followed by neuronal death which evolves in a very delayed fashion.[26] Following 10 minutes of global ischemia, numbers of normal small neurons in the dorsolateral striatum began to decline significantly only at 4–10 weeks following the insult, although increases in reactive microglia were maximal even at 1 week and were sustained at 2–8 weeks. This gradual emergence of striatal ischemic cell change contrasted with the situation in CA1 hippocampus, in which, although a similar microglial pattern was apparent, numbers of normal pyramidal neurons were nonetheless already decreased by 80% at 1 week postischemia. Interestingly, a minority of rats at 4–10 weeks showed a more severe histopathological response with large confluent necrotic lesions. These changes were accompanied by occasional large thrombi within lenticulostriate arteries and by focal endothelial damage, hypertrophic microvessels, and enlarged perivascular spaces—seen after 4-week survival.[26] Thus, both microglial responses[21,27] as well as secondary endothelial alterations may play important roles in inducing delayed neuronal pathology—another fertile area for study.

The Conundrum of Glutamate Receptor Subtype Downregulation Ischemia— Selective, Nonselective, or Both?

Chapter 23 recapitulates evidence supporting the hypothesis that the GluR2 gene, one of four genes encoding AMPA receptors, is selectively downregulated following ischemia. Because the GluR2 subunit renders the AMPA receptor-mediated ion channel impermeable to calcium ions, GluR2 downregulation might lead to calcium-permeable AMPA receptors, facilitating excessive intracellular calcium influx, and, by implication, contributing to delayed neuronal death. The initial evidence supporting this hypothesis stemmed from the work of Pellegrini-Giampietro et al.[28] in rats subjected to 10-minutes of forebrain ischemia by four-vessel occlusion. In the hippocampal CA1 sector at 24 hours postischemia, their results appeared to show that GluR2 mRNA was significantly more downregulated than were the GluR1 or GluR3 subtypes. However, closer inspection of their graphical data reveals that in fact all GluR subtypes showed some degree of downregulation (GluR1 by about 25%; GluR3 by about 50%; and GluR2 by about 70%).

The molecular biology and electrophysiology underlying the GluR2 hypothesis in neurological disorders has been comprehensively reviewed.[29] Although it is well established that AMPA receptors lacking the GluR2 subunit are permeable to calcium ions while AMPA receptors containing this subunit are not, the essential point of contention revolves around the *degree of selectivity* of GluR2 downregulation following ischemia. Other groups have not consistently confirmed the findings of Zukin and collaborators. Thus, Frank, Diemer and their colleagues,[30] using two different models of global ischemia (neck cuff inflation, and four-vessel occlusion plus hypotension), showed that all GluR mRNA species were downregulated to approximately the same degree. We have also been unable to confirm selective GluR2 downregulation in ischemia.[31] In rats studied 1 day after 10-minute normothermic global ischemia by two-vessel occlusion plus hypotension, the expression of all three AMPA receptor mRNAs—GluR1, GluR2, and GluR3—was markedly suppressed in the vulnerable CA1 sector, and the NMDA receptor NR1 message was also mildly suppressed. By contrast, 1 day following a comparable intraischemic hypothermic insult (30°C), all four mRNAs remained at or near control levels throughout the hioppocampus.

Monyer emphasizes that the reliable comparative assessment of the relative abundance of different messages (eg, the various GluR subtypes) requires that measurements be made *in the same individual cell*. In a study carried out with Monyer and Choi, Ying et al.[32] subjected hippocampal neurons to sublethal oxygen-glucose deprivation and then amplified mRNA from individual neurons. The abundance of the GluR2 subunit was not affected.

This study and those of other groups also support the view that the vulnerability of various neuronal populations cannot be predicted on the basis of their GluR2 subunit expression alone. For example,

NOS-positive interneurons have low GluR2 subunit expression and yet are resistant to ischemia and neurodegeneration, suggesting that glutamate receptor-mediated calcium influx is not sufficient of itself to explain neuronal vulnerability.[33] Other workers have shown that GluR2 and/or GluR3 subunits are absent in both vulnerable and resistant types of hippocampal interneurons, again supporting the view that a knowledge of receptor subunit composition is insufficient to predict neuronal vulnerability.[34]

Discrepant findings serve importantly as stimuli to further studies to resolve perplexing issues. Chapter 24 in this section adds an additional dimension of complexity to the consideration of delayed cell death by the novel suggestion that intracellular calcium depletion (rather than excess) may be a culprit. One awaits with great interest further explorations of the nature and causes of delayed cell death.

References

1. Dietrich WD, Busto R, Valdes I, et al. Effects of normothermic versus mild hyperthermic forebrain ischemia in rats. *Stroke* 1990;21:1318-1325.
2. Baena RC, Busto R, Dietrich WD, et al. Hyperthermia delayed by 24 hours aggravates neuronal damage in rat hippocampus following global ischemia. *Neurology* 1997;48:768-773.
3. Kim Y, Busto R, Dietrich WD, et al. Delayed postischemic hyperthermia in awake rats worsens the histopathological outcome of transient focal cerebral ischemia. *Stroke* 1996;27:2274-2281.
4. Lin B, Globus MY-T, Dietrich WD, et al. Differing neurochemical and morphological sequelae of global ischemia: Comparison of single- and multiple-insult paradigms. *J Neurochem* 1992;59:2213-2223.
5. Busto R, Dietrich WD, Globus MY-T, et al. Small differences in intraischemic brain temperature critically determine the extent of ischemic neuronal injury. *J Cereb Blood Flow Metab* 1987;7:729-738.
6. Dietrich WD, Busto R, Alonso O, et al. Intraischemic but not postischemic brain hypothermia protects chronically following global forebrain ischemia in rats. *J Cereb Blood Flow Metab* 1993;13:541-549.
7. Morse JK, Davis JN. Regulation of ischemic hippocampal damage in the gerbil: Adrenalectomy alters the rate of CA1 cell disappearance. *Exp Neurol* 1990;110:86-92.
8. Perez-Pinzon MA, Zu G-P, Dietrich WD, et al. Rapid preconditioning protects rats against ischemic neuronal damage after 3 but not 7 days of reperfusion following global cerebral ischemia. *J Cereb Blood Flow Metab* 1997;17:175-182.
9. Corbett D, Crooks P. Ischemic preconditioning: A long term survival study using behavioural and histological end-points. *Brain Res* 1997;760:129-136.
10. Nurse S, Corbett D. Neuroprotection following several days of mild, drug-induced hypothermia. *J Cereb Blood Flow Metab* 1996;16:474-480.
11. Belayev L, Zhao W, Busto R, Ginsberg MD. Transient middle cerebral artery occlusion by intraluminal suture: I. Three-dimensional autoradiographic

image- analysis of local cerebral glucose metabolism - blood flow interrelationships during ischemia and early recirculation. *J Cereb Blood Flow Metab* 1997;17:1266- 1280.

12. Zhao W, Belayev L, Ginsberg MD. Transient middle cerebral artery occlusion by intraluminal suture: II. Neurological deficits, and pixel-based correlation of histopathological alterations with local blood flow and glucose utilization. *J Cereb Blood Flow Metab* 1997;17:1281-1290.

13. Strong AJ, Tomlinson BE, Venables GS, et al. The cortical ischaemic penumbra associated with occlusion of the middle cerebral artery in the cat: 2. Studies of histopathology, water content, and in vitro neurotransmitter uptake. *J Cereb Blood Flow Metab* 1983;3:97-108.

14. Lassen NA. Incomplete cerebral infarction—focal incomplete ischemic tissue necrosis not leading to emollision. *Stroke* 1982;13:522-523.

15. Markgraf CG, Kraydieh S, Prado R, et al. Comparative histopathologic consequences of photothrombotic occlusion of the distal middle cerebral artery in Sprague-Dawley and Wistar rats. *Stroke* 1993;24: 286-292.

16. Nedergaard M. Transient focal ischemia in hyperglycemic rats is associated with increased cerebral infarction. *Brain Res* 1987;408:79-85.

17. Nedergaard M. Neuronal injury in the infarct border: A neuropathological study in the rat. *Acta Neuropathol (Berl)* 1987;73:267-274.

18. Alexis NE, Back T, Zhao W, et al. Neurobehavioral consequences of induced spreading depression following photothrombotic middle cerebral artery occlusion. *Brain Res* 1996;706:273-282.

19. Back T, Ginsberg MD, Dietrich WD, et al. Induction of spreading depression in the ischemic hemisphere following experimental middle cerebral artery occlusion: Effect on infarct morphology. *J Cereb Blood Flow Metab* 1996;16:202- 213.

20. Du C, Hu R, Csernansky CA, et al. Very delayed infarction after mild focal cerebral ischemia: A role for apoptosis? *J Cereb Blood Flow Metab* 1996;16:196-201.

21. Banati RB, Rothe G, Valet G, et al. Respiratory burst in brain macrophages: A flow cytometric study on cultured rat microglia. *Neuropathol Appl Neurobiol* 1991;17:223-230.

22. Corbett D, Nurse S. The problem of assessing effective neuroprotection in experimental cerebral ischemia. *Prog Neurobiol* 1998;54:531-548.

23. Dietrich WD, Lin B, Globus MY-T, et al. Effect of delayed MK-801 (dizocilpine) treatment with or without immediate postischemic hypothermia on chronic neuronal survival after global forebrain ischemia in rats. *J Cereb Blood Flow Metab* 1995;15:960-968.

24. Green EJ, Pazos AJ, Dietrich WD, et al. Combined postischemic hypothermia and delayed MK-801 treatment attenuates neurobehavioral deficits associated with transient global ischemia in rats. *Brain Res* 1995;702:145-152.

25. Globus MY-T, Ginsberg MD, Busto R. Excitotoxic index—a biochemical marker of selective vulnerability. *Neurosci Lett* 1991;127:39-42.

26. Lin B, Ginsberg MD, Busto R, et al. Sequential analysis of subacute and chronic neuronal, astrocytic and microglial alterations after transient global ischemia in rats. *Acta Neuropathol* 1998;95(5):511-523.

27. Kreutzberg GW. Microglia: A sensor for pathological events in the CNS. *Trends Neurosci* 1996;19:312-318.

28. Pellegrini-Giampietro DE, Zukin RS, et al. Switch in glutamate receptor subunit gene expression in CA1 subfield of hippocampus following global ischemia in rats. *Proc Natl Acad Sci USA* 1992;89:10499-10503.

29. Pellegrini-Giampietro DE, Gorter JA, Bennett MVL, et al. The GluR2 (GluR-B) hypothesis: Ca2++-permeable AMPA receptors in neurological disorders. *Trends Neurosci* 1997;20:464-470.

30. Frank L, Diemer NH, Kaiser F, et al. Unchanged balance between levels of mRNA encoding AMPA glutamate receptor subtypes following global cerebral ischemia in the rat. *Acta Neurol Scand* 1995;92:337-343.

31. Friedman LK, Ginsberg MD, Lin B, et al. Intraischemic hypothermia prevents non-selective downregulation of hippocampal AMPA and NMDA receptor gene expression in rat. *Soc Neurosci Abstr* 1998.

32. Ying HS, Weishaupt JH, Grabb M, et al. Sublethal oxygen-glucose deprivation alters hippocampal neuronal AMPA receptor expression and vulnerability to kainate-induced death. *J Neurosci* 1997;17:9536-9544.

33. Catania MV, Tolle TR, Monyer H. Differential expression of AMPA receptor subunits in NOS-positive neurons of cortex, striatum, and hippocampus. *J Neurosci* 1995;15:7046-7061.

34. Leranth C, Szeidemann Z, Hsu M, et al. AMPA receptors in the rat and primate hippocampus: A possible absence of GluR2/3 subunits in most interneurons. *Neuroscience* 1996;70:631-652.

Section VII

Cortical Reorganization and Post-Acute Stroke Treatment

Chapter 26

Introduction

Alexander W. Dromerick, MD and
Larry B. Goldstein, MD

There have now been significant advances in secondary and tertiary stroke prevention based on the results of a series of well-conducted clinical trials. For example, meta-analysis has shown that the use of aspirin in patients with transient ischemic attack (TIA) or stroke is associated with an overall reduction of 37 fewer vascular events for every 1000 treated patients.[1] Other platelet antiaggregants offer alternatives to aspirin for selected patients. A series of studies show that the careful use of warfarin reduces the risk of stroke in high-risk patients with atrial fibrillation.[2] The performance of carotid endarterectomy can decrease stroke risk in selected individuals with high-grade stenosis of the extracranial carotid artery.[3,4] Much of the recent excitement in clinical stroke therapeutics has been generated by the advent of hyper-acute treatment with rt-PA as a means of reducing stroke-related disability.[5] Despite these advances, it is clear that preventive strategies cannot be universally effective and that only a relatively small group of patients with acute stroke are candidates for treatment with rt-PA. The poststroke recovery period represents a third potential "window of opportunity" for therapeutic intervention. The central issues underlying the session on cortical reorganization and the second plenary lecture is whether the post-acute period represents a viable treatment window and which research priorities should be pursued in this area.

In an introduction, Dr. Goldstein framed the session by posing three questions: what are the changes that occur in the brain that underlie late functional recovery?; how may these changes be facili-

From: Choi D, Dacey RG, Hsu CY. Powers WJ. *Cerebrovascular Disease: Momentum at the End of the Second Millennium.* Armonk, NY: Futura Publishing Company, Inc., © 2002.

tated?; and will these manipulations result in enhanced functional recovery? Brain responses to injury responsible for clinically observed spontaneous poststroke functional improvements are complex. Simply viewing stroke as the sum of injuries to individual neuronal or glial cells may underestimate both the effects of injury and the ability of the brain to respond to injury. Recovery is influenced by the pathologic sequellae to acute brain injury, the brain's adaptive responses to injury, and by a variety of potential neuronal rearrangements.[6] Focal injuries can cause distant effects on cell populations and on cortical representations. Such higher order effects may occur on a time scale of weeks to months, thus extending the treatment window much longer than the hyperacute window currently being exploited.

One major theme of the session is presented by Dr. Schallert and Dr. Nudo. Dr. Schallert reviews the interaction between postinjury behavioral experience and degenerative events.[7] Dr. Nudo's presentation of changes in primate motor cortex representation after stroke and the effects of various motor training paradigms in changing that representation suggests that current rehabilitation techniques may be altering cortical representation in stroke patients.[8] Several members of the audience presented data suggesting that changes in cortical representation does occur in humans. New initiatives in physical rehabilitation after stroke[9,10] may take advantage of insights gained from these and other basic studies.

A variety of other novel approaches to improving poststroke recovery may also have therapeutic potential. Dr. Goldstein's review of his work and others' highlights the notion that pharmacological agents used in routine stroke treatment may positively or negatively affect motor recovery.[11] Such pharmacological effects may represent a real opportunity for stroke treatment. Dr. Gage presents work suggesting that undifferentiated cells may be recruited during the brain's response to injury, and may thus represent an exploitable treatment approach.[12,13] Dr. Finklestein describes the role of beta fibroblast growth factor, demonstrating the role that growth factors may play in such responses and implying that the molecular and cellular responses to injury can be unraveled.[14] A greater understanding of how the brain responds to focal injury at the cellular and the motor and sensory system level may uncover new treatment opportunities.

There was general agreement that, relative to other areas of stroke research, postacute events and potential interventions remain underinvestigated. From the presentations, the discussion session afterwards and the summary session, a consensus emerged regarding the research priorities in this area:

The brain's response to focal injury in the days to years following injury:

- What responses take place at the level of motor, sensory, and language systems?
- What cellular and molecular events underlie these responses?
- What is the time course of such responses?
- Do the changes in cortical representation reported in the literature underlie clinical recovery or are these changes epiphenomena?

Can the brain's subacute response to focal injury be modified?

- How can modifications be effected?
- Do different motor training paradigms affect cortical reorganization in humans and are such changes clinically significant?
- Can pharmacological agents affect recovery?
- Are there deleterious responses that can be suppressed?

With over 3 million stroke survivors with varying levels of disability in the United States, the potential to develop treatments to enhance poststroke recovery must be rigorously explored.

References

1. Antiplatelet Trialists' Collaboration. Collaborative overview of randomised trials of antiplatelet therapy—I: Prevention of death, myocardial infarction, and stroke by prolonged antiplatelet therapy in various categories of patients. *BMJ* 1994;308:81-106.
2. Shivkumar K, Jafri SM, Gheorghiade M. Antithrombotic therapy in atrial fibrillation: A review of randomized trials with special reference to the Stroke Prevention in Atrial Fibrillation II (SPAF II) trial. *Prog Cardiovasc Dis* 1996;38:337-344.
3. Goldstein LB, Hasselblad V, Matchar DB, et al. Comparison and meta-analysis of randomized trials of endarterectomy for symptomatic carotid artery stenosis. *Neurology* 1995;45:1965-1970.
4. Executive Committee for the Asymptomatic Carotid Atherosclerosis Study. Endarterectomy for asymptomatic carotid artery stenosis. *JAMA* 1995;273:1421-1428.
5. Marler JR, Brott T, Broderick J, et al. Tissue plasminogen activator for acute ischemic stroke. *N Engl J Med* 1995;333:1581-1587.
6. Goldstein LB. Basic and clinical studies of pharmacologic effects on recovery from brain injury. *J Neural Transplant Plast* 1993;4:175-192.
7. Schallert T, Kozlowski DA, Humm JL, et al. Use-dependent structural events in recovery of function. *Adv Neurol* 1997;73:229-238.
8. Nudo RJ, Wise BM, SiFuentes F, et al. Neural substrates for the effects of rehabilitative training on motor recovery after ischemic infarct. *Science* 1996;272:1791-1794.

9. Taub E, Crago JE, Burgio LD, et al. An operant approach to rehabilitation medicine: Overcoming learned nonuse by shaping. *J Exper Analysis Behav* 1994;61:281-293.

10. Visintin M, Barbeau H, Korner-Bitensky N, et al. A new approach to retrain gait in stroke patients through body weight support and treadmill stimulation. *Stroke* 1998;29:1122-1128.

11. Goldstein LB. Potential effects of common drugs on stroke recovery. *Arch Neurol* 1998;55:454-456.

12. Aubert I, Ridet JL, Gage FH. Regeneration in the adult mammalian CNS: Guided by development. *Current Opinion Neurobiol* 1995;5:625-635.

13. Gage FH, Coates PW, Palmer TD, et al. Survival and differentiation of adult neuronal progenitor cells transplanted to the adult brain. *Proc Natl Acad Sci USA* 1995;92:11879-11883.

14. Kawamata T, Speliotes EK, Finklestein SP. The role of polypeptide growth factors in recovery from stroke. *Adv Neurol* 1997;73:377-382.

Chapter 27

Functional Remodeling of Motor Cortex After Stroke

Randolph J. Nudo, PhD, Jeffrey A. Kleim, PhD, and Kathleen M. Friel, MS

A stroke or other injury to the motor cortex results in paralysis or weakness in the contralateral musculature. However, most individuals who survive a stroke experience some functional recovery in the weeks to months following the injury. Some degree of motor recovery is seen even in patients with dense hemiplegia but the time course of recovery is highly variable.[1] Stroke patients are often left with permanent weakness in the contralateral musculature, especially of the hand so that dexterous movements often are not possible. A number of studies over the past decade suggest that the most dramatic motor recovery occurs early, within the first 30 days after stroke.[2] It is becoming increasingly clear that the ultimate level and time course of recovery is a function of the initial level of stroke severity. Thus, recovery can be protracted in patients with severe stroke, reaching a plateau at 6 months or more after injury.[3]

Throughout this century, neuroscientists have attempted to understand the neurological bases for functional recovery after brain injury.[4-6] But until a few years ago neural models for recovery of function were vague notions based on poorly understood processes such as diaschisis and substitution.[7] However, neurophysiological studies in animals and neuroimaging and noninvasive stimulation

This research was supported by grants from the National Institute of Neurological Diseases and Stroke (NS30853), the Kansas Claude D. Pepper Center for Independence in Older Americans (National Institute on Aging grant AG14635), the Natural Sciences and Engineering Research Council of Canada and the American Heart Association.

From: Choi D, Dacey RG, Hsu CY, Powers WJ. *Cerebrovascular Disease: Momentum at the End of the Second Millennium.* Armonk, NY: Futura Publishing Company, Inc., © 2002.

studies in humans over the past 10-15 years have begun to shed light on the neurological bases of motor recovery in greater detail. A common theme in many of these recent studies is that the cerebral cortex undergoes significant alterations in functional organization after peripheral or central damage.[8,9] The intense interest in these plasticity studies stems from the assumption that the time course and extent of functional recovery is related to the time course and extent of cortical remodeling.

In the early 1980s a number of studies were performed in the somatosensory cortex of nonhuman primates that suggested that the functional organization of the cerebral cortex was plastic in adult animals. For example, when functional "maps" of the somatosensory cortex are derived in a normal monkey, a regular topographic arrangement of the representation of the fingers and thumb is found. However, if one of the digits, for example, digit 3, is amputated, the neurons in the digit 3 region of the cerebral cortex become responsive to stimuli presented to the adjacent digits.[10] This remodeling of cortical tissue that had been functionally deafferented is one of many examples that the functional organization of the cerebral cortex can be experimentally modified. Numerous studies in both sensory and motor cortical areas of experimental animals have now demonstrated that the cerebral cortex can be modified by peripheral and central nervous system injury, electrical stimulation, and by specific behavioral experiences.[11-19] Further, a number of recent studies using noninvasive techniques in humans, including positron emission tomography, magnetic resonance imaging, transcranial magnetic stimulation and others have confirmed that functional plasticity can occur in the human cortex as well.[8,9,20-25]

In this chapter, the changes that occur in the functional arrangement of the mammalian motor cortex are described. These results are based on neurophysiologic studies in experimental animals. It will be argued that plasticity after injury to the cortex, as might occur in stroke, is the result of two interacting variables. First, the cerebral cortex can be altered functionally based on specific motor experiences of the animal. As animals acquire new motor skills there are compensatory alterations in the physiologic and anatomic organization of the motor cortex. Second, after stroke, compensatory changes inevitably occur in the functional organization of the uninjured, surrounding cortical tissue in the weeks to months after the injury. And finally, these two variables, motor experience and injury, interact such that behavioral use can modulate the effects of injury. The relevance of these studies for understanding the effects of physical therapy after stroke is also discussed.

Techniques to Derive Maps of Motor Representations in Motor Cortex

The results described below are based on cortical stimulation techniques, not unlike those used to derive maps of the motor homunculus in the human motor cortex by Wilder Penfield half a century ago and still illustrated in many neurological textbooks.[26] Penfield's results were derived from stimulation experiments in locally anesthetized human subjects in which the surface of the cerebral cortex was electrically stimulated. These surface stimulation techniques required several milliamps of current to evoke an observable contraction in skeletal musculature, and thus the volume of activated tissue was relatively large. Nevertheless, these techniques were sufficient for demonstrating the normal topography of motor cortex organization with exaggerated representations of hand and face.

The technique used in our laboratory to electrically stimulate the motor cortex in adult primates is similar to this method in many respects, except that the tip of the stimulating electrode is very fine (10-15μ), and is introduced into deep laminae of the cortex (about 1.8 mm below the surface). The squirrel monkey was chosen for these studies for a number of reasons. First, this species has reasonable manual dexterity when picking up small objects; we are primarily interested in recovery of hand function after stroke. Second, the squirrel monkey has a relatively smooth cortex. The primary motor hand representation is located on an exposed, flat, unfissured sector of the cortex just anterior to the central sulcus (Figure 1). In these experiments animals are first anesthetized (surgical procedure under halothane/nitrous oxide; physiological procedure under ketamine/acepromazine) and then over the course of 15-20 hours a map of the motor representations of the hand are derived by microelectrode stimulation techniques. A microelectrode is introduced into each site down into the deep layers of the cerebral cortex so that the tip is located in the vicinity of the corticospinal cell bodies. Using these microelectrode stimulation techniques, it is relatively easy to evoke movements in an anesthetized animal at current levels (10-20μA) an order of magnitude below those used by Penfield with surface stimulation.

The mosaical arrangement of the resulting maps of evoked movements is due to the overlapping pattern of individual muscle representations in the motor cortex. At any given site a number of muscles are represented. In fact, a single corticospinal neuron may influence several motor neurons in the spinal cord.[27] When movement maps are derived, a characteristic mosaical pattern of interdigitating digit and wrist/forearm movements are evident. These so-called evoked-movement

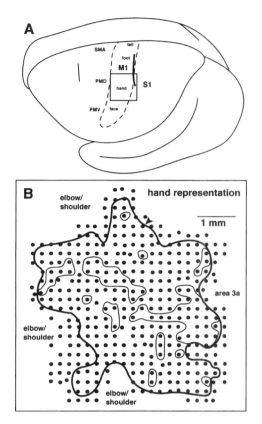

Figure 1. Techniques used to derive detailed maps of movement representations in primary motor cortex of squirrel monkeys. Monkeys are anesthetized and the primary motor cortex (M1) is exposed. Then microelectrodes are introduced sequentially into hundreds of sites approximately 250 μm apart. At each site, a small train of current pulses (< 30 μA) is delivered and the evoked movement is recorded. The representations of movements in M1 are arranged in a topographic fashion on a global scale, but in an interdigitated mosaic pattern on a local scale.

A. Cartoon of a lateral view of a squirrel monkey brain showing the location of the primary motor cortex (dotted line) and its relation to somatosensory cortex (S1), premotor cortex (PMV, PMD) and the supplementary motor area (SMA). The thick line is the central sulcus, a shallow dimple in this species.

B. Results of a cortical stimulation experiment derived from 375 cortical sites. Sites at which electrical stimulation resulted in movements of the hand (fingers, thumb, wrist, forearm) are enclosed by the thick line. Sites at which stimulation resulted in movements of the digits (fingers and thumb) are enclosed by the thin line. The hand representation is surrounded on three sides by representations of more proximal body parts (elbow and shoulder), and on one side (posterior border) by a separate cortical area (area 3a) that is less responsive to electrical stimulation. Abbreviations: M1: primary motor cortex; S1: primary somatosensory cortex; SMA: supplementary motor area; PMD: dorsal premotor area; PMV: ventral premotor area.

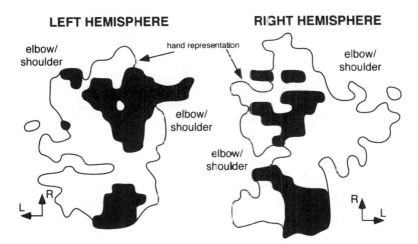

Figure 2. Representation of finger flexion movements (in black) in the left and right hemispheres of an individual squirrel monkey. Despite large variations in movement topography between individuals, the representation of a given hand movement in one hemisphere is a rough mirror-image of its representation in the opposite hemisphere. In each map, the finger flexion movements were evoked in the contralateral hand. White regions within the hand representation include representations of wrist, forearm and thumb.

maps reveal that motor cortical organization is functionally topographic on a global scale: that is, the leg is represented medially, the hand lateral to the leg, and the face lateral to the hand. However, on a more local scale, the overlapping muscle representations result in mosaical movement representations.

Evoked-movement maps are highly idiosyncratic across individuals.[28] Because of this individual variation, it is necessary to derive maps at different points in time in the same animal, ie, before and after one or another manipulation, rather that compare maps between different experimental groups. These so-called map/re-map experiments are very important for addressing issues of use-dependent and injury-dependent changes. By utilizing a repeated-measures statistical design, it is possible to use a relatively small number of animals (usually four to five per group) and still achieve statistical significance. Since the cost of primate subjects is continually rising, repeated-measures designs are becoming increasingly important.

Despite idiosyncratic differences among individuals, the representation of a given movement in one hemisphere is roughly a mirror image of its representation in the opposite hemisphere (Figure 2). However, representations of hand movements contralateral to the animal's dominant, or preferred, hand are typically larger and spatially more complex; that is, more interdigitated and mosaical.[28] This systematic difference between the "dominant" and "nondominant" hemispheres suggest that motor maps may be modifiable by experience.

Effects of Motor Learning on Functional Representations in Motor Cortex

To examine use dependent features of motor cortex organization more directly, squirrel monkeys were trained on a task requiring dexterous use of the digits. In this task, food pellets were placed into different sized wells in a Plexiglas board and the animals were required to retrieve them. The largest well was large enough for insertion of the entire hand. The smallest well required the insertion of one or two fingers to retrieve the pellet. Figure 3 depicts the results of a monkey who underwent such training on the smallest well for 11 days. Over a course of several days the number of pellets that were retrieved within a single, 1-hour session increased, so that by the end of training the animal was retrieving over 800 pellets per day. Likewise, motor efficiency, as defined by the number of finger flexions per retrieval decreased so that near optimal performance was achieved by day 8. When motor maps were examined in these same monkeys systematic changes were evident that were predictable based on the movements that were used in the task.[29]

In the motor maps depicted in Figure 3, it is clear that the digit (finger and thumb) representations expanded significantly at the expense of wrist/forearm representations. In another monkey that was trained on a task requiring forearm supination and pronation, the opposite result was seen: wrist/forearm representations expanded at the expense of digit representations. Motor maps also undergo more specific alterations after training. These more specific changes are related to the specific movements that the monkey uses to accomplish the task. During the course of training, monkeys become highly stereotyped in the movement sequences and combinations that are used to extract pellets, typically a finger flexion in combination with wrist extension. These results showed that there was not only a specific expansion of the finger representation but an expansion of multijoint regions. When these multijoint regions were stimulated during motor mapping experiments, contraction of multiple joints was observed (eg, finger flexion and wrist extension) at the same current level. There was a striking parallel between the specific multijoint movement representations that expanded in the post-training maps and the actual multijoint movements that were used during pellet retrieval. Thus, it appears that representations of joint movements that are used together or in close temporal synchrony during a motor learning task expand after

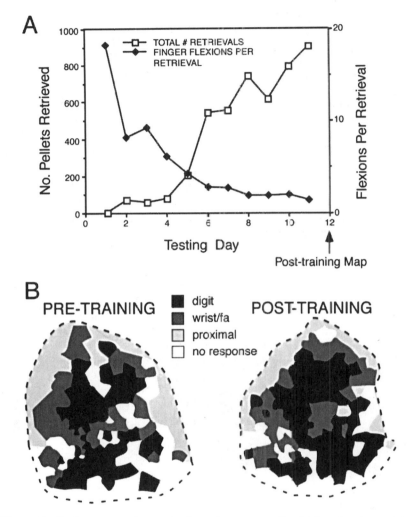

Figure 3. Performance of a squirrel monkey on a pellet retrieval task requiring skilled use of the fingers. **A.** Total number of successful retrievals per day (open squares) and average number of finger flexions per retrieval (filled diamonds). **B.** Representation of hand movements before and after training on the retrieval task. Digit representations expanded significantly at the expense of wrist/forearm movement representations. Dotted line indicates limits of map exploration.

training. This is not unlike the hypothesis that has been proposed for sensory areas to explain map changes induced by use.[30] Temporally correlated inputs result in functional modules with common features within the cortex.

It is also important to note that these changes are driven by acquisition of new motor skills and not simply by motor use. In a recent experiment in our laboratory, monkeys were required to repetitively retrieve pellets out of the largest well of the Plexiglas board, in contrast to retrieval from the smallest well, as described above. Motor activity levels, estimated by the total number of finger flexions performed during training, were matched between the small and large well groups. Detailed analysis of the motor behavior of the monkeys indicates that their retrieval behavior was highly successful and stereotypical throughout the training period, suggesting that no new motor skills were learned during the performance of the large well retrieval task. Comparisons between pre- and post-training maps of movement representations revealed no task-related changes in the areal extent of distal forelimb movement representations. We conclude that repetitive motor activity alone does not produce functional reorganization of cortical maps. Instead, we propose that motor skill acquisition, or motor learning, is a prerequisite factor in driving representational plasticity in motor cortex.[31,32]

Aside from the theoretical importance of these results for understanding the role of motor cortex in motor learning, these results may also be relevant for developing optimum rehabilitation strategies after stroke. If physiologic plasticity in cortical maps is critical for functional recovery, then it follows that tasks requiring progressively increasing motor skill are more important than tasks that simply requiring the patient to repetitively move the limb in the absence of skill acquisition.

Effects of Cortical Injury on Functional Representation in Motor Cortex

Numerous animal studies of stroke and recovery have shed light on the immediate events which occur within the ischemic core and the penumbra or peri-infarct zone adjacent to the injury.[33] Interventions have focused on the neuroprotective effects of various pharmacologic agents after stroke or other cortical injury in an attempt to rescue as many vulnerable neurons as possible. Until recently very little attention had been devoted to the long-term (weeks to months) neurophysiologic and neuroanatomic consequences of neuronal death. By contrast, our own studies have focused on the remaining intact motor cortex and its ability to functionally reorganize after ischemic injury to motor cortex, and to determine whether compensatory changes in cortical motor organization are correlated with functional motor recovery. It is now known that there are a number of physiologic, pharmacologic and anatomic events that occur in much more wide spread regions and these remote effects may occur over much longer time periods.[34] Remote effects are not surprising given that neurons in any damaged

Infarct

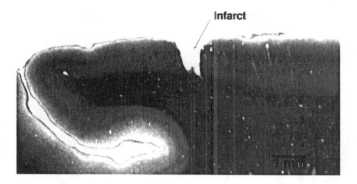

Figure 4. Histologic parasagittal section through primary motor cortex of a squirrel monkey three months after a focal ischemic infarct showing the typical extent of the lesion. Tissue was processed with a silver stain for the presence of myelin. The infarcted region extends from the surface to layer six. The adjacent tissue appears indistinguishable from normal tissue in this and other stains.

region of cortex have reciprocal synaptic connections with neurons with other cortical (and subcortical) brain regions. For example, the primary motor cortex has reciprocal connections with the premotor cortex and the supplementary motor area.[35] Thus, a stroke in primary motor cortex would necessarily result in a partial deafferentation of these other cortical motor areas. It follows that the physiology and anatomy of these remote areas would be altered by ischemic injury in primary motor cortex.

We have begun to model the effects of a focal injury in the motor cortex of squirrel monkeys.[36] The injury is created by bipolar electrocoagulation of a vascular bed over the physiologically characterized region cortex within the motor hand area. This procedure is not intended to mimic stroke, per se since it is a vascular coagulation that involves primarily venous drainage and to a lesser extent, small end-arteries supplying the targeted tissue. The infarcted vessels include very fine capillaries as well as larger vessels. We specifically avoid any bypassing arterial supply to other areas. This technique was chosen because it can induce a very focal injury in a localized region with very sharp borders. Figure 4 shows an example of a histologic section through one of these lesions about 3 months after the injury. The actual injury is somewhat larger than shown here because of necrosis that occurs after injury. This fiber stain shows the extent of the infarct from the surface through layer six. Histological examination suggests that the tissue adjacent to the injury is structurally indistinguishable from normal tissue.

Figure 5A illustrates the neurophysiologic results of a focal infarct created in a small portion of the hand area of motor cortex. The extent

A

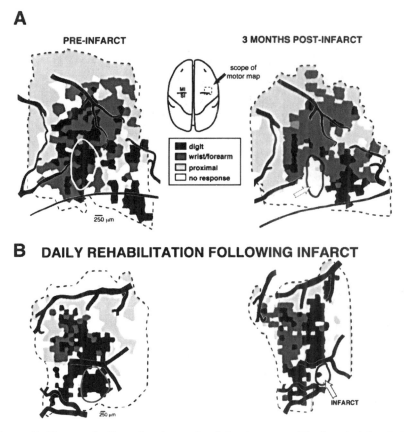

Figure 5. Reorganization of motor cortex following a small ischemic infarct. **A.** In the absence of rehabilitation, the adjacent, intact tissue undergoes a further loss of digit representation. **B.** With rehabilitation, spared digit representations are maintained. These results demonstrate that motor experience after cortical injury modulates the functional changes that inevitably occur in the surrounding, undamaged tissue.[36, 37]

of the cortical injury in absolute size is only 2-3 mm². However, this represents about 25%-30% of the squirrel monkey's hand representation. When we examined the motor cortex 3 months later we found that there was a reduction in the remaining, spared hand representation. Behaviorly, these animals are mildly impaired. Within a few days after injury, they use both hands to climb the cage bars and to manipulate monkey chow. However, when they are tested on a task requiring some digital skill such as retrieving pellets out of small food wells the deficit is quite apparent (as defined by the number of finger flexions required for retrieval). This deficit in manual skill persists for several weeks. Eventually they achieve normal levels of skill even in this spontaneous recovery paradigm.[36]

If the lesion is made larger the effects on the spared hand representation are more substantial. In one monkey with an infarct affecting over 40% of the hand representation, the remaining hand representation was completely replaced by elbow and shoulder representations.[36] It is important to point out that the motor maps shown are based on the movement that is evoked at threshold current levels and that if the current is increased a second movement is evoked. This is probably due to a) spread of current to a larger volume of tissue, and b) neurons in the original volume of activated tissue that have a higher threshold for depolarization. However, prior to the infarct, thresholds for evoking digit and wrist movements are quite low in the hand area, whereas thresholds for evoking elbow and shoulder movements are high. Thus, it is difficult to evoke elbow and shoulder movements in the hand area prior to infarct even with relatively high current levels. However, after the injury digit movements cannot be evoked even with higher current levels, whereas elbow and shoulder movements can be evoked at very low current levels. Thus, these changes in movement representations adjacent to the lesion appear to be qualitative.

Interactive Effects of Cortical Injury and Motor Learning on Functional Reorganization in Motor Cortex

The monkeys undergoing spontaneous recovery as described above tend to use their unimpaired hand to perform tasks requiring manual dexterity. Therefore, to study the effects of use of the impaired hand after injury it is necessary to restrict the movement of the unimpaired hand. This can be accomplished by placing animals in a jacket with a long sleeve extending the length of the unimpaired limb.[37] The sleeve contains a mitten over the unimpaired hand. Monkeys wearing these jackets can still climb the cage bars, support themselves with the unimpaired hand and even pick up large pieces of monkey chow. However, they must use their impaired hand for dexterous tasks, such as small pellet retrieval. Because we specifically examined the effects of repetitive use after injury, it was possible to track motor performance daily throughout the recovery period. After a small ischemic injury to the motor cortex, motor performance on the pellet retrieval task declines. Eventually these animals return to the normal range of motor performance and remain within this range until the postinfarct mapping procedure is conducted. When the physiology of these monkeys was examined after recovery (a few weeks after infarct), it was found that the spared hand representa-

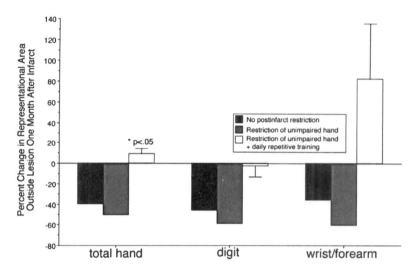

Figure 6. Change hand representation area after spontaneous recovery (no postinfarct intervention), postinfarct restriction of the unimpaired hand, and postinfarct restriction of the unimpaired hand in combination with daily repetitive training. The results demonstrate that restriction of the unimpaired hand is not sufficient to retain spared hand representations after focal ischemic injury.[38]

tion was retained (Figure 5B). In some cases the digit representation expanded into former elbow and shoulder territories. This is in contrast to the spontaneous recovery group in which the spared hand area contracted (Figure 5A). Increased use of the impaired hand after injury appears to have a modulatory effect on plasticity in the surrounding tissue.

Finally, in a more recent study we attempted to determine whether restriction of the unimpaired hand was sufficient to retain spared hand area after cortical injury or if retention of spared hand representation required repetitive use of the impaired limb. Following an infarct to the hand area of M1 in adult squirrel monkeys, the unimpaired hand was restrained as above. However, these monkeys did not receive additional rehabilitative training. One month after the lesion, the size of the total hand representation and the sizes of finger and wrist/forearm representations had decreased (Figure 6). Areal changes were significantly lower than in the group that had received daily repetitive training after infarct (P < 0.05). Areal changes were not different from animals that did not receive rehabilitative intervention or hand restraint after cortical injury. Taken together with previous findings, these results suggest that retention of hand representational area within M1 after cortical injury requires repetitive use of the impaired hand after injury.[38]

Relevance of Animal Models of Recovery to Human Stroke Patients

These results demonstrating the effects of rehabilitative training after stroke utilizing restraint of the unimpaired arm parallel a series of studies ongoing in humans. These studies have shown that forced use of the affected limb for 14 days (by constraint of the unaffected limb) resulted in long-term improvement of motor function of the impaired limb.[39] The improvements were seen in a 2-week intervention period, during a 4-week follow-up period, and in a 2-year follow-up after the forced use was ended. It would appear that forced use of the impaired limb has significant functional benefit as well as a modulatory effect on the physiology of the undamaged cortex. It is provocative to suggest that the recovery may be due to cortical reorganization in the adjacent, undamaged sector of the cortex.

Comparison of Primate and Rodent Models for Studying Neural Compensation After Stroke

All of the neurophysiological mapping data described above have been derived from studies in squirrel monkeys. Since much of the research into cerebral ischemia has been directed towards generating animal models which produce motor impairments comparable to those seen in human patients, it would seem that nonhuman primate models of stroke are highly desirable. However, primate models of stroke and recovery are relatively uncommon, primarily due to the cost of the animals. In most studies of neural response to stroke, such as those utilizing utrastructural or immunocytochemical analyses, it is not possible to use a repeated-measures statistical design as in the neurophysiological procedures described above. Thus, a much larger number of animals is required, limiting the feasibility of performing these experiments in primates.

While the choice of species must be guided by the requirements of each particular experiment, the most prevalent model for studies of neural response to ischemia is the rat. Occlusion of the middle cerebral artery (MCA) in the rat is believed to closely resemble certain types of stroke in humans.[33] Transient or permanent MCA occlusion produces impairments on several behavioral tasks including the rotor rod[40] foot fault[41] and grip strength tests.[42] These deficits have also been positively correlated with the volume of damaged neural tissue[41] and can be ameliorated by various pharmacological manipulations.[43,44] Despite these results, the rodent model has sometimes been criticized because it is believed that rats: a) lack the ability to produce complex movements, b) lack complex motor representations within the motor cortex, c) do not posses premotor areas, and 4) fail to exhibit long-lasting deficits following cortical injury.

Contrary to these criticisms, numerous studies have shown rats to possess a highly developed motor system that both supports an extensive motor repertoire and when damaged by ischemic insult, produces robust motor impairments. The rat motor cortex, like that of primates, is defined by the presence of large layer V pyramidal cells whose axons form an extensive corticospinal tract including direct corticomotoneuronal projections.[44] Studies using ICMS techniques have also revealed a complex topography of movement representations that is characterized by a fractured somatotopy not unlike that seen in the primate.[45] In addition to a large caudal forelimb area, a completely separate, rostral forelimb representation has also been identified.[45,46] This rostral forelimb area has been suggested to function as a premotor or supplementary motor area given its connectivity with subcortical and cortical regions,[46] its apparent lack of sensory input[47] and the presence of movement related activity which precedes that of the caudal forelimb area.[48] This highly developed motor system also appears to support the production of complex movements. Rats are capable of fine object manipulation[49] skilled target reaching[50] and even the ability to obtain food rewards by manually recoiling a length of string.[51] Detailed kinematic analysis of these movements has also revealed that they closely resemble those used by primates, including humans.[52]

In addition to the anatomical and behavioral characteristics described above, there is evidence that rat and primate motor cortex exhibit similar functional and structural plasticity in response to experience. Motor skill learning has been shown to increase pyramidal cell dendritic material within the motor cortex of both rats[53,54] and monkeys.[55] Furthermore, recent work in our laboratory has shown that the functional organization of the rat motor cortex, like the primate, is sensitive to experience. In a normal rat microelectrode stimulation experiments reveal a contiguous forelimb representation in which the component evoked movements are comprised primarily of wrist, elbow, and shoulder movements. However, if we compare a normal motor map to that derived in a litter-mate control that has been trained to retrieve pellets from a rotating disk, significant training-related changes are seen. First there is a large expansion of the wrist representation and a reduction in the size of the elbow/shoulder representation (Figure 7). Second, and perhaps more importantly, there is an emergence of several sites at which movement evokes specific digit responses, primarily digit flexion responses. This differentiation of the

SKILLED REACHING CONDITION

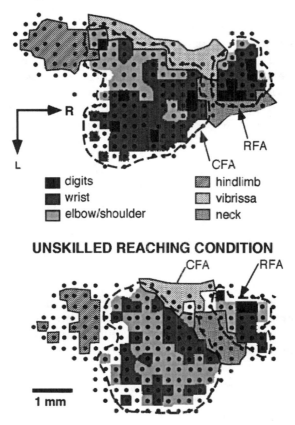

Figure 7. Reorganization of motor representations following skilled-reach training in a rat. Animals in the skilled reaching condition exhibited an increase in wrist and digit representations and a decrease in elbow/shoulder representations in the caudal forelimb area (CFA) in comparison to animals in the unskilled reaching condition (URC). No differences in movement topography were found in the rostral forelimb area (RFA).[62]

motor cortex is reminiscent of the results just shown for the primate motor cortex.[29]

In summary, rats possess a highly developed motor system that is alterable by motor experience, are capable of complex movements and exhibit enduring motor impairments following ischemia. The advantages of rodent ischemia models are the number and complexity of the experiments that can be performed. Rodent studies have already provided the foundation for research into the effectiveness of different pharmacological therapies which have had obvious benefits for guiding similar interventions in human patients.[33] Thus, in terms of the functional reorganization of motor cortex it is clear that the rat displays the same kinds of plastic changes in its physiology as the monkey. Thus, the rat is an appropriate model in many respects for some of the pharmacological manipulations and anatomical tests that require a larger number of animals. Each model obviously has its own unique set of advantages and disadvantages. It has been suggested that the primate motor system possesses some unique anatomical features, especially in the organization of the premotor cortex.[56] However, for many experiments the rat model may be highly desirable.

Mechanisms of Plasticity in Motor Cortex

The synaptic mechanisms underlying adaptive plasticity in sensory and motor cortex are currently under investigation in a number of different laboratories. A thorough review of this literature is beyond the scope of the present chapter. However, it should be noted that these mechanisms are thought to be similar to those proposed for the hippocampus. That is, both long-term potentiation and long-term depression can be produced in the motor cortex of intact animals or in slice preparations and may provide a mechanism for modulating motor maps.[57,58] After a cortical injury, remote physiological changes can be demonstrated as well. Cortical injury induces a prolonged but reversible depression of neuronal activity (diaschisis), blood flow and glucose metabolism in the surrounding tissue (cortical spreading depression). Further, neuronal hyperexcitability has recently been reported in cortical regions remote from the site of focal ischemia and is accompanied by down-regulation of GABA receptor activity.[34]

In addition to these neurophysiologic and metabolic changes after injury, anatomic changes occur in the intact, contralateral hemisphere of rats after cortical lesions.[59-61] As overuse of the impaired limb after injury results in exaggeration of neuronal injury, some concerns have been raised regarding the safety of forced-use paradigms after stroke. On the surface, this would seem to contradict the results presented in monkeys regarding the benefits of forced use after stroke. However, it is important to note that the rat and monkey models are quite different. Since rats are quadrupeds the effects of a body cast and restriction of all movements of the unimpaired limb are much more severe. The casted rat is forced to rely on its impaired limb not only for grasping and manipulation, but also for locomotion and balance. It is an extreme example of overuse that is qualitatively different from the restrictive use we see in a monkey or human with a sling-type restraint. However, the use dependent exaggeration of injury is an important phenomenon that needs extensive further study.

Future Directions

While the plasticity studies of the past decade have suggested provocative hypotheses regarding the neural bases for recovery of function, several important issues still need to be addressed. First, while the current data is compelling, the functional meaning of plastic change after injury is not yet clear. The changes over long time courses after cortical injury may be either adaptive or maladaptive, and the distinction between the two may not always be obvious. There is an immediate need for more and better correlational studies in animals and humans that relate neurophysiological and neuroimaging data with functional outcome. Second, while primary motor cortex provides a handy window into the spatial distribution of movement representations in the motor system, a more integrative picture of reorganization in other cortical and subcortical motor regions is needed. Third, the interactive effects of various other modulators of plasticity (behavioral, pharmacologic, etc.) need to be addressed in more detail. It is now clear that specific behavioral experiences have a modulatory effect on cortical function after injury and may be as potent as pharmacological agents in improving motor function after stroke. Fourth, dynamic processes triggered by neuronal injury occur for long periods of time after the injury. It is important to address the issue of critical, or sensitive, periods for each of these modulators. While these challenges are significant, the tools are now available to address the complex questions of neural recovery in detail from the molecular to the behavioral level.

References

1. Nakayama H, Jorgenson HS, Raaschou HO, et al. Compensation in recovery of upper extremity function after stroke: The Copenhagen study. Arch Phys Med Rehabil 1994;75:852-857.
2. Wade DT, Wood VA, Langston-Hewer R. Recovery after stroke: The first three months. J Neurol Neurosurg Psychiat 1985;48:7-13.
3. Duncan PW, Lai SM. Stroke recovery. Top Stroke Rehabil 1997;4(3):51-58.
4. Ogden R, Franz SI. On cerebral motor control: The recovery from experimentally produced hemiplegia. Psychobiol 1917;1:33-50.
5. Leyton ASF, Sherrington CS. Observations on the excitable cortex of the chimpanzee, orang-utan and gorilla. Quart J Exp Physiol 1917;11:135-222.
6. Lashley KS. Factors limiting recovery after central nervous system lesions. J Nerv Ment Dis 1938;88:733-755.
7. Bach-y-Rita P. Process of recovery from stroke. In Brandstater ME, Basmajian JV (eds): Stroke Rehabilitation. Baltimore: Williams and Wilkins, 1987:80-108.
8. Seitz RJ, Huang Y, Knorr U, et al. Large-scale plasticity of the human motor cortex. Neuroreport 1995;6:742-744.

9. Chollet F, DiPiero V, Wise RJ, et al. The functional anatomy of motor recovery after stroke in humans: A study with positron emission tomography. Ann Neurol 1991;29(1):63-71.

10. Merzenich MM, Nelson RJ, Stryker MP, et al. Somatosensory cortical map changes following digit amputation in adult monkeys. J Comp Neurol 1984;224:591-605.

11. Donoghue JP, Sanes JN. Peripheral nerve injury in developing rats reorganizes representation pattern in motor cortex. Proc Nat Acad Sci USA 1987;84(4):1123-1126.

12. Jenkins WM, Merzenich MM. Reorganization of neocortical representations after brain injury: A neurophysiological model of the bases of recovery from stroke. Prog Br Res 1987;71:249-266.

13. Kaas JH, Krubitzer LA, Chino YM, et al. Reorganization of retinotopic cortical maps in adult mammals after lesions of the retina. Science 1990;248:229-231.

14. Merzenich MM, Kaas JH, Wall J, et al. Topographic reorganization of somatosensory areas 3b and 1 in adult monkeys following restricted deafferentation. Neurosci 1983;8:33-55.

15. Nudo RJ, Jenkins WM, Merzenich MM. Repetitive microstimulation alters the cortical representation of movements in adult rats. Somatosens Mot Res 1990;7(4):463-483.

16. Recanzone GH, Allard TT, Jenkins WM, et al. Receptive field changes induced by peripheral nerve stimulation in S-I of adult cats. J Neurophysiol 1990;63:1213-1225.

17. Recanzone GH, Schreiner GE, Merzenich MM. Plasticity in the frequency representation of primary auditory cortex following discrimination training in adult owl monkeys. J Neurophysiol 1993;13:87-103.

18. Sanes JN, Wang J, Donoghue JP. Immediate and delayed changes of rat motor cortical output representation with new forelimb configurations. Cereb Cortex 1992;2(2):141-152.

19. Jenkins WM, Merzenich MM, Ochs MT, et al. Functional reorganization of primary somatosensory cortex in adult owl monkeys after behaviorally controlled tactile stimulation. J Neurophysiol 1990;63:82-104.

20. Karni A, Meyer G, Jezzard P, et al. Functional MRI evidence for adult motor cortex plasticity during motor skill learning. Nature 1995;377:155-158.

21. Grafton ST, Mazziotta JC, Presty S, et al. Functional anatomy of human procedural learning determined with regional cerebral blood flow and PET. J Neurosci 1992;12:2542-2548.

22. Cohen LG, Brasil-Neto JP, Pascual-Leone A, et al. Plasticity of cortical motor output organization following deafferentation, cerebral lesions, and skill acquisition. Adv Neurol 1993;63:187-200.

23. Elbert T, Sterr A, Flor H, et al. Input-increase and input-decrease types of cortical reorganization after upper extremity amputation in humans. Exp Brain Res 1997;117(1):161-164.

24. Weiller C, Chollet F, Friston KJ, et al. Functional reorganization of the brain in recovery from striatocapsular infarction in man. Ann Neurol 1992;31:463-472.

25. Seitz RJ, Freund H-J. Plasticity of the human motor cortex. Adv Neurol 1997;73:321-333.

26. Penfield W, Boldrey E. Somatic motor and sensory representation in the cerebral cortex of man as studied by electrical stimulation. Brain 1937;60:389-443.

27. Cheney PD, Fetz EE. Comparable patterns of muscle facilitation evoked by individual corticomotoneuronal (CM) cells and by single intracortical microstimuli in primates: Evidence for functional groups of CM cells. J Neurophysiol 1985;53:786-804.

28. Nudo RJ, Jenkins WM, Merzenich MM, et al. Neurophysiological correlates of hand preference in primary motor cortex of squirrel monkeys. J Neurosci 1992;12(8):2918-2947.

29. Nudo RJ, Milliken GW, Jenkins WM, et al. Use-dependent alterations of movement representations in primary motor cortex of adult squirrel monkeys. J Neurosci 1996;16(2):785-807.

30. Clark SA, Allard T, Jenkins WM, et al. Receptive fields in the body-surface map in adult cortex defined by temporally correlated inputs. Nature 1988;332:444-445.

31. Nudo RJ, Plautz EJ, Milliken GW. Adaptive plasticity in primate motor cortex as a consequence of behavioral experience and neuronal injury. Sem Neurosci 1997;9:13-23.

32. Plautz EJ, Milliken GW, Nudo RJ. Differential effects of skill acquisition and motor use on the reorganization of motor representations in area 4 of adult squirrel monkeys. Soc Neurosci Abst 1995;21:1902.

33. Hunter JA, Mackay KB, Rogers DC. To what extent have functional studies of ischaemia in animals been useful in the assessment of potential neuroprotective agents? Tr Pharmacol Sci 1998;19:59-66.

34. Schiene K, Bruehl C, Zilles K, et al. Neuronal hyperexcitability and reduction of GABAA-receptor expression in the surround of cerebral thrombosis. J Cereb Blood Flow Metab 1996;16:906-914.

35. Stepniewska I, Preuss TM, Kaas JH. Architectonics, somatotopic organization, and ipsilateral cortical connections of the primary motor area (M1) of owl monkeys. J Comp Neurol 1993;330(2):238-271.

36. Nudo RJ, Milliken GW. Reorganization of movement representations in primary motor cortex following focal ischemic infarcts in adult squirrel monkeys. J Neurophysiol 1996;75:2144-2149.

37. Nudo RJ, Wise BM, SiFuentes F, et al. Neural substrates for the effects of rehabilitative training on motor recovery after ischemic infarct. Science 1996;272:1791-1794.

38. Friel KM, Nudo RJ. Restraint of the unimpaired hand is not sufficient to retain spared primary motor hand representation after focal cortical injury. Neurorehabilitation Neural Repair 2000;14:187-198.

39. Taub E, Miller NE, Novack TA, et al. Technique to improve chronic motor deficit after stroke. Arch Phys Med Rehabil 1993;74:347-354.

40. Borlongan CV, Cahill DW, Sandberg PR. Locomotor and passive avoidance deficits following occlusion of the middle cerebral artery. Physiol Beh 1995;58:909-917.

41. Rogers DC, Campbell CA, Stretton JL, et al. Correlation between motor impairment and infarct volume after permanent and transient middle cerebral artery occlusion in the rat. Stroke 1997;28:2060-2065.

42. Wood NI, Sopesen BV, Roberts JC, et al. Motor dysfunction in a phootothrombotic focal ischaemia model. Beh Br Res 1996;78:113-120.

43. Sharkey J, Crawford JH, Butcher SP, et al. Tacrolimus (FK506) ameliorates skilled motor deficits produced by middle cerebral artery occlusion. Stroke 1996;27:2282-2286.

44. Liang FY, Moret V, Wiesendanger M, et al. Corticomotoneuronal connections in the rat: Evidence from double-labeling of motoneurons and corticospinal axon arborizations. J Comp Neurol 1991;311(3):356-366.

45. Neafsey EJ, Bold EL, Haas G, et al. The organization of rat motor cortex: A microstimulation mapping study. Br Res Rev 1986;11:77-96.

46. Roullier EM, Moret V, Liang F. Comparison of the connectional properties of the two forelimb areas of the rat sensorimotor cortex: Support for the presence of a premotor or supplementary motor cortical area. Somatosens Mot Res 1993;10:269-289.

47. Sievert CF, Neafsey EJ. A chronic unit study of the sensory properties of neurons in the forelimb areas of rat sensorimotor cortex. Br Res 1986;381:15-23.

48. Donoghue JP. Contrasting properties of neurons in two parts of the primary motor cortex of the awake rat. Br Res 1985;333:173-177.

49. Whishaw IQ, Coles BLK. Varieties of paw and digit movement during spontaneous food handling in rats: Postures, bimanual coordination, preferences and the effect of forelimb cortex lesions. Beh Br Res 1996;77:135-148.

50. Whishaw IQ, Pellis SM. The structure of skilled forelimb reaching in the rat: A proximally driven movement with a single distal rotary component. Beh Br Res 1990;41:49-59.

51. Tomie J, Whishaw IQ. New paradigms for tactile discrimination studies with the rat: Methods for simple, conditional and configural discriminations. Physiol Beh 1990;48:225-231.

52. Whishaw IQ, Pellis SM, Gorny PG. Skilled reaching in rats and humans: Evidence for parallel development or homology. Beh Br Res 1992;47:59-70.

53. Withers GS, Greenough WT. Reach training selectively alters dendritic branching in subpopulations of Layer II/III pyramids in rat motor-somatosensory forelimb cortex. Neuropsychologia 1989;27:61-69.

54. Greenough WT, Larson JR, Withers GS. Effects of unilateral and bilateral training in a reaching task on dendritic branching of neurons in the rat motor-sensory forelimb cortex. Behav Neurol Biol 1985;44:301-314.

55. Stell M, Riesen A. Effects of early environments on monkey cortex neuroanatomical changes following somatomotor experience: Effects on layer III pyramidal cells in monkey cortex. Behav Neurosci 1987;101:341-346.

56. Nudo RJ, Masterton RB. Descending pathways to the spinal cord, III: Sites of origin of the corticospinal tract. J Comp Neurol 1990;296(4):559-583.

57. Aroniadou VA, Keller A. The patterns and synaptic properties of horizontal intracortical connections in the rat motor cortex. J Neurophysiol 1993;70(4):1553-1569.

58. Hess G, Donoghue JP. Long-term potentiation of horizontal connections provides a mechanism to reorganize cortical motor maps. J Neurophysiol 1994;71(6):2543-2547.

59. Jones TA, Schallert T. Overgrowth and pruning of dendrites in adult rats recovering from neocortical damage. Br Res 1992;581:156-160.

60. Kozlowski DA, James DC, Schallert T. Use-dependent exaggeration of neuronal injury after unilateral sensorimotor cortex lesions. J Neurosci 1996;16(15):4776-4786.

61. Jones TA, Schallert T. Use-dependent growth of pyramidal neurons after neocortical damage. J Neurosci 1994;14:2140-2152.

62. Kleim JA, Barbay S, Nudo RJ. Functional reorganization of the rat motor cortex following motor skill learning. J Neurophysiol 1998 Dec;80(6): 3321-3325.

Chapter 28

Growth Factors and Stroke Recovery

JingMei Ren, MD, John Markman, MD, and Seth P. Finklestein, MD

Growth factors are endogenous proteins that influence the cascade of molecular and cellular responses underlying recovery after stroke.These endogenous proteins act as signaling molecules to initiate and sustain cellular processes resulting in cell survival, growth, and differentiation. Through interaction with cell surface (and intracellular) high-affinity receptors, growth factors promote new gene expression and protein synthesis. Neurotrophic growth factors stimulate neuronal survival and differentiation, while gliotrophic and angiogenic growth factors modulate glial and vascular survival and proliferation, resectively.[1] The upregulation of growth factor production in the brain following stroke suggests that these proteins are instrumental in neurorecovery.[2,3]

Cerebrovascular disease (stroke) remains a major cause of morbidity and mortality worldwide. More than 550,000 Americans suffer a new stroke each year, making it the third largest cause of death and disability in the US.[4] The mechanism of injury in 85% of these cases is ischemic, that is to say, thromboembolic occlusion of an extra- or intracranial cerebral artery that leads to the localized death of brain tissue (infarction). Depending on the size and location of infarction, neurological disability ensues—including disturbances of motor and sensory function, vision, coordination, speech, and cognition, among others. Stroke is generally nonlethal; only one-third of patients die

This work is supported by NS10828

From: Choi D, Dacey RG, Hsu CY, Powers WJ. *Cerebrovascular Disease: Momentum at the End of the Second Millennium*. Armonk, NY: Futura Publishing Company, Inc., © 2002.

within the first year, the remainder live for an average of 7 years.[5] As a consequence, stroke is the leading cause of adult disability, and costs the US economy in excess of $30 billion per year.[4]

Recovery from stroke commonly occurs, but is often incomplete. Some neurological deficits (eg, inability to walk or swallow, mild limb weakness, aphasia, neglect, etc.) tend to improve, whereas others (eg, dense hemiplegia, hemianopia) may not.[5] Since infarcted brain tissue does not regenerate, recovery must emanate from the remaining intact brain. Possibilities include "reawakening" of intact but "stunned" brain tissue ("diaschisis"), as well as new structural and functional reorganization of the remaining intact brain.[6] Indeed, a considerable amount of evidence both in animals and man show neural reorganization in intact brain tissue following focal brain wounds or infarcts that appears to be correlated with functional recovery.

In human stroke patients, functional imaging techniques (positron-emission tomography and magnetic resonance imaging) show increased cerebral blood flow and metabolism (reflecting increased neuronal activity) in tissue surrounding focal brain infarcts and in homologous regions contralateral to infarcts as patients recover from ischemic stroke.[7,8] In primates, there is extensive synaptic and functional reorganization in cerebral cortex surrounding focal brain lesions, effectively "remapping" sensory and motor fields.[9] In rats, there is axonal and dendritic sprouting in cortex surrounding focal wounds or infarcts to sensorimotor cortex, as well as in sensorimotor cortex contralateral to lesions.[10-12] The time course of such sprouting parallels that of functional recovery of the impaired limbs. Moreover, both sprouting in the intact contralateral hemisphere and functional recovery of the impaired limbs can be blocked by splinting (forced disuse) of the intact limbs.[11] These data suggest that intact brain regions can "learn" to "take over" some of the function of damaged brain regions, provided that the intact regions receive appropriate stimulation. In the case of the intact contralateral hemisphere, the neural pathways mediating recovery may be direct (eg, uncrossed pathways from intact hemisphere to impaired limbs) or indirect (eg, transcallosal pathways from intact hemisphere to intact regions of damaged hemisphere to impaired limbs).

We have investigated the role of growth factors in animal models of focal cerebral infarction, especially basic fibroblast growth factor (bFGF), a factor that supports neuronal survival and axonal outgrowth, and osteogenic protein-1 (OP-1, BMP-7), a factor that supports dendritic outgrowth. The endogenous expression of both of these factors is increased in the brain after focal stroke.[13] If recombinant bFGF is administered exogenously (intracerebrally or intravenously) within a few hours after the onset of ischemia, infarct size is reduced, presumably due to protection of cells at the borders of infarcts. On the other hand, if bFGF or OP-1 are administered intracerebrally (intracisternally) at later times (≥ 24 hours) after stroke, infarct size is not reduced, but neurological recovery is enhanced, presumably due to stimulation of new neuronal sprouting and synapse formation in the remaining intact brain.

Basic fibroblast growth factor is a 154 amino acid, 18 kiloDalton (kDa) member of the fibroblast growth factor (FGF) superfamily.[14,15] It has at least four high-affinity tyrosine kinase receptors. Named initially because of its mitogenic effects on fibroblasts, bFGF and its receptors are widely distributed in the body, including the brain. In the brain, bFGF has multipotential effects with neurotrophic, gliotrophic, and angiogenic properties.[14,16,17] Specifically, bFGF is a potent neurotrophic factor that supports the survival and outgrowth of a wide variety of brain neurons, and protects neurons against a number of toxins and insults, including anoxia, hypoglycemia, excitatory amino acids, free radicals, nitric oxide, and programmed cell death (apoptosis).[18-22] Basic fibroblast growth factor also selectively promotes axonal outgrowth from a wide variety of brain neurons both in vitro and in vivo.[18,23,24] The bFGF gene lacks a classical "leader" sequence, so that this protein is not freely secreted from cells.[25] However, bFGF is released from damaged cells and from intact cells by nonclassical pathways.[26]

Osteogenic protein-1 (OP-1, or BMP-7) is a member of the bone morphogenetic protein (BMP) subfamily of the transforming growth factor-β (TGF-β) superfamily. It is a 35 kDa homodimeric glycoprotein that has at least three high-affinity serine/threonine kinase receptors.[27-29] OP-1 is freely secreted from cells. Initially named because of its effects on stimulating bone growth from osteoblasts, OP-1 and its receptors are also found in the developing, mature, and injured brain.[30-33] In cultured neurons, OP-1 appears to have a selective effect in enhancing dendritic outgrowth. Specifically, in sympathetic and embryonic hippocampal neurons, OP-1 promotes dendritic outgrowth in a dose-dependent manner, without effects on axonal outgrowth or neuronal survival.[34,35] This property distinguishes OP-1 from virtually all other identified growth factors (including bFGF), that promote axonal outgrowth. Basic fibroblast growth factor and OP-1 were chosen specifically for our studies on stroke recovery because of the probable important role of axonal and dendritic sprouting, respectively, in the recovery process.

Previous studies by ourselves and others have shown upregulation of bFGF and OP-1 expression in brain following focal brain wounds or infarcts. Basic fibroblast growth factor mRNA, and bFGF protein are widely localized within astroglia and in a few select neuronal populations in the mature rat brain.[36,37] Following focal infarction, bFGF, mRNA, and protein expression are markedly increased in tissue surrounding focal infarcts during the few days after stroke.[13] Basic fibroblast growth factor mRNA levels peak at 1 day, and bFGF protein levels peak at 3 days after infarction.[13] Increased bFGF expression occurs largely in reactive astroglia surrounding infarcts.[13] Other investigators have shown upregulation of high-affinity bFGF receptors in neurons, glia, and endothelia surrounding focal infarcts.[38] In other preliminary studies, we found increased OP-1 mRNA expression in tissue surrounding focal infarcts, peaking at 3 days after infarction (Caday, Charette and Finklestein, unpublished observations). The cell types expressing increased OP-1 mRNA have yet to be identified. Other investigators have reported upregulation of high-affinity OP-1 receptors in brain neurons following traumatic injury.[32] Increased bFGF and OP-1 expression in tissue surrounding focal infarcts may have both local and distant effects. Locally released bFGF may promote local neuronal survival and axonal outgrowth as well as glial and endothelial survival and proliferation.[13] Moreover, bFGF may be taken up by local neuronal processes and undergo retrograde transport to distant cell bodies of origin. Likewise, locally secreted OP-1 may exert local dendritic-promoting effects and also be transported retrogradely to distant neuronal cell bodies. Thus, locally expressed bFGF and OP-1 may have important effects on both local and distant axonal and dendritic sprouting, respectively.

Stimulation of neuronal sprouting by increased endogenous expression of bFGF and OP-1 may play an important role in functional recovery after stroke. The availability of recombinant growth factors has enabled testing of this hypothesis, which we have done in recent studies. In a previous series of studies,[39-43] we showed that recombinant bFGF, delivered intracerebrally or intravenously before or within hours after the onset of ischemia, reduced infarct volume in models of focal cerebral ischemia in rats, mice, and cats. In the case of intravenously administered bFGF, the mechanism of infarct reduction appears to depend on penetration across the damaged blood brain barrier and direct receptor-mediated protection of cells at the borders ("penumbra") of focal infarcts.[40] Basic fibroblast growth factor is likely to initiate a signal transduction cascade in these cells, resulting in the expression of neuroprotective genes and their products, including free radical scavenging enzymes, calcium binding proteins, and anti-apoptotic genes.[16,22,44]

In subsequent studies, we examined the effects of growth factor treatment given long after the onset of ischemia to enhance functional recovery after stroke. In these studies, focal infarcts were made by unilateral MCA occlusion, producing focal infarction in the contralateral dorsolateral cortex and underlying striatum, and resulting in deficits of sensorimotor function in the contralateral limbs. We found that if bFGF was administered intracerebrally (intracisternally) starting 24 hours after the onset of ischemia, infarct size was not reduced, but animals recovered more rapidly and to a greater extent on tests of sensorimotor function of the impaired limbs.[45,46] Basic FGF was delivered intracisternally in these studies to ensure access to the intact as well as damaged cerebral cortex. Initial studies used 8 intracisternal injections during the first month after stroke,[45,46] but recent preliminary studies suggest that as few as two injections are also effective. Immunostaining studies using an antibody to a neuronal protein that is selectively upregulated during new axonal growth ("growth associated protein-43," GAP-43) showed enhancement of GAP-43 immunoreactivity (IR) in the intact sensorimotor cortex contralateral to focal infarcts, consistent with stimulation of axonal sprouting by bFGF.[46] Moreover, we found that co-injection of GAP-43 antisense oligonucleotide blocked both enhancement of neurological recovery, as well as increased brain GAP-43 expression following bFGF administration (Kawamata and Finklestein, unpublished observations). In other recent preliminary studies, we found that as few as 1–2 intracisternal injections of OP-1, starting at 24 hours after stroke, also enhanced recovery of sensorimotor function of the impaired limbs in a dose-dependent fashion.[47,48] This enhancement of behavioral recovery persists for at least 3 months after stroke.

Other investigators have also shown that the exogenous administration of trophic growth factors can enhance functional recovery and neural sprouting after mechanical brain injury. Specifically, Kolb and colleagues[49] have shown that the intracerebroventricular (i.c.v.) administration of nerve growth factor (NGF) enhances recovery of sensorimotor function and stimulates dendritic sprouting in the intact ipsilateral cortex following unilateral cortical damage in mature rats. Moreover, Kolb et al.[50] found that i.c.v. NGF promoted increased dendritic branching and spine density in the cortex of intact young adult rats.

In summary, neurotrophic factors are potentially useful tools in the promotion of recovery from stroke. The therapeutic window appears to be substantially larger than with the many agents currently being tested for the treatment of acute stroke.

References

1. Ren JM, Finklestein SP. Trophic factor treatment for stroke. In Welch KMA, Caplan L, Reis DJ, et al. (eds): Primer on Cerebrovascular Diseases. San Diego: Academic Press; 1997:269-271.
2. Berlove DJ, Finklestein SP. Growth Factors and Brain Injury. In Moody TW (ed): Growth Factors, Peptides and Receptors. New York: Plenum Press; 1993:137-143.

3. Finklestein SP. Growth Factors in Stroke. In Caplan LR (ed): Brain Ischemia: Basic Concepts and Clinical Relevance. London: Springer-Verlag; 1995:37-41.

4. Barnett HJM, Mohr JP, Stein BM, et al. Stroke: Pathophysiology, Diagnosis, and Management. New York: Churchill Livingstone, 1992.

5. Cramer S, Finklestein SP. Stroke Recovery. In Rosenberg RN (ed): The Atlas of Clinical Neurology. Philadelphia: Current Medicine; 1998.

6. Kawamata T, Speliotes EK, Finklestein SP. The role of polypeptide growth factors in recovery from stroke. In Freund H-J, Sabel BA, Witte OW (eds): Brain Plasticity. Philadelphia: Lippincott-Raven; 1997:73,377-382.

7. Weiller C, Ramsay S, Wise RJ, et al. Individual patterns of functional reorganization in the human cerebral cortex after capsular infarction. Ann Neurol 1993;33:181-189.

8. Cramer SC, Nelles G, Benson RR, et al. A functional MRI study of subjects recovered from hemiparetic stroke. Stroke 1997;28:2518-2527.

9. Nudo RJ, Wise BM, SiFuentes F, et al. Neural substrates for the effects of rehabilitative training on motor recovery after ischemic infarct. Science 1996;272:1791-1794.

10. Jones TA, Schallert T. Overgrowth and pruning of dendrites in adult rats recovering from neocortical damage. Brain Research 1992;581:156-160.

11. Jones TA, Schallert T. Use-dependent growth of pyramidal neurons after neocortical damage. J Neurosci 1994;14:2140-2152.

12. Stroemer RP, Kent TA, Hulsebosch CE. Neocortical neural sprouting, synaptogenesis, and behavioral recovery after neocortical infarction in rats. Stroke 1995;26:2135-2144.

13. Speliotes EK, Caday CG, Do T, et al. Increased expression of basic fibroblast growth factor (bFGF) following focal cerebral infarction in the rat. Mol Brain Research 1996;39:31-42.

14. Baird A. Fibroblast growth factors: Activities and significance of non-neurotrophin neurotrophic growth factors. Curr Opin Neurobiol 1994;4:78-86.

15. Baird A, Klagsbrun M. The Fibroblast Growth Factor Family. New York: Annals New York Acad. Sci., 1991.

16. Ay I, Finklestein SP. Preclinical trials of basic fibroblast growth factor (bFGF) in animal models of stroke. In Mattson MP (ed): Neuroprotective Signal Transduction. Totowa, NJ: Humana Press, Inc.; 1997:111-118.

17. Lin D, Finklestein SP. Basic fibroblast growth factor as a treatment for stroke. Neuroscientist 1997;3:247-250.

18. Walicke PA. Basic and acidic fibroblast growth factors have trophic effects on neurons from multiple CNS regions. J Neurosci 1988;8:2618-2627.

19. Mattson MP, Murrain M, Guthrie PB, et al. Fibroblast growth factor and glutamate: Opposing roles in the generation and degeneration of hippocampal neuroarchitecture. J Neurosci 1989;9:3728-3740.

20. Finklestein SP, Kemmou A, Caday CG, et al. Basic fibroblast growth factor protects cerebrocortical neurons against excitatory amino acid toxicity in vitro. Stroke 1993;24[suppl I]:I-141-I-143.

21. Cheng B, Mattson MP. NGF and bFGF protect rat hippocampal and human cortical neurons against hypoglycemic damage by stabilizing calcium homeostasis. Neuron 1991;7:1-20.

22. Mattson MP, Barger SW. Programmed cell life: Neuroprotective signal transduction and ischemic brain injury. In Moskowitz MA, Caplan LR (eds): Cerebrovascular Diseases: The 19th Princeton Stroke Conference. Newton, MA: Butterworth Heinemann; 1995:271-290.

23. Aoyagi A, Nishikawa K, Saito H, et al. Characterization of basic fibroblast growth factor-mediated acceleration of axonal branching in cultured rat hippocampal neurons. Brain Res 1994;661:117-126.

24. Otto D, Unsicker K. Basic FGF reverses chemical and morphological deficits in the nigrostriatal system of MPTP-treated mice. J Neurosci 1990;10: 1912-1921.

25. Abraham JA, Mergia A, Whang JL, et al. Nucleotide sequence of a bovine clone encoding the angiogenic protein, basic fibroblast growth factor. Science 1986;233:545-548.

26. Ku P-T, D'Amore PA. Regulation of basic fibroblast growth factor (bFGF) gene and protein expression following its release from sublethally injured endothelial cells. J Cellular Biochem 1995;58:328-343.

27. Griffith DL, Keck PC, Sampath TK, et al. Three-dimensional structure of recombinant human osteogenic protein 1: Structural paradigm for the transforming growth factor beta superfamily. Proc Natl Acad Sci 1996;93: 878-883.

28. tenDijke P, Yamashita H, Sampath TK, et al. Identification of type I receptors for osteogenic-protein 1 and bone morphogenetic protein-4. J Biol Chem 1994;269:16985-16988.

29. Yamashita H, TenDijke P, Heldin CH, et al. Bone morphogenetic protein receptors. Bone 1996;19:569-574.

30. Sampath TK, Maliakal JC, Hauschka PV, et al. Recombinant human osteogenic protein-1 (hOP-1) induces new bone formation in vivo with a specific activity comparable with mature bovine osteogenic protein and stimulates osteoblast proliferation and differentiation in vitro. J Biol Chem 1992;267: 20352-20362.

31. Ozkaynak E, Rueger DC, Drier EA, et al. Cp-1 cDNA encodes an osteogenic protein in the TGF-b family. EMBO J 1990;9:2085-2093.

32. Lewen A, Soderstrom S, Hillered L, et al. Expression of serine/threonine kinase receptors in traumatic brain injury. Neuroreport 1997;8:475-479.

33. Soderstrom S, Bengtsson H, Ebendal T. Expression of serine/threonine kinase receptors including the bone morphogenetic factor type II receptor in the developing and adult rat brain. Cell Tissue Res 1996;286:269-279.

34. Lein P, Johnson M, Guo X, et al. Osteogenic protein-1 induces dendritic growth in rat sympathetic neurons. Neuron 1995;15:597-605.

35. Lein P, Guo X, Hedges AM, et al. The effects of extracellular matrix and osteogenic protein-1 on the morphological differentiation of rat sympathetic neurons. Int J Dev Neurosci 1996;14:203-215.

36. Emoto N, Gonzalez A-M, Walicke PA, et al. Basic fibroblast growth factor (FGF) in the central nervous system: Identification of specific loci of basic FGF expression in the rat brain. Growth Factors 1989;2:21-29.

37. Gomez-Pinilla F, Lee JW-K, Cotman CW. Basic FGF in adult rat brain: Cellular distribution and response to entorhinal lesion and fimbria-fornix transection. J Neurosci 1992;12:345-355.

38. Sakaguchi T, Yamada K, Wanaka A, et al. Expression of basic fibroblast growth factor receptor messenger RNA in the periinfarcted brain tissue. Rest Neurol Neurosci 1994;7:29-36.

39. Koketsu N, Berlove DJ, Moskowitz MA, et al. Pretreatment with intraventricular basic fibroblast growth factor (bFGF) decreases infarct size following focal cerebral ischemia in rats. Ann Neurol 1994;35:451-457.

40. Fisher M, Meadows M-E, Do T, et al. Delayed treatment with intravenous basic fibroblast growth factor reduces infarct size following permanent focal cerebral ischemia in rats. J Cereb Blood Flow Metab 1995;15:953-959.

41. Jiang N, Finklestein SP, Do T, et al. Delayed intravenous administration of basic fibroblast growth factor reduces infarct volume in a model of focal cerebral ischemia/reperfusion (abstr.). Stroke 1995;26:165.

42. Huang Z, Chen K, Huang PL, et al. bFGF ameliorates focal ischemic injury by blood flow-independent mechanisms in eNOS mutant mice. Amer J Physiol 1996;272:H1401-H1405.

43. Bethel A, Kirsch JR, Koehler RC, et al. Intravenous basic fibroblast growth factor decreases brain injury resulting from focal ischemia in cats. Stroke 1997;28:609-615.

44. Mattson MP, Lovell MA, Furukawa K, et al. Neurotrophic factors attenuate glutamate-induced accumulation of peroxides, elevation of intracellular Ca2+ concentration, and neurotoxicity and increase antioxidant enzyme activities in hippocampal neurons. J Neurochem 1995;65:1740-1751.

45. Kawamata T, Alexis NE, Dietrich WD, et al. Intracisternal basic fibroblast growth factor (bFGF) enhances behavioral recovery following focal cerebral infarction in the rat. J Cereb Blood Flow Metab 1996;16:542-547.

46. Kawamata T, Dietrich WD, Schallert T, et al. Intracisternal basic fibroblast growth factor (bFGF) enhances functional recovery and upregulates the expression of a molecular marker of neuronal sprouting following focal cerebral infarction. Proc Natl Acad Sci 1997;94:8179-8184.

47. Kawamata T, Ren J, Chan TCK, et al. Intracisternal osteogenic protein-1 enhances functional recovery following focal stroke. NeuroReport 1998; 9:1441-1445.

48. Kawamata T, Charette MF, Finklestein SP. Single administration of osteogenic protein-1 improves recovery following stroke (abstr.). Soc Neurosci Abstr 1997;23:573.

49. Kolb B, Cote S, Ribeiro-Da-Silva A, et al. Nerve growth factor treatment prevents dendritic atrophy and promotes recovery of function after cortical injury. Neuroscience 1996;76:1139-1151.

50. Kolb B, Gorny G, Cote S, et al. Nerve growth factor stimulates growth of cortical pyramidal neurons in young adult rats. Brain Research 1997;751: 289-294.

Chapter 29

Activity-Associated Growth Factor Expression and Related Neural Events in Recovery of Function after Brain Injury

Timothy Schallert, PhD, J. Leigh Humm, MA, Sondra Bland, BA, Theresa Jones, PhD, Bryan Kolb, PhD, Jaroslaw Aronowski, PhD, and James Grotta, MA

Introduction

Direct manipulation of motor behavior after brain injury can modify mechanisms linked to neuroplasticity, neurodegenerative events, and functional outcome in rats after focal cortical injury.[1-8] Evidence for these relationships in animal models includes experiments in which motor behavior after brain damage was examined closely in relation to anatomical or electrophysiological changes and then directly manipulated at different postinjury time points.[6-13] This chapter summarizes the effects of <u>extreme</u> manipulations of movement and the structural events in the brain that follow.

After brain injury, some neural events may require motor experience (use-dependency), and this use-dependency may be time-dependent, unfolding in definable phases, during which the brain may be differentially sensitive to modification. For example, it has been shown that there is a period soon after sensorimotor cortex injury when neural

Supported by the Texas Advanced Research Program, MH55525, MH52361 and NS23979

From: Choi D, Dacey RG, Hsu CY, Powers WJ. *Cerebrovascular Disease: Momentum at the End of the Second Millennium.* Armonk, NY: Futura Publishing Company, Inc., © 2002.

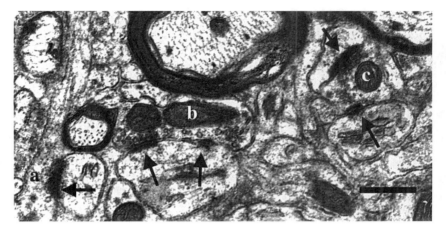

Figure 1. Use-dependent synaptic events in homotopic layer V motor cortex, 30 days following electrolytic damage to the FL-SMC. Arrows point to post-synaptic densities (PSD's). **A.** Bouton forming a single non-perforated synapse with a dendritic spine, **B.** Bouton forming a perforated synapse with a dendritic spine, **C.** Bouton forming synapses with two different dendritic spines (a multiple synaptic bouton (MSB)). Scale bar = 0.5 μm.

plasticity may be optimal, perhaps because injury primes surviving tissue.[11-16] A number of plasticity-associated events occur as recovery of function progresses over several weeks, including dendritic arborization, expression of growth-correlated markers, NMDA-dependent hyperexcitability, pruning, increases in spine density and synaptogenesis.[8,14,17-21] In the intact sensorimotor cortex, dendritic arborization appears to depend on movement because it can be prevented by restricting use of the "crutch" forelimb during the period of dendritic growth.[6,8,11-12] However, movement alone is not sufficient to cause extensive arborization. Thus, in nonlesioned animals with one limb restricted, there is no detectable increase in dendritic growth in the hemisphere opposite the nonrestricted forelimb.[11]

In lesioned animals, analysis of synapse density and morphology using electron microscopy reveals a dramatic increase in so-called multiple axodendritic synapses and perforated postsynaptic receptors in the intact sensorimotor cortex[19,22] (see Figures 1 and 2). These synapses are similar to those formed after long-term potentiation (LTP) in the hippocampus, an established activity-related model of learning and memory.

Limb-Specific Impairment, Rehabilitation, and Plasticity

Damage to the motor cortex in humans and other mammals causes transient disruption of function of the contralateral limb. Although

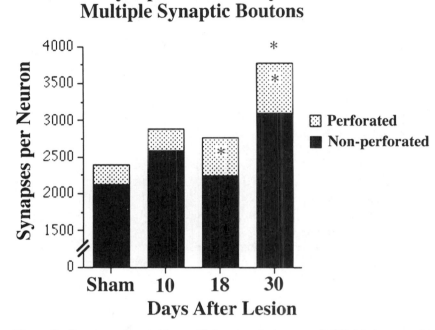

Synapses Formed by Multiple Synaptic Boutons

Figure 2. Synapses formed by multiple synaptic boutons (MSBs) in homotopic layer V motor cortex 10, 18, and 30 days following electrolytic lesion of the FL-SMC, and in nonlesioned animals. Shaded bars represent nonperforated synapses, stippled bars represent perforated synapses.
*(inside bar) P < 0.05 significantly more perforated MSBs relative to sham.
**(above bar) P < 0.05 significantly more total MSBs relative to sham.

gradual recovery of function occurs, residual impairment can be observed.[8,13,23-24]

Taub et al.[25] suggest that at least some of the residual impairment is due to "learned non-use" of the contralateral forelimb. It is well known that animals readily learn to adopt alternative motor strategies after injury or drugs in order to compensate for dysfunction. If these strategies are immediately effective, then the animal may fail to demonstrate its maximum potential for function during a sensitive period soon after injury. Thus, it might be useful to apply moderate rehabilitative pressure that focuses preferentially on the impaired forelimb, which often is *disused* in clinical situations when the patient fails to be self-motivated or when the affected limb is either broken or has been fitted with an intravenous catheter. Taub and his colleagues showed that months after unilateral stroke, immobilizing the good arm of patients, together with physical rehabilitation of the bad limb, detectably improved the function of the bad limb.[26]

Basic Fibroblast
Growth Factor and Brain Injury

Neurotrophic factors are frequently increased after brain injury and have long been thought to contribute to neural, glial and other cell survival, maintenance and plasticity.[27-29] Among the most studied of these is basic fibroblast growth factor (bFGF). Shortly after injury, bFGF expression and its mRNA expression is found prominently in the nuclei and cell bodies of reactive astrocytes surrounding the damage.[18,30-33]

As Rowntree and Kolb found after suction ablation lesions,[33] we have shown that after electrolytic lesions of the forelimb representation area of the sensorimotor cortex (FL-SMC), both bFGF-positive and glial fibrillary acid protein (GFAP)-positive astrocyte numbers are increased in the region surrounding the injury.[32]

A representative electrolytic lesion is shown in Figure 3. This section was typical of the extent of damage at the rostro-caudal midpoint of unilateral FL-SMC lesions. Note that tissue in the peri-lesion zone largely survives the primary injury, unlike stroke models,[6] as indicated using triphenyl tetrazolium chloride (TTC) for mitochondria. At this 21-hour time point, no differences were found between casted and uncasted animals using TTC.

Figure 3 also shows suction ablation of similar size and location at 7 days post-injury, with the distribution of bFGF expression represented in the peri-lesion zone. bFGF immunoreactivity was observed in the peri-lesion area by day 2 (the earliest time evaluated), peaked at day 7, and was still detectable at day 21.[33] GFAP-positive astrocytes also were increased. In collaboration with Kolb, we observed a similar increase in the number of both GFAP- and bFGF-positive astrocytes in the peri-lesional zone at day 10 postlesion in our electrolytic lesion model.[32]

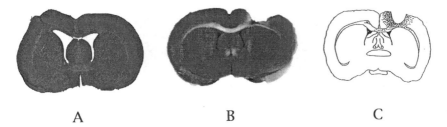

A   B   C

Figure 3. **(A)** illustrates a representative FL-SMC lesion, **(B)** depicts a lesioned brain processed with TTC, **(C)** shows a suction lesion of similar size and location to the FL-SMC lesions in A; the stippled region illustrates the area in which expression of bFGF is found on postinjury day 2.

Restraint of Impaired Forelimb after Injury Inhibits Astrocytic Expression of bFGF in the Peri-Lesional Zone

Rowntree and Kolb also examined layer V pyramidal neurons in remaining cortex in animals in which reactive bFGF expression had been eliminated by neutralizing antibodies. Blockade of bFGF expression caused dendritic atrophy and decreased spine density in surviving cortical neurons.[33] We examined surviving Golgi-Cox stained neurons in the peri-lesional zone, and found them to be normal in extent of dendritic arborization when examined several weeks after the injury. Immobilization of the impaired forelimb for the first 15 days after injury reduced the extent of dendritic branches in Layer V pyramidal neurons of the peri-lesion zone and disturbed recovery of function (see Figure 4).

In sum, bFGF-positive astrocytes and GFAP-positive astrocytes are clearly visible in the vicinity of an FL-SMC lesion soon after brain injury, and the bFGF-positive astrocytes appear to be important for maintaining the structural integrity of surviving neurons surrounding the injury.

We examined bFGF and GFAP expression after electrolytic cortical lesions. In the injured brains there was an increase of bFGF immunoreactivity around the cortical lesions (Figure 5A). This increase was due to the dense accumulation of small bFGF-reactive cells. The morphological characteristics and pattern of immunohistochemistry with anti-GFAP (a useful marker for identifying astrocytes) and anti-bFGF antibodies on alternate sections clearly identified these cells as astrocytes.

Immobilization of the contralateral forelimb with a cast for 10 days postlesion reduced bFGF expression, as indicated by little or no immunoreactivity (Figure 5B). GFAP expression in astrocytes also was increased in the peri-lesional area (sections not shown), but we found no effect of casting on GFAP immunoreactivity.

These data suggest that the use of the contra-lesion forelimb is necessary for the normal expression of endogenous bFGF, but not GFAP, in the vicinity of FL-SMC lesions. Moreover, these data may explain why casting the contralateral forelimb for the first 7-15 days after injury interferes with the rate of recovery of function:[6,12] 1) bFGF expression after injury promotes the integrity of surviving neurons in the peri-lesional region; 2) bFGF expression depends on minimal levels of motor behavior involving the impaired forelimb; and 3) bFGF expression after injury may be important for functional outcome. Establishing that an animal's motor response to the injury can influence neurotrophic expression and related events has implications for studies of

Lesion + No Cast   **Lesion + Contra Cast**

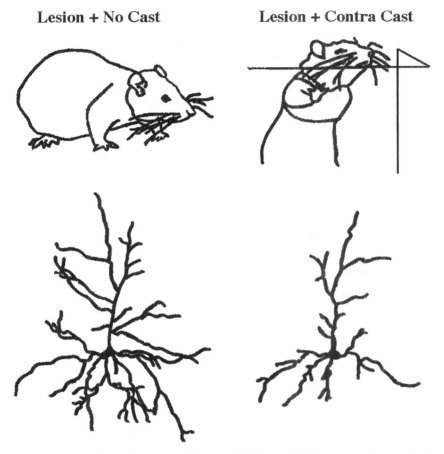

Figure 4. Drawings of neurons observed in the peri-lesion area of noncasted rats and rats that were forced to rest the impaired forelimb following injury.

recovery of function in which motor behavior might be changed directly by pharmacological interventions.[34-35]

Electrolytic FL-SMC lesions cause transient deficits in overall use of the impaired (contralateral) forelimb during exploration for limb-placing, and for walking on grid surfaces (foot-fault impairment). Impairment and recovery of other sensorimotor functions are detailed in published papers.[6,8,12] In order to hypothesize that bFGF expression is use-linked, it is important to have evidence that uncasted animals with FL-SMC lesions actually *use* the impaired forelimb spontaneously, albeit dysfunctionally, during the period of bFGF expression. (Casted animals, of course, cannot use the impaired forelimb at all because it is immobilized). Accordingly, four 1-minute samples of spontaneous limb-use activity in the home cage were taken, during the dark portion

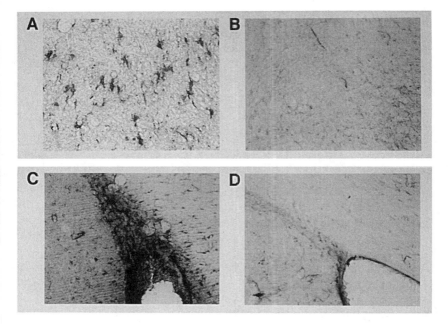

Figure 5. bFGF immunoreactivity in cortical tissue sampled from Layer V of the peri-lesional region and dorsolateral subependymal zone (SEZ) 10 days after electrolytic lesions of the FL-SMC. **(A)** represents tissue from the peri-lesion area of uncasted rats, while **(B)** represents tissue from the peri-lesion zone of rats that had the contralateral forelimb immobilized for 10 days after surgery. **(C)** shows bFGF expression in the dorsolateral SEZ of a non-casted animal, while **(D)** shows the same region from an animal that underwent immobilization of the contralateral forelimb for 10 days following injury.

Table 1.

Impaired forelimb movements/minute

	pre-surgery	post-surgery
Lesion + no cast	5.89 + 3.1	3.02 + 0.6
Lesion + contra cast	6.67 + 2.9	0.00 (casted limb)
Sham	5.78 + 2.7	6.71 + 1.0

of the light/dark cycle, on days 2, 4, and 7 after FL-SMC lesions or sham operations in casted versus non-casted rats. These data are pooled and shown in Table 1. The data indicate that uncasted rats made about three movements of the impaired forelimb per minute versus none in casted rats. Although the number of movements is less than that of either forelimb of uncasted sham-operated rats, clearly the total number of movements over an entire week after injury was substantial.[6,12] Thus, casting the impaired forelimb represents an impressive motor intervention that reasonably could have a considerable influence on neural events in the damaged hemisphere.

In the context of the present discussion, which focuses on use-related bFGF expression, a brief summary of spontaneous use of the impaired forelimb immediately after the injury and chronic functional outcome is relevant. Although lesioned rats show functional impairment of the forelimb contralateral to the lesion, they continue to use the limb during exploratory movements.[6,12] For the first day or so after the injury, the contralateral forelimb is used together with the intact forelimb for locomotion on the floor of the home cage and elsewhere, but it is used rarely for landing after rearing up on the hind limbs, and not at all for vertical exploration along the walls. Instead, the animal relies on the intact forelimb preferentially for landing and for initiating weight-shifting movements. During the next several weeks, as placing recovers, the impaired forelimb is used increasingly to assist the intact forelimb for landing after a rear and for vertical exploration and other movements.[8] If direct striatal damage is minimal, the impaired forelimb is gradually used independently of the intact forelimb for landing, but is almost never used independently to initiate weight-shifting movements along a vertical surface.[6,8] Thus, rebound recovery of forelimb use occurs, but certain limb-use functions do not recover even up to 60 days after injury, such as a lasting impairment in use of that forelimb for weight-shifting movements during vertical exploratory movements.[6]

For example, chronic deficits result from unilateral lesions of the FL-SMC, as lesioned animals demonstrate a strong and persistent reliance on the unimpaired limb for *lateral* weight-shifting movements along a wall, relative to independent use of the contralateral forelimb. Animals are slightly better, but still chronically impaired, in using their impaired limb to make vertical (nonlateral) movements on a wall.

Implications

These data augment the literature in terms of the role of experience after brain injury. Thus, motor behavior can affect not only the morphological characteristics of neurons and synapses,[11,13,19] but may also be necessary for the expression of bFGF in astrocytes. bFGF and perhaps other molecular precursor events may prepare the tissue for plasticity expressed more specifically in neuronal structure, organization and function.[27]

Motor behavior is changed substantially after injury to the central nervous system as well as during the aging process. Moreover, exercise, taming and enrichment techniques may prime the brain for improved outcome during aging and after brain injury. The possibility that structural events might be use- or disuse-sensitive could have implications for understanding key molecular events associated with neuroplasticity, treatment, and perhaps preventive behavioral medicine as well.

Overuse of the Impaired Forelimb: Implications for bFGF Expression

In contrast to the subtle astrocytic bFGF inhibition caused by *restraint* of the impaired forelimb after injury, forced *overuse* of the impaired forelimb in rats with FL-SMC damage results in expansion of the damage into the surrounding tissue.[6,8,36] Figure 6 represents use-dependent exaggeration of damage in rats with unilateral FL-SMC lesions (rats were sacrificed 40 days after surgery). Forced overuse of the impaired forelimb during the 2 weeks after surgery caused a dramatic increase in lesion size.

Overuse-related exaggeration of injury has been shown also after unilateral fluid percussion injury[37] and after moderate focal ischemia.[38] Forced overuse following unilateral middle cerebral artery/common carotid artery (MCA/CCA) occlusion for 90 minutes resulted in an increase in infarct volume (Figure 7). Exacerbation of the infarct was found as early as 3 days after casting in this model, and a similar increase in infarct size was found when animals were casted for 14 days and sacrificed at day 28.

Forced overuse of the contralateral forelimb following a more severe MCA occlusion, however, did not result in increases in infarct volume. Unilateral MCA and bilateral CCA occlusion for 90 minutes resulted in large infarcts which included the forelimb sensorimotor cortex and substantial involvement of the underlying striatum. Furthermore, pathology scores representing secondary degeneration in striatum and thalamus were the same in both casted and uncasted animals. It is possible that if the extent of infarct is severe, extreme physical training regimens may not exaggerate the extent of injury further.

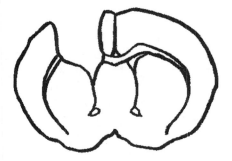

Figure 6. Representative drawing of the extent of lesion damage in animals forced to rely exclusively on the impaired forelimb for the first postoperative week.

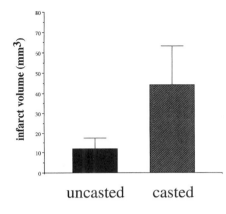

Figure 7. Infarct volume after 90 minute MCA/CCA occlusion 72 hours after reperfusion.

It may be that early rehabilitative training in human patients may lead to damage to vulnerable tissue surrounding limited focal injury to the cortex. It is also likely that infarct location and the extent to which the rehabilitative repertoire exerts pressure specifically on vulnerable tissue will be influential. However, systematic manipulation of physical therapy in human brain damaged patients is rare. In one study presented at an aphasiology conference in 1993, Holland and colleagues reported that following thrombolytic stroke in human patients, performance in Kertesz's Western Aphasia Battery was worse when patients received several weeks of extreme didactic training than when they were allowed to simply engage in brief (15 minute) conversation[39] (see Figure 8).

Disuse of Impaired Forelimb Extends Window of Vulnerability to Overuse

When the impaired forelimb is immobilized during the first 7 days after injury (which inhibits bFGF expression in astrocytes), a window of vulnerability to forced overuse of the impaired forelimb is extended to later periods. Figure 9 describes data from rats receiving unilateral FL-SMC lesions or sham operations. Limb use was manipulated with unilateral casts, as previously described. The animals were sacrificed at 40 days postsurgery, and the remaining tissue in the lesioned hemisphere was quantified using stereologic analysis. Forced overuse of the impaired forelimb for the *first* 7 days after surgery results in expansion of the lesion, while forced overuse only for the *second* 7 days does not.[40] However, completely restricting use of the impaired limb for the first 7 days, followed by forced overuse for the second 7 days, results in expansion of the lesion. This last manipulation thus extended the window of vulnerability into the formerly "safe" period (ie, the *second*

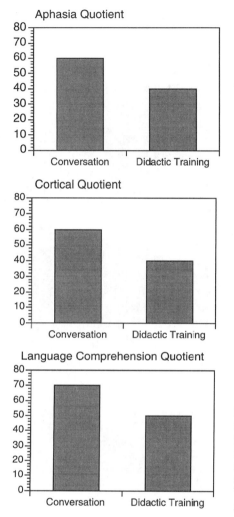

Figure 8. Effects of early (within 3 days) daily rehabilitative training in thrombolytic stroke patients on performance in Kertesz's Western Aphasia Battery. Mild (15 minute conversation only) versus Extensive Training (pushing to the limit). Adapted from Holland et al.[39]

7 days post-lesion). Time-dependent stereological[6] and degenerative histological methods (including an amino-cupric-silver stain), as well as within-groups brain imaging (by MRI) analysis revealed that cortical, striatal, and substantia nigra pars reticulata were particularly affected by the manipluation.[41]

Thus, *complete disuse* of the impaired forelimb via casting during the first postinjury week appears to extend the time frame during which overuse causes extensive tissue loss into the second (previously "safer") week. Thus, it is possible that minimal forelimb use (ie, as observed in *uncasted* animals) initiates at least partial plasticity that may provide significant neural protection against later, more aggressive,

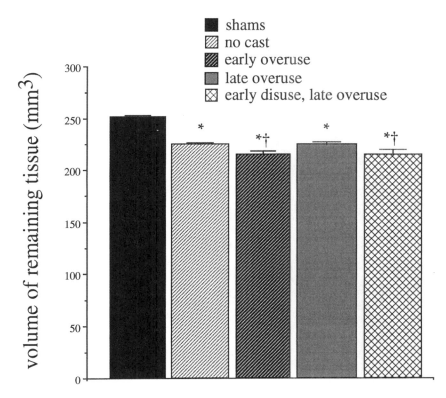

condition

Figure 9. Volume of remaining (intact) tissue after unilateral FL-SMC lesion, 40 days postinjury. The solid bar represents the volume of remaining tissue from sham-operated rats (controls). Next to it, for comparison, is a bar depicting the volume of remaining tissue in lesioned, noncasted animals. The third bar shows exaggerated tissue loss in lesioned rats forced to overuse the impaired limb via casting for 7 days post-lesion, while the fourth bar illustrates the finding that overuse of the impaired limb for the *second* week following injury (a "safer" period) does not result in exaggerated tissue loss. The last bar shows that lesioned rats forced to *disuse* the impaired limb for the first 7 days postlesion, and then forced to *overuse* it immediately thereafter do show exaggerated tissue loss, signifying a shift of the window of vulnerability into the formerly "safe" period.
* $P < 0.01$ significantly different from shams.
† $P < 0.01$ significantly different from noncasted lesions.

rehabilitative intervention. Conceivably, in uncasted rats bFGF-reactive astrocytes in the tissue surrounding the injury may provide a trophic influence that could protect the tissue from later insults. Furthermore, 7 days of forelimb disuse decreases levels of extracellular glutamate in the affected FL-SMC when compared to uncasted animals, while

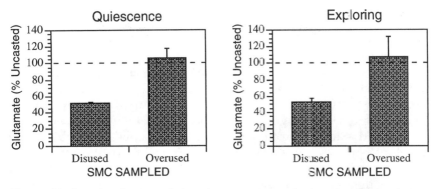

Figure 10. Levels of extracellular glutamate in nonlesioned animals during behavioral quiescence and exploratory activity. During both periods, levels of extracellular glutamate in the hemisphere corresponding to the overused limb exceeded those found in the hemisphere corresponding to the disused limb.

forelimb overuse does not affect levels of extracellular glutamate in the affected FL-SMC (see Figure 10). Note that mild or brief periods of forced exercise or training during the first week after FL-SMC lesions does not exaggerate the deficit.[7,32,42]

Thus, it may be dangerous to completely rest the impaired limb early after injury, particularly when this is followed by intense physical therapy once the patient's neurological outcome has become stable. The effects of encouraging the patient to avoid total disuse prior to eventual behavioral therapy may be worth investigating.

Summary

We have found that injury causes time-dependent anatomical events in rats that may be alterable. Some of these events may be related to neuroplasticity (eg, trophic factor expression and synaptogenesis) while others may be associated with tissue loss and degeneration. Plasticity and degenerative events both are modified by manipulating behavioral demand. Moderate physical therapy has not been shown to be harmful and may improve functional outcome, depending on the timing of the intervention and the injury model. Early after injury there may be a window of opportunity during which the beneficial effects of motor rehabilitation might be potentiated by endogenous trophic factor expression. Extreme disuse of the affected forelimb can prevent plasticity-related events, including bFGF expression and dendritic arborization in the peri-lesional area. It is as though complete motor quiescence during the first week or so after injury is detrimental. On the other hand, extreme forced overuse of the affected forelimb can exaggerate the injury. In stroke models, the extent of the initial infarct and the timing of the intervention can be significant factors in determining whether extreme rehabilitative pressure has an adverse effect on outcome. Use-dependent extracellular glutamate and the NMDA receptor may interact with other factors associated with excessive movement, to degrade peri-lesional tissue, which appears to be vulnerable during the first week or so after injury. Importantly, however, total disuse during the vulnerable period, followed immediately by delayed extreme forced overuse of the impaired forelimb (during the "safe" period) yields severe exaggeration of injury. It is conceivable that preventing endogenous bFGF expression by forced "resting" of the impaired forelimb may have extended the window of vulnerability to extreme behavioral demand, suggesting that minimal motor activity has long-term adaptive value, perhaps via its effects on trophic factor expression. Finally, it may be possible to re-open a window of opportunity long after brain injury despite the progressive disappearance of trophic factors, by combining exogenous trophic factors with functional rehabilitation.

References

1. Greenough WT, Fass B, DeVoogd T. The influence of experience on recovery following brain damage in rodents: Hypotheses based on developmental research. In Walsh R, Greenough W, (eds): *Environments as Therapy for Brain Dysfunction*. New York: Plenum Press;1976:10-5O.

2. Rosenzweig MR. Animal models for effects of brain lesions and for rehabilitation. In Bach-y-Rita P (ed): *Recovery of Function: Theoretical Considerations For Brain Injury Rehabilitation* . Baltimore: University Park Press;1980.

3. Withers GS, Greenough WT. Reach training selectively alters dendritic branching in subpopulations of layer II-III pyramidals in rat motor-somato-sensory forelimb cortex. *Neuropsychologia* 1989;27:61-69.

4. Johansson BB. Functional recovery after brain infarction. *Cerebrovas Dis* 1995;5: 271-278.

5. Freund HJ. Remapping the brain. *Science* 1996;272:1754.

6. Kozlowski DA, James DC, Schallert T. Use-dependent exaggeration of neuronal injury following unilateral sensorimotor cortex lesions. *J Neurosci* 1996;16:4776-4786.

7. Nudo RJ, Wise BM, SiFuentes F. Neural substrates for the effects of rehabilitative training on motor recovery after ischemic infarct. *Science* 1996;272: 1791-1794.

8. Schallert T, Kozlowski, DA, Humm JL, et al. Use-dependent events in recovery of function. In Freund H-J, Sabel BA, Witte OW, (eds): *Brain Plasticity, Advances in Neurology*. Philadelphia: Lippencott-Raven; 1996; 229-238.

9. Castro-Alamancos MA, Garcia-Segura LM, Borrell J. Transfer of function to a specific area of the cortex after induced recovery from brain damage. *Eur J Neurosci* 1992;4:853-863.

10. Castro-Alamancos MA, Borrell J. Functional recovery of forelimb response capacity after forelimb primary motor cortex damage in the rat is due to the reorganization of adjacent areas of cortex. *Neurosci* 1995;68:793-805.

11. Schallert T, Jones TA. "Exuberant" neuronal growth after brain damage in adult rats: The essential role of behavioral experience. *J Neural Trans Plast* 1993;4:193-198.

12. Jones TA, Schallert T. Use-dependent growth of pyramidal neurons after neocortical damage. *J Neurosci* 1994;14:2140-2152.

13. Kolb B. *Brain Plasticity and Behavior.* New York: Erlbaum & Associates; 1995.

14. Jones TA, Schallert T. Overgrowth and pruning of dendrites in adult rats recovering from neocortical damage. *Brain Res* 1992;581:156-160.

15. Jones TA, Kleim JA, Greenough WT. Synaptogenesis and dendritic growth in the cortex opposite unilateral sensorimotor cortex damage in adult rats: A quantitative electron microscopic examination. *Brain Res* 1996;733:142-148.

16. Cramer SC, Nelles G, Benson RR, et al. A functional MRI study of subjects recovered from hemiparetic stroke. *Stroke* 1997;28:2518-2527.

17. Stroemer RP, Kent TA, Hulsebosch CE. Neocortical neural sprouting, synaptogenesis, and behavioral recovery after neocortical infarction in rats. *Stroke* 1995;26:2135-2144.

18. Finklestein SP. The potential use of neurotrophic factors in the treatment of cerebral ischemia. *Adv Neurol* 1996;71:1413-1417.

19. Jones TA, Klintsova AY, Kilman VL, et al. Induction of multiple synapses by experience in the visual cortex of adult rats. *Neurobiol Learn & Mem* 1997;68:13-20.

20. Kawamata T, Schallert T, Dietrich WD, et al. Intracisternal basic fibroblast growth factor (bFGF) enhances functional recovery and upregulates the expression of a molecular marker of neuronal sprouting following focal cerebral infarction. *Proc Nat Acad Sci USA* 1997;94:8179-8184.

21. Witte OW, Stoll G. Delayed and remote effects of focal cortical infarctions: Secondary damage and reactive plasticity. 1997;73:207-227.

22. Chu C, Gregory A, Grande L, et al. Motor skills training effects on behavioral and neocortical structural plasticity following unilateral sensorimotor cortex lesions in adult rats. *Soc Neurosci Abtrs* 1997;95:18.

23. Fulton JF, Kennard MA. A study of flaccid and spastic paralysis produced by lesions of the cerebral cortex in primates. *Res Pub Assoc Ment Dis* 1934;13:158-210.

24. Whishaw IQ, Pellis SM, Gorny BP, et al. The impairments in reaching and the movements of compensation in rats with motor cortex lesions: An endpoint, videorecording, and movement notation analysis. *Behav Brain Res* 1991;42:77-91.

25. Taub E, Crago JE, Burgio LD, et al. An operant approach to rehabilitation medicine: Overcoming learned non-use by shaping. *J Exp Anal Behav* 1994;61:281-293.

26. Taub E, Pidikiti D, DeLuca SC, et al. Effects of motor restriction of an unimpaired upper extremity and training on improving functional tasks and altering brain/behaviors. In Toole JF, Good DC (eds): *Imaging in Neurologic Rehabilitation.* New York: Demos Vermande; 1996;133-154.

27. Nieto-Sampedro M, Cotman CW. Growth factor induction and temporal order in central nervous system repair. In Cotman CW (ed): *Synaptic plasticity*. New York: Guilford Press, 1985;407-456.

28. Mattson MP, Scheff S. Endogenous neuroprotection factors and truamatic brain injury: Mechanisms of action and implications for therapy. *J Neurotr* 1994;11:3-33.

29. Speliotes EK, Caday CG, Do T, et al. Increased expression of basic fibroblast growth factor (bFGF) following focal cerebral infarction in the rat. *Molec Brain Res* 1996;39:31-42.

30. Finklestein SP, Apostolides PJ, Caday CG, et al. Increased basic fibroblast growth factor (bFGF) immunoreactivity at the site of focal brain wounds. *Brain Res* 1988;460:23-29.

31. Humpel C, Chadi G, Lippoldt A, et al. Increase in basic fibroblast growth factor (bFGF, GFG-2) messenger RNA and protein following implantation of a microdialysis probe into rat hippocampus. *Exp Brain Res* 1994;98:229-237.

32. Humm JL, James DC, Gibb R, et al. Forced disuse of the impaired forelimb by restraint after sensorimotor cortical injury inhibits expression of endogenous bFGF in astrocytes and adversely affects behavioral function. *Soc Neurosci Abstr* 1997;95:5.

33. Rowntree S, Kolb B. Blockade of basic fibroblast growth factor retards recovery from motor cortex injury. *Eur J Neurosci* 1997;9:2432-2441.

34. Schallert T, Hernandez TD. GABAergic drugs and neuroplasticity after brain injury: Impact of functional recovery. In Goldstein L (ed): *Restorative Neurology: Advances in the Pharmacotherapy of Recovery after Stroke*. Armonk, NY: Futura Publishing; 1998:91-120.

35. Walker-Batson D, Smith P, Curtis S. Amphetamine paired with physical therapy accelerates motor recovery after stroke. Further evidence. *Stroke* 1995;26:2254-2259.

36. Schallert T, Kozlowski DA. Brain damage and plasticity: Use-related neural growth and overuse-related exaggeration of injury. In Ginsberg, MD, Bogousslavsky J (eds): *Cerebrovascular Disease: Pathology, Diagnosis, and Management*. Cambridge, MA: Blackwell Science;1998;611-619.

37. Kozlowski DA, von Stuck SL, Lee SM, et al. Behaviorally-induced contusions following raumatic brain injury: Use-dependent secondary insults. *Soc Neurosci Abstr* 1996;744:17.

38. Bland S, Humm JL, Kozlowski DA, et al. Forced overuse of the contralateral forelimb increases infarct volume following a mild, but not a severe, transient cerebral ischemic insult. *Soc Neurosci Abstr* 1998;774:14.

39. Holland AL. In Brookshire RK (ed): *Clinical Aphasiology Conference Proceedings*. Minneapolis: BRK Publishers; 1993:44-48.

40. Humm JL, Kozlowski DA, James DC, et al. Use-dependent exacerbation of brain damage occurs during and early post-lesion vulnerable period. *Brain Res* 1998;783:286-292.

41. Humm JL, Kozlowski DA, Bland ST, et al. Use-dependent exaggeration of brain damage: NMDA receptor mechanism. *Natl Neurotr Soc Abstr* 1996;152.

42. Hart CL, Davis GW, Barth TM. Forced activity facilitates recovery of function following cortical lesions in rats. *Natl Neurotr Soc Abstr* 1997;101.

Section VIII

Clinical Treatment Trials

Chapter 30

Recent Clinical Trials of Neuroprotective Agents and Thrombolytic Therapy for Acute Stroke

Gregory W. Albers, MD

Major scientific advances have elucidated many of the basic molecular and cellular mechanisms that mediate ischemic brain injury. These discoveries, coupled with substantial progress in clinical trial design and methodology, have led to increasing expectations that safe and effective stroke therapies will soon be available. An impressive array of neuroprotective agents, first demonstrated to be effective in animal stroke models, are now being tested in human stroke patients. Early clinical trials, using neuroprotective agents administered within 6 hours of stroke onset, have produced generally disappointing results. Newer agents, many with excellent safety profiles, have recently produced more encouraging results. In addition, in June of 1996, the Food and Drug Administration (FDA) approved tissue plasminogen activator (t-PA) as the first therapy with an indication for treatment of acute ischemic stroke. At present, thrombolytic therapy with t-PA is only indicated for highly selected patients who can receive therapy within three hours of stroke onset. There continues to be great hope that combination therapy with both a thrombolytic agent, as well as a neuroprotective strategy, will ultimately provide safe and effective therapy that will be available to a substantial percentage of ischemic stroke patients.

From: Choi D, Dacey RG, Hsu CY, Powers WJ. *Cerebrovascular Disease: Momentum at the End of the Second Millennium.* Armonk, NY: Futura Publishing Company, Inc., © 2002.

Neuroprotective Agents

Neuroprotective agents are often categorized based on their presumed mechanism of action. Some agents have several potential mechanisms, others were discovered by screening large numbers of compounds in experimental ischemia models, and their mechanisms of action are often less clear. Agents that are undergoing clinical investigation in stroke patients were first established to possess significant neuroprotective efficacy in animal models of cerebral ischemia. Major categories of neuroprotective agents include: glutamate antagonists, modulators of other neuronal receptors, inhibitors of ischemic injury cascade, membrane stabilizers, inhibitors of leukocyte adhesion, and growth factors.

Glutamate Antagonists

Glutamate is the most common excitatory neurotransmitter in the central nervous system and the ischemic neuronal injury cascade appears to begin with excessive activation of glutamate receptors. Therefore, glutamate antagonists have been extensively studied as potential neuroprotective agents in acute brain ischemia. Glutamate receptor pharmacology is complex; three major families of ionophore-linked receptors and metabotropic receptors have been identified. Among the ionotropic receptors, the N-methyl-D-aspartate (NMDA) receptor has received the most attention because of its high calcium conductance. In addition, numerous experimental studies performed in the late 1980s documented that NMDA antagonists were highly effective for reducing hypoxic neuronal injury in cell culture models and ischemic brain injury in animal stroke models.[1] These trials typically showed a substantial reduction in brain injury if the NMDA antagonist was administered either prior to the onset of ischemia, or within one or two hours after the ischemic event. In the animal stroke models, maximum neuroprotection (often up to a 50% or 60% reduction in infarct volume) was obtained in the cortex; however, minimal or no benefit was typically seen in the striatum. Poor collateral blood flow to the striatum, or the higher concentration of NMDA receptors in the cortex, may explain these experimental findings.

Based on the encouraging results from animal stroke models, NMDA antagonists moved into active clinical trials in human stroke patients. The noncompetitive NMDA antagonist dextrorphan, which is the major metabolite of the commonly used antitussive dextromethorphan, was the first NMDA antagonist to be evaluated in stroke patients.[2] Unfortunately, very high doses of dextrorphan were required to obtain potentially neuroprotective serum levels, and significant toxicity was encountered. Hallucinations and agitation were seen in a substantial number of patients, mimicking the effects of phencyclidine, which is also a noncompetitive NMDA antagonist. The most concerning side effect was sudden hypotension, which is particularly dangerous in stroke patients. Subsequently, the clinical development of this agent was aborted.

It was hoped that targeting an NMDA antagonist to the glutamate binding site on the NMDA receptor might produce less toxicity than the noncompetitive NMDA antagonists that bind to the ion channel associated with the NMDA receptor. This strategy was tested with the competitive NMDA antagonist, selfotel. Unfortunately, in Phase II trials involving stroke patients, escalating doses of selfotel were found to produce a side effect profile that was very similar to the noncompetitive NMDA antagonists. Therefore, a low dose of selfotel (1.5 mg/kg) was chosen for further clinical investigation, despite the fact that this dose level did not produce plasma levels in humans comparable to the levels required for neuroprotection in animal stroke models. A pair of large Phase III trials, in which a single intravenous dose of selfotel was administered within six hours of stroke onset, were initiated.[3] The first of these studies was primarily based in Europe, but was terminated by the Safety Monitoring Committee after 389 patients had been enrolled. A similar study in the United States and Israel was also terminated, although this study had only enrolled 87 patients. A combined analysis of the two trials indicated a trend toward more deaths in selfotel-treated patients and a substantial increase in brain-related mortality (death related to cerebral edema or stroke progression) in the selfotel-treated patients. In addition, there was no hint of a beneficial effect of the therapy to counterbalance the increase in brain-related mortality. Therefore, clinical development of selfotel was abandoned.

Two other NMDA antagonists were evaluated in large Phase III trials. Eliprodil was tested in a large European trial. Although the results of this study have not been published, further development of this agent has apparently been abandoned because of lack of efficacy. Aptiganel (Cerestat, CNS 1102) had a better safety profile than previously tested noncompetitive NMDA antagonists and encouraging efficacy results from a small Phase II trial. Unfortunately, a large Phase III trial that enrolled 628 patients was stopped prematurely by the Safety Committee, apparently because of a trend toward increased mortality in aptiganel-treated patients.

Because of safety concerns and clinical failures of early NMDA antagonists, alternative approaches to blocking the NMDA receptor have been pursued. Since glycine binding to the NMDA receptor is required for glutamate to open the ion-channel associated with the

NMDA receptor, glycine site antagonists have been investigated. In experimental models, these agents are highly effective for reducing infarct volume and, in preliminary clinical trials, they appear to have a favorable safety profile.[4] Two of these agents, ACEA-1021 and GV150526, are undergoing clinical investigation.

Modulators of Other Neuronal Receptors

The most intensely studied neuroprotective agent in clinical stroke trials is the voltage-gated calcium channel antagonist nimodipine. Numerous trials have been performed with this agent, enrolling more than 3,500 patients. Most of these studies involved oral administration of nimodipine more than 12 hours after stroke onset. Meta-analysis of these trials indicates that there was no clear evidence of efficacy, however, there was a suggestion of benefit among patients who were treated within 12 hours of symptom onset.[5] Currently, a Dutch trial is evaluating oral nimodipine therapy in patients who can be treated within 6 hours of stroke onset.[6]

Kappa opiate receptors appear to modulate ischemic neuronal injury. Therefore, opiate antagonists have also been evaluated for acute stroke therapy. Several small studies investigated the use of naloxone for stroke treatment; however, no significant benefits were noted.[7] More recently, nalmefene (Cervene), which is an opiate antagonist with a higher affinity for kappa receptors and a longer half-life than naloxone, has been evaluated. Patients treated with nalmefene within six hours of stroke onset had no difference in outcome from placebo-treated patients in a recent study.[8] However, a subgroup analysis indicated possible benefit among the patients who were less than 70 years of age. A larger Phase III trial involving nalmefene has been completed, but the results have not yet been reported.

Because excessive excitatory neurotransmission appears to mediate ischemic neuronal injury, agents that facilitate inhibitory neurotransmission have been evaluated for stroke treatment. Clomethiazole, a GABA agonist, has been used therapeutically in humans because of its sedative properties. This agent appears to have a good safety profile; however, significant sedation and hypotension can occur at high doses. A large Phase III trial, in which ischemic stroke patients were treated within 12 hours of symptom onset, failed to reveal beneficial effects with this agent. However, a subgroup analysis found that patients with large hemispheric strokes had substantially better outcomes in the clomethiazole-treated group.[9] This finding is being investigated in a large ongoing study. Another agent under clinical investigation that modulates neuronal receptors is fos-phenytoin, a sodium channel antagonist.

Inhibitors of Neuronal Ischemic Injury Cascade

Following excessive activation of excitatory amino acid receptors, levels of intracellular calcium rise dramatically and trigger a cascade of harmful biochemical events. The details of these complex cellular reactions are currently being elucidated; however, synthesis of intra-neuronal nitric oxide and activation of lipid peroxides and free radical generation appear to be critical events. Clinical strategies, aimed at attenuating the intra-neuronal ischemic injury cascade, have been evaluated in stroke patients.

Tirilazad, a 21-amino steroid, is a potent inhibitor of lipid peroxidation. A large study treated patients who were within 6 hours of stroke onset with tirilazad or a placebo. Although tirilazad was not found to have any significant toxicity, there was no evidence of clinical benefit with this agent.[10] It is unclear, however, whether adequate doses of tirilazad were tested.

More encouraging results were obtained with lubeluzole, which is an agent that appears to attenuate cellular injury mediated by intracellular nitric oxide. Following an encouraging Phase II trial,[11] the results of two large Phase III trials of lubeluzole were recently reported.[12,13] These trials had very similar study designs; however, they reached different conclusions regarding the efficacy of lubeluzole. In the North American trial, lubeluzole-treated patients had a modest but significant improvement in functional recovery and a trend toward decreased mortality. The European trial, however, found no beneficial effects on neurologic outcome or mortality. Lubeluzole had an excellent safety profile in both studies. This agent was administered by continuous IV infusion for 5 days and was initiated within 6 hours of stroke symptom onset. A much larger, international Phase III trial has recently been completed; however, the results have not yet been reported.

Membrane Stabilizers

Several additional neuroprotective agents are thought to have beneficial effects on neuronal membranes. Although their mechanisms of action remain speculative, these agents may enhance repair of damaged neuronal membranes and facilitate recovery following a stroke. The most extensively evaluated of these agents is GM 1 ganglioside. Numerous randomized studies have been performed with this agent in stroke patients; however, to date no convincing evidence of efficacy has been documented. More encouraging results were seen in recent trials with citicoline. Also known as CDP-choline, citicoline is a precursor for phosphatidyl choline. Because this agent may facilitate repair of injured membranes, it has been administered within 24 hours of stroke onset in several recent trials. Three different doses of citicoline were tested in a Phase II study.[14] Both a 500 mg per day dose and a 2,000 mg per day dose appeared to provide beneficial effects on stroke outcome without causing any significant toxicity. A larger Phase III trial, involving 394 patients, failed to document statistically significant benefits using a 500 mg per day dose. Unfortunately, randomization error resulted in a larger number of mild stroke patients in the placebo group, making interpretation of this study more difficult. In a subgroup analysis that included only patients with moderate or severe strokes, citicoline appeared to have beneficial effects. At present, a much larger trial, which will evaluate the efficacy of a 2,000 mg per day dose of citicoline, is planned.

Inhibitors of Leukocyte Adhesion

During reperfusion of ischemic brain tissue, leukocytes adhere to endothelial cells and can substantially impair the microcirculation. In addition, leukocyte migration into ischemic brain parenchyma can promote additional neuronal injury. Therefore, antibodies directed at endothelial sites of neutrophil adhesion have been studied, both in experimental stroke models and stroke patients. The largest clinical experience using this strategy involved a murine monoclonal antibody against the human ICAM-1 endothelial receptor. A commercial preparation of this antibody (Emlimomab) was recently tested in a large acute stroke trial. Patients were treated within 6 hours of stroke onset with a daily infusion of the antibody for 5 days.[15] Unfortunately, among the 625 patients enrolled, those treated with Emlimomab had worse neurologic outcomes and a higher mortality rate than the placebo-treated patients. A partial explanation for the poor results in this study may relate to the fact that the murine antibody may have led to complement activation and a local inflammatory response. Of note, there was a significant increase in the number of patients who experienced fever among the Emlimomab-treated patients. However, even among patients who did not develop fevers, Emlimomab treatment was associated with a poorer outcome. Therefore, further development of Emlimomab for stroke treatment has been abandoned. A Phase II clinical trial using a humanized antibody directed against a receptor on the surface of a neutrophil (Hu23F2G) has recently been completed; however, results are not yet available.

Thrombolytic Agents

Both intra-arterial and intravenous administration of thrombolytic agents are under active clinical investigation. Experience with intra-arterial therapy is primarily limited to uncontrolled case series which document that recanalization can be achieved in approximately 60%-70% of patients, often associated with dramatic clinical improvement. Although intra-arterial thrombolytic therapy has a number of potential advantages (such as direct visualization of thrombus dissolution, use of lower doses of thrombolytic agents, and the option of mechanical disruption of the thrombus with the catheter tip), the requirement for angiography usually results in significant treatment delays. Patients who suffer a stroke during angiography or while hospitalized for another disorder may be ideal candidates. Ongoing randomized trials should help clarify the role of intra-arterial thrombolysis.

Large randomized trials of intravenous thrombolytic therapy have produced mixed results. The three large randomized multi-center trials of streptokinase treatment for acute stroke were all stopped prematurely by the safety monitoring committees because of excess brain hemorrhage and death in the streptokinase-treated patients. Two of the studies were European[16,17] and the other was conducted in Australia.[18] All three studies used a streptokinase dose of 1.5 million units. The two European trials both enrolled patients within 6 hours of stroke onset and one of these trials included the combination of aspirin and streptokinase in one of the treatment groups. The risk of intracranial hemorrhage was highest in the streptokinase plus aspirin treated group. In the Australian trial, a 4-hour treatment window was chosen. The trial was modified when an interim analysis revealed poor outcomes in patients treated between 3 and 4 hours after stroke onset. Subsequently, the entire study was aborted. The reasons for the unsatisfactory results in the streptokinase stroke trials is unclear, however, a number of factors, including the choice of the thrombolytic agent, dose selection, and timing of administration, have all been implicated.

The results of the two large randomized t-PA trials are much more favorable. The European Cooperative Acute Stroke Study (ECASS) enrolled patients with an acute middle cerebral artery distribution infarct within 6 hours of stroke onset.[19] Patients were randomized to therapy with 1.1 mg/kg of t-PA versus placebo. No significant difference in functional outcome was found at 3 months, however, a large number of the patients enrolled in this trial did not meet the inclusion criteria for the study. The most common protocol violation was the inclusion of patients who had substantial early infarct signs on their baseline CT scan. A particularly high rate of brain hemorrhage and death occurred in these patients. When these "protocol violation" patients were removed from the analysis, the t-PA-treated patients had significantly improved functional outcomes compared with the patients who received placebo.

The NINDS t-PA stroke trial enrolled 624 patients with an acute anterior or posterior circulation ischemic stroke within 3 hours of symptom onset.[20] A lower dose of t-PA (0.9 mg/kg, maximum dose 90 mg) than used in the ECASS trial was chosen for this study based on dose escalation trials that suggested doses greater than 0.9 mg/kg were associated with higher rates of cerebral hemorrhage. Ten percent of the total dose was given as a bolus with the remainder infused over 1 hour. Strict patient selection criteria were used in this study. Patients were excluded if they had significant hypertension (blood pressure > 185/110 mmHg), recent stroke, head trauma, or major surgery. In addition, patients who were taking oral anticoagulants or who had received heparin within the last 48 hours were also excluded. Mild antihypertensive therapies could be used to reach the pretreatment blood pressure goal of less than 185/110 mmHg, however, aggressive measures to reduce blood pressure were not allowed.

The study documented a highly significant 30% increase in the number of patients who had a full recovery or only minimal disability at three months in the t-PA-treated group. This degree of benefit was seen despite a 6.4% rate of symptomatic intracranial hemorrhage in the t-PA group compared with only a 0.6% rate in the placebo group. Approximately half of the patients who suffered symptomatic brain hemorrhage died. Patients with very severe deficits or early evidence of cerebral edema on their pretreatment CT scan had a higher incidence of symptomatic brain hemorrhage. Therapy with t-PA appeared to have similar benefits for patients with all major subtypes of ischemic stroke. Mortality was also slightly (but not statistically significantly) reduced in t-PA-treated patients (17% vs. 21%). Based on the results of this trial, t-PA was approved by the FDA for treatment of acute stroke in June of 1996.

As indicated above, specific inclusion and exclusion criteria were used to select patients for this trial; thousands of patients were screened for the study and most were determined to be ineligible, usually because of presentation beyond 3 hours after stroke onset. Because of the serious risks of thrombolytic therapy in acute stroke patients, this treatment must be used with great caution and only in patients who are clearly documented to be within 3 hours of stroke onset. It should be administered by clinicians who are knowledgeable of the appropriate clinical and radiographic selection criteria.

Conclusions

A wide range of neuroprotective and thrombolytic agents have now been evaluated in human stroke trials. Unfortunately, many agents that were highly effective in animal stroke models were either too toxic for use in humans or were ineffective in large-scale clinical trials. Despite the disappointing results in many of these early trials, there continues to be substantial reason to believe that safe and effective stroke therapy is still an obtainable goal. Beneficial effects of neuroprotective agents were noted in specific subgroups of several recent trials. These results suggest that more effort is required to identify the types of patients who are most likely to benefit from specific agents and selectively enroll these patients into clinical trials. Recent advances in neuroimaging techniques, such as diffusion weighted imaging, may allow rapid and accurate identification of stroke subtypes within minutes of stroke onset. In addition, more rapid enrollment of patients into clinical trials may be required. Most animal models suggest that neuroprotective agents are effective only if administered within 1 to 2 hours after stroke onset; however, these agents were typically administered 4 to 6 hours after symptom onset in the clinical trials. With the recent approval of t-PA for selected stroke patients, ongoing trials are now evaluating combinations of neuroprotective agents and t-PA. This "cocktail therapy" approach may be the most efficacious strategy for stroke treatment.

References

1. Albers GW, Goldberg NP, Choi DW. N-methyl-D-aspartate antagonists: Ready for clinical trial in brain ischemia? *Ann Neurol* 1989;25:398-403.
2. Albers GW, Atkinson RP, Kelley RE, et al., on behalf of the Dextrorphan Study Group. Safety, tolerability, and pharmacokinetics of the N-Methyl-D-Aspartate antagonist dextrorphan in patients with acute stroke. *Stroke* 1995;26:254-258.
3. Davis SM, Albers GW, Diener HC, et al. Termination of acute stroke studies involving selfotel treatment. *Lancet* 1997;349:32.
4. Albers GW, Clark WM, Atkinson RP, et al. Dose escalation study of the NMDA glycine-site antagonist ACEA 1021 in acute ischemic stroke. *Stroke* 1997;28:233.
5. Mohr JP, Orgogozo JM, Hennerici M. Meta-analysis of nimodipine trials in acute ischemic stroke. *Cerebrovasc Dis* 1994;4:197-203.

6. Very Early Nimodipine Use in Stroke (VENUS). Major ongoing stroke trials. *Stroke* 1998;29:553..

7. Dorman PJ, Counsell CE, Sandercock P. Recently developed neuroprotective therapies for acute stroke. A qualitative systematic review of clinical trials. *CNS Drugs* 1996;6:457-474.

8. Clark WM, Ertag E, Orecchio EJ, et al. Cervene in acute ischemic stroke: Results of a double-blind, placebo-controlled, dose-comparison study. *Stroke* 1997;28:233.

9. Wahlgren NG. The Clomethiazole Acute Stroke Study (CLASS): Efficacy results in a subgroup of 545 patients with total anterior circulation syndrome. *Stroke* 1998;29:287.

10. The RANTTAS Investigators. A Randomized Trial of Tirilazad Mesylate in Patients With Acute Stroke (RANTTAS). *Stroke* 1996;27:1453-1458.

11. Diener HC, Hacke W, Hennerici M, et al, for the Lubeluzole International Study Group. Lubeluzole in acute ischemic stroke: A double-blind, placebo-controlled phase II trial. *Stroke* 1996;27: 76-81.

12. Diener HC, Kaste M, Hacke W, et al. Lubeluzole in acute ischemic stroke. *Stroke* 1997;28:271.

13. Grotta J, Hantson L, Wessel T. The efficacy and safety of lubeluzole in patients with acute ischemic stroke. *Stroke* 1997;28:271.

14. Clark WM, Warach SJ, Pettigrew LC, et al, for the Citicoline Stroke Study Group. A randomized dose-response trial of citicoline in acute ischemic stroke patients. *Neurology* 1997;49(3):671-678.

15. Sherman DG, The Enlimomab Acute Stroke Trial Investigators. The Enlimomab Acute Stroke Trial: Final Results. *Neurology* 1997;48:A270-A271.

16. Multicenter Actue Stroke Trial Europe Study Group: Thrombolytic therapy with steptokinase in acute ischemic stroke. *N Engl J Med* 1996;335:145-150.

17. Multicentre Acute Stroke Trial-Italy (MAST-I) Group: Randomized controlled trial of streptokinase, aspirin, and combination of both in treatment of acute ischemic stroke. *Lancet* 1995;346:1509-1514.

18. Donnan GA, Davis SM, Chambers BR, et al. Trials of streptokinase in severe acute ischaemic stroke. *Lancet* 1995;345:578-579.

19. Hacke W, Kaste M, Fieschi C, et al., for the ECASS Study Group. Intravenous thrombolysis with recombinant tissue plasminogen activator for acute hemispheric stroke. The European Cooperative Acute Stroke Study (ECASS). *JAMA* 1995;274:1017-1025

20. The NINDS rt-PA Stroke Study Group. Tissue plasminogen activator for acute ischemic stroke. *N Engl J Med* 1995;333:1581-1587.

Chapter 31

Debate: MRI is a Good Endpoint for Determining the Efficacy of Stroke Treatment Trials:

Affirmative Position

Steven Warach, MD, PhD

This discussion of magnetic resonance imaging (MRI) as a tool in stroke trials is timely as we continue to see the failure of clinical trials, particularly for neuroprotective agents, to definitively prove a beneficial effect in patients. Re-evaluations of approaches to trial design are underway. There has been a great deal of interest in the potential of new MRI methods as tools in stroke clinical trials. A body of evidence that speaks to and supports this potential has accumulated over the last several years and has been reviewed in detail elsewhere.[1] In this chapter I will summarize the rationale and premises for proposing MRI as a surrogate measure in stroke trials and highlight the data that supports this position. I will use examples from my own group's work, but similar results have been reported independently from many groups. Support for the role of diffusion and perfusion MRI as a surrogate marker has recently been confirmed in the first prospective multicenter stroke trial using MRI as an inclusion and primary outcome measure, the citicoline MRI stroke trial.[2]

---

[1]Baird AE, Warach S: Magnetic Resonance Imaging of Acute Stroke. J Cereb Blood Flow Metab 1998; 18:583-609.

[2]S Warach et al., Lesion volume as a surrogate marker in stroke trials. *The Lancet Conference Abstracts*, 1998: 7.

From: Choi D, Dacey RG, Hsu CY, Powers WJ. *Cerebrovascular Disease: Momentum at the End of the Second Millennium*. Armonk, NY: Futura Publishing Company, Inc., © 2002.

The potential uses of MRI are logical extensions of fundamental principles in clinical trial design aimed at reducing statistical variance and linking outcome measures to the pathology that the treatments are hypothesized to affect MRI, particularly diffusion (DWI) and perfusion (PWI) imaging, has been an attractive tool because it can rapidly provide quantifiable information about brain perfusion and tissue injury in the first hours after a stroke, a time scale compatible with use in acute trials.

To fully establish diffusion and perfusion MRI as a useful tool and validated surrogate in stroke trials several conditions need to be met:

1. DWI and PWI are biologic markers of the disease process in ischemic stroke.
2. The tests are sensitive and specific for the diagnosis of stroke in patients.
3. Lesion volumes correlate with clinical function as measured by clinical rating scales, predict outcome, and covary over time with clinical severity.
4. Rational covariates affecting lesion volumes have been identified.
5. Utility in identifying effective treatments in trials has been proven.

The first four of these requirements have been met.[1] Nearly 10 years of research using DWI and PWI in animal models and acute human stroke have established that DWI delineates a region of early ischemic injury within minutes after onset of ischemia. This region appears relatively hyperintense due to a drop in the apparent diffusion coefficient of water to approximately 60% of normal. This change corresponds, in the earliest hours, to the effects of critically low cerebral blood flow, sodium-potassium ATPase failure, and excitotoxic agonists. Untreated, the tissue progresses from this stage of early cytotoxic edema seen with DWI to infarction. Early reperfusion or neuroprotection can potentially reverse some or all of the abnormality seen with DWI. Chronic infarction is best delineated with T2-weighted MRI. In clinical practice, acute strokes are readily diagnosed by DWI at the earliest time points with high sensitivities and specificities.[3] Approval of DWI by the FDA as an effective diagnostic method for acute stroke, superior to T2-weighted MRI, has led to widespread availability on clinical scanners, refuting the notion that the technology is not sufficiently available to use in trials. In one study, for example, acute lesion volumes by DWI in 50 patients correlated significantly with acute clinical severity on NIH stroke scale scores ($r = 0.56$) and with chronic lesion volume ($r = 0.84$); the chronic lesion volume by T2-weighted MRI significantly correlates with chronic NIH stroke scale score ($r = 0.86$).[4]

---

[3]Lovblad KO,.et al. Clinical experience with diffusion weighted MR in patients with acute stroke. Am J Neuroradiol 1998; 19:1061-1066.

Perfusion MRI has demonstrated hemodynamic abnormalities consistent with ischemic penumbra and predictive of lesion progression. Combining diffusion with perfusion imaging gives correlations of volume of tissue at risk with clinical severity by NIH Stroke Scale much stronger (r = 0.91) than the DWI lesion alone and shows correlation of the change in abnormal tissue volume with the change in stroke scale score (r = 0.82).[5]

Confirmation of these features of DWI and PWI in acute stroke has come from the first prospective multicenter stroke trial using MRI as an inclusion and primary outcome measure, the citicoline MRI stroke trial.[2] In this study identical MRI hardware and software were used in 17 centers across the United States to study 100 patients with ischemic stroke within 24 hours from onset. Patients were randomly assigned to citicoline 500 mg per day or placebo. Diffusion and perfusion MRI were obtained prior to treatment, at 1 week, and at 12 weeks. Image data processing and volumetric analysis were performed at a single central lab using a single expert reader blinded to patients" clinical severity and treatment assignment. The primary MRI inclusion criterion was a lesion of volume 1–120 cc in middle cerebral artery territory gray matter. The primary efficacy endpoint was a change in lesion volume from pretreatment to week 12. Although the primary efficacy endpoint of an effect of citicoline on lesion growth was numerically different (181% increase in lesion volume in placebo patients versus 34% increase for citicoline treated patients), it was not statistically significant. However, the study replicated the findings of other investigations regarding the relationship of MRI-derived lesion volumes to patients" clinical status. Acute lesion volumes by DWI in 100 patients correlated significantly with acute clinical severity on NIH stroke scale scores (r = 0.64) and with chronic lesion volume (r = 0.79); the chronic lesion volume by T2-weighted MRI significantly correlated with chronic NIH stroke scale score (r = 0.63). The strongest predictor of change in lesion size from baseline in the 81 patients who completed their week 12 assessment was the size of the perfusion abnormality (P < 0.0001 by covariance analysis). The volume change over the 12 weeks of observation was significantly related to the patients clinical improvement. Patients meeting the protocol specified criterion of clinical improvement (improvement on the NIH stroke scale of seven points or more) had a significantly more favorable response on the lesion

[4]Lovblad KO, et al. Ischemic lesion volumes in acute stroke by diffusion weighted MRI correlate with clinical outcome. Ann Neurol 1997; 42:164-170.

[5]Baird AE, et al. Correlation of diffusion perfusion abnormalities and clinical outcome in acute stroke. Neurology 1997; 48 (suppl 2): A205.

volume change outcome variable than those who did not improve. The differentiation of improved from not improved was present whether the lesion volume change was assessed as an absolute decrease [74% vs. 36%], median change [−2.8 cc vs. 3.7 cc], or mean (SE) change [3.8 (3.8) cc vs. 25.5 (6.8) cc]. This prospective multicenter, centrally analyzed trial confirmed the value of MRI as a marker of disease severity and progression in stroke trials, and indicated that the change in MRI lesion size is likely to predict clinical improvement in clinical trials.

Confirmation or rejection of the fifth condition for proving validity awaits the results of further therapeutic trials that use MRI. The validity of MRI as a surrogate is supported by the available data but needs to be tested in the context of treatment trials. Proposed uses of DWI with PWI as a tool in clinical trials have been in three areas.

Patient Selection for Inclusion into Trials

A goal of patient selection in any clinical experiment is a sample sufficiently diverse to be representative of the disease, yet as homogeneous as possible to minimize statistical variance. All stroke trials follow this principle, although they differ in the acceptable range of inclusion variables and the relative importance placed on the generalizibility versus homogeneity of the sample. In proposing MRI as a selection criterion, the goal would be a sample based upon a positive imaging diagnosis of a pathology rationally linked to the drug's mechanisms of action. Requiring a positive diagnosis of acute ischemic injury by DWI would assure that no patients with diagnoses mimicking stroke are included in the sample, a desirable objective unachievable in trials using bedside impression and normal computed tomography (CT) findings as the basis of inclusion. Furthermore, every drug by design treats a specific aspect of schemic pathology – eg, arterial occlusions and perfusion defects for reperfusion strategies, ischemic cortical neurons for NMDA antagonists. Selection of patients with the appropriate pathology increases the power of the design by excluding patients (eg, normal perfusion for reperfusion treatments, white matter lacunes for NMDA antagonists) who could not benefit from an effective therapy and would thereby dilute group differences based on treatment.

Selection of patients by DWI is also optimally suited for using change in lesion volume as a surrogate outcome variable. This variable is discussed below.

Proof of Pharmacological Principle Using MRI as a Marker of Response to Therapy: The Rat Experiment in Patients

Before an experimental stroke therapy is brought from the laboratory to clinical trial it is necessary to demonstrate that the treatment causes reduction in lesion volume in experimental models. The fundamental premise of drug discovery and development in acute stroke is that treatments that reduce lesion size are those most likely to lead to clinical benefit. In clinical trial programs that depend solely on clinical endpoints as indices of benefit, drugs may be brought to Phase III testing – costing several years and tens of millions of dollars—without the slightest evidence that the drug will have the therapeutic effect observed in the experimental model. Only a safe and acceptable dose must be demonstrated by the end of Phase II. However, the question of whether the treatment causes reduction of lesion volume may be answerable in the study of one to two hundred patients in Phase II, whereas five to ten times as many patients are typically tested in Phase III studies in order to evaluate the treatment with clinical endpoints. Thus, a Phase II MRI endpoint trial may be the most rational and cost effective basis of deciding whether or not to proceed with Phase III testing. Only drugs that reproduce the laboratory findings of a beneficial pharmacological effect on lesion volume, it is proposed, would proceed for large clinical endpoint trials.

Arguments about the limitations of CT-derived volumes as surrogates are not applicable in considering MR-derived lesion volume as an outcome variable, since CT is less sensitive than MRI in lesion detection and a pretreatment assessment of lesion volume using CT is not possible in acute trials. It is this potential for measurement of change in lesion volume pre- and post treatment that makes MRI most appealing as a surrogate measure. Because the acute and chronic lesion volumes are highly correlated, the variance – and therefore the required sample size—must necessarily be smaller using a within subject change in volume as the outcome measure rather than the more variable final volume. For example, in the citicoline trial results, the standard deviation of the week 12 lesion volumes was 61.5 and 41.1 for placebo and citicoline groups, respectively, whereas the standard deviation of the *change* in volume was 44.8 and 27.8, a reduction in variance of about 30%. The exact sample size required for detecting the effect of lesion volume change with MRI will depend upon many factors in the design of a trial. The citicoline trial, with approximately 40 patients to evaluate per group, approached but did not reach significance. Estimates based on natural history data are that 50 to 100 patients per treatment arm will be sufficient, a size compatible with typical Phase II sample sizes.

Surrogate Endpoint in Phase III Trials to Support Drug Registration

There have been concerns raised that the use of MRI in clinical trails is impractical for technical and logistical reasons (eg, scan duration and availability). The practical limitations have disappeared with the widespread availability of ultrafast echoplanar imaging on commercial MRI scanners. A highly motivated, well-coordinated center can perform emergency diffusion and perfusion MRI with a latency to scan and scanning session duration comparable to that of emergency head CT.

The concept that improvement on a measure of brain lesion volume is a proper surrogate outcome for destructive central nervous systme (CNS) diseases has been already accepted by academic and regulatory communities alike. Approval of beta interferon for the treatment of multiple sclerosis was based in part upon lesion volume as a surrogate marker of disease activity even though the surrogate was not considered fully validated.

A surrogate outcome measure in clinical trials does not need to be fully validated as a condition of drug approval. Recent changes to the Federal Food Drug and Cosmetic Act, which regulates the FDA approval process, have specified a fast track drug designation to expedite review for drugs that have "the potential to address unmet medical needs for serious and life-threatening conditions."[6] Drugs to treat stroke have fallen under this designation. Ordinarily a drug must have a beneficial effect on a clinical endpoint or on a validated surrogate endpoint to demonstrate effectiveness. The new regulations codify what had been ambiguously defined for expedited approval and state that a drug "may be approved if it has an effect on a surrogate endpoint that is *reasonably likely to predict clinical benefit*. Such surrogate endpoints are considered *not to be validated* because, while suggestive of clinical benefit, their relationship to clinical outcomes, such as morbidity and mortality, is not proven" [italics mine].[6] The issue with regard to MRI as a surrogate in stroke trials is whether it is *reasonably likely to predict clinical benefit*. The hypothesis that neuroprotection—the restriction of infarct volume – is reasonably likely to be clinically beneficial to patients is the premise of virtually all acute stroke drugs being developed. The clinical data discussed above supports its value as a surrogate.

---

[6]Prescription Drug User Fee Reauthorization and Drug Regulatory Modernization Act of 1997. House of Representatives Report, 105th Congress, 1st session, Report 105-310, Section 4, pp. 54-56, 1997.

Strict validation must eventually be proven, but as we see from FDA regulations it is no longer required in order to use lesion volume by MRI as a surrogate outcome in stroke trials. The question, therefore, is no longer *whether* MRI surrogates should be used in trials, but *how* they should be used. Proponents on either side of this debate agree that the ultimate validity must come from the performance of these surrogate markers in clinical trials. Only by continuing to use MRI as a surrogate measure in clinical trials will its ultimate validity be established or refuted. Discouraging its use in trials risks inhibiting the very research that is needed to test its validity.

The pharmaceutical industry has taken the initiative investigating this final step in validation. The results of several industry-sponsored drug trials using MRI as a surrogate will be known over the next several years, and those studies should provide the most decisive information regarding the utility of MRI as a surrogate outcome measure in stroke trials.

References

1. Baird AE, Warach S. Magnetic resonance imaging of acute stroke. *J Cereb Blood Flow Metab* 1998;18:583-609.
2. Warach S, et al., Lesion volume as a surrogate marker in stroke trials. *The Lancet Conference Abstracts*, 1998:7.
3. Lovblad KO, et al. Clinical experience with diffusion weighted MR in patients with acute stroke. *Am J Neuroradiol* 1998;19:1061-1066.
4. Lovblad KO, et al. Ischemic lesion volumes in acute stroke by diffusion weighted MRI correlate with clinical outcome. *Ann Neurol* 1997;42:164-170.
5. Baird AE, et al. Correlation of diffusion perfusion abnormalities and clinical outcome in acute stroke. *Neurology* 1997;48(suppl 2):A203.
6. Prescription Drug User Fee Reauthorization and Drug Regulatory Modernization Act of 1997. House of Representatives Report, 105th Congress, 1st session, Report 105-310, Section 4, pp. 54-56, 1997.

Chapter 32

Debate: MRI is a Good Endpoint for Determining the Efficacy of Stroke Treatment Trials:
Arguments Against

Joseph Broderick, MD

I have been asked to give the negative argument regarding the use of magnetic resonance imaging (MRI) as the primary outcome measure in stroke treatment trials. But before I champion the use of clinical scales as the most sensitive current measure of a drug's activity at present, I need to provide a little bit of history about our research group in Cincinnati.

First of all, we are major proponents of brain imaging in the use of clinical stroke research. Our group in Cincinnati, along with colleagues at the University of Iowa, was the first to measure cerebral infarction volumetrically as part of a pilot Phase I Study of naloxone in the 1980s and was the first to correlate the volume of infarction with the neurologic deficit as measured by the NIH Stroke Scale Score (NIHSSS).[1,2] The overall correlation between the volume of cerebral infarction and the NIHSSS was good (Table 1). Yet, the actual plot of the computed tomograph (CT) volume versus NIHSSS showed that the volume of infarction did not correspond well with the amount of neurologic deficit in a substantial number of the patients (Figure 1).

From: Choi D, Dacey RG, Hsu CY, Powers WJ. *Cerebrovascular Disease: Momentum at the End of the Second Millennium.* Armonk, NY: Futura Publishing Company, Inc., © 2002.

Table 1

Spearman's Rank-Order correlation of
Infarction Volume (cm³) to Neurologic Deficit

Time of CT	Neurologic exam on Admission (r)	Neurologic exam at 1 week (r)	Neurologic exam at 3 months (r)
< **48** hours from stroke onset	0.35	0.28	0.38
7–10 days from stroke onset	0.78	0.79	0.68
3 months from stroke onset	0.76	0.70	0.62

CT computed tomography.
$p<0.0001$.

Reprinted with permission from Stroke 1989;20:864-875.

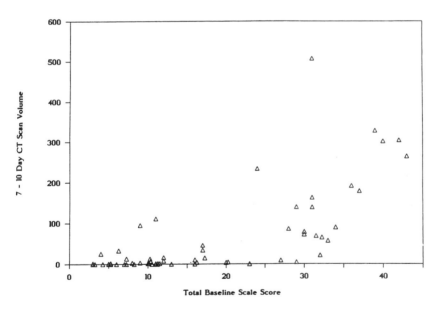

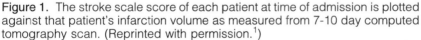

Figure 1. The stroke scale score of each patient at time of admission is plotted against that patient's infarction volume as measured from 7-10 day computed tomography scan. (Reprinted with permission.[1])

Our group has published extensively on the volumetric measurement of intracerebral hemorrhage as part of a prospectively defined cohort study of patients with spontaneous intracerebral hemorrhage and have shown how the volume of hemorrhage is the most important predictor of outcome.[3,4] We have been very active in the analysis of the CT measurements of infarction in the NINDS t-PA Stroke Trial.[5]

Finally, we were the coordinating center for a multicenter MR imaging study which was part of a randomized treatment trial of patients with vascular dementia.[6,7] In this MR study, we showed that change in ventricular volume over a year was a more sensitive measure of change in this group of patients than changes in the clinical scale during the same year.[7] Having said this, I wish to illustrate the substantial limitations of brain imaging as a surrogate endpoint of outcome in acute stroke trials.

The potential advantages of imaging endpoints as compared to clinical endpoints are depicted in Table 2. In particular, the use of an actual biological measure of brain damage is quite attractive and looks to be a "harder" endpoint than clinical scale.

Yet, the disadvantages of brain imaging endpoints are often minimized (Table 3 and 4). Of the six primary disadvantages or limitations of brain imaging endpoints, probably the most important are variability and the failure to account for missing imaging data in the analysis at completion of the study.

The sources of variability in the measurement of brain lesions are numerous (Table 4). When brain imaging can be performed at a single center using a standard protocol, variability is less. Most acute stroke trials require many centers which increases the variability of how the study is performed. Variability also occurs in the actual measurement of the brain lesions at the image analysis center and is often minimized by proponents of a particular protocol.

Even if the performance of the study and measurement of stroke volume are perfect, the volume of cerebral infarction varies substantially among the population of stroke patients. In addition, the distribution of the volume of cerebral infarction is skewed as depicted in

---

Table 2

Proposed Potential
Advantages of Imaging Compared to Clinical Measurement

1. Use as a biological marker
2. Elimination of the potential bias in clinical measurements made by the treating physician
3. Greater sensitivity to brain pathology than clinical measures
4. Decrease variability of brain measurement as compared to variability among physicians performing clinical scales
5. Potential detection of a treatment effect with a smaller sample size
6. Ability to use more powerful statistical tests since lesion and brain volumes can be treated as continuous variable rather than a categorical variable as for clinical measurement scales.

Table 3

Disadvantages of Imaging Endpoints

---

1. The more cognitively impaired the patient, the less likely the MRI study will be performed with high quality or without the risks of sedation.
2. The newer the technology (e.g. MR perfusion and diffusion), the less likely most centers in a multi-center study will have the technology available or will perform the study consistently and with high quality.
3. The more severe the disease and the longer the period between imaging studies, the less likely the second imaging study will be performed at all or will be performed using the same hardware and imaging protocol (Issues of missing endpoints because of death or severe disability).
4. Variability in the measurements of lesion or brain volumes, particularly at two time points, may actually be greater than the variability in measurements using clinical scales and make it more difficult to detect a treatment effect than using clinical scales.
5. Inclusion of MRI imaging in a randomized treatment study is much more expensive than the cost of the performance of a clinical scale.
6. How to account for missing imaging data in the analysis of imaging endpoints in randomized treatment studies has not been satisfactorily addressed.

Table 4

Sources of Variability

---

1. Variation in head positioning
2. Variability in magnetic fields
3. Movement artifact (even with echo-planar imaging)
4. Variability in lesion measurement (image-edge identification)
5. Abnormal brain already present (one advantage young MS patients have over stroke patients)
6. Errors in overlapping data sets during image analysis (T-2 weighted, diffusion, etc.)
7. If films are used – film processing
8. Variations in imaging protocols and data storage
9. Technician variability even if same technician does it
10. Stroke is quite variable in terms of volume
11. Stroke is often patchy

Figure 1 and statistical analysis usually require data transformation or nonparametric statistical tests.

The area which has received least attention in the literature is how to handle missing imaging data in the analysis of imaging endpoints in a randomized treatment study. In randomized studies that use clinical scales as the primary endpoint, patients with missing scale data are often assigned the worst possible scale score or the score of the patient at the last evaluation.[8] For example, in the NINDS t-PA Stroke Trial, a patient who died before the 3-month NIHSSS evaluation was assigned an NIHSSS of 42 (maximum deficit). In an intent-to-treat analysis, this approach to missing data prevents potential biases. If a treatment arm has a high mortality rate, and if the NIHSSS score of all the patients who died prior to 3 months are not included in the final analysis, this treatment arm will appear to have a better outcome as measured by the mean NIHSSS at 3 months as compared to the treatment group which had few deaths.

Similarly, excluding imaging data patients who have died or who can't be imaged could lead to biased result. For example, consider that one of two treatment arms in an acute stroke trial has a very high mortality rate. Patients who die soon after onset of stroke usually have large cerebral infarcts. If the imaging data of patients who died during the first 3 months are not accounted for in the analysis of the volume of infarction at 3 months, the treatment arm with a higher mortality will likely have a smaller mean volume of CT infarction as compared to the other treatment arm with a lower mortality. Proponents of imaging endpoints for acute stroke trials must prospectively determine how to deal with missing imaging data in patients who have died or can't be imaged for any other reason. Thus far, only the NINDS t-PA Stroke Trial prospectively designed an approach to handle missing imaging data in the analysis of the volume of cerebral infarction at 3 months (a secondary study endpoint).[5]

The primary goal of clinical stroke trials is to find an agent that improves long-term functional outcome. Because of the relatively small and finite number of stroke patients who can be treated within a time window that is likely to be beneficial, we need to identify methods to screen new therapies more efficiently. A surrogate endpoint is an endpoint which correlates well to the primary endpoint of interest but hopefully is a more sensitive measure of a drug's effectiveness. In stroke trials, we predominantly focus upon the functional outcome of patients at 3 months, 6 months, or a year. Ideally, we would like a surrogate measure of a drug's effectiveness that requires a smaller number of patients than our current functional outcome measures at 3 months, 6 months, and a year. Both clinical scales, such a as the NIHSSS, as well as volumetric measures of cerebral infarction correlate reasonably well with 3-month functional outcome. Yet, I would argue that changes in the NIHSSS or a composite clinical measure at 3 months may be a more sensitive measure of a treatment effect in randomized treatment trials of acute ischemic stroke than current imaging measures of brain infarction of ischemia.

An excellent comparison between the clinical and imaging approaches can be found in the NINDS t-PA Stroke Trial.[5,8] In the two studies of the NINDS t-PA Stroke Trial, the clinical measures of improvement were a change in the NIHSSS from baseline to 24 hours and 3-month outcome as defined by four clinical scales (a Rankin of 0-1, an NIHSSS of 0-1, a Barthel of 95 or 100, and a Glasgow Outcome Scale of 1). A secondary outcome measure in the two studies was the volume of cerebral infarction at 3 months. Both studies included a very detailed protocol for CT imaging at each of the study sites with a very clearly defined protocol. Both film and tape data was collected and analyzed. The analysis of the images included detailed image-analysis methodology and the first use of an intent-to-treat approach for management of missing CT imaging data.

A highly significant benefit for t-PA was clearly demonstrated using the global statistic for the four clinical measures at 3 months (P = 0.005).[8] A clinical benefit was seen whether one looked at the 3-month measures as tested by the global statistic or at the change in the NIHSSS from baseline to 24 hours (Figure 2).[9] Yet, the analysis of the median volume of cerebral infarction in the t-PA (15.2 cm^3) and placebo-treated

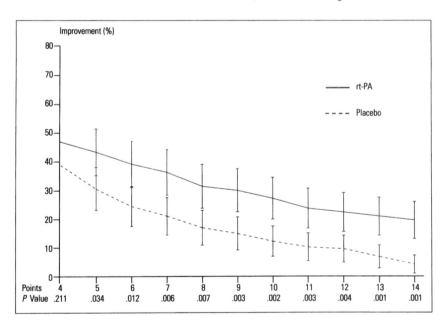

Points	4	5	6	7	8	9	10	11	12	13	14
P Value	.211	.034	.012	.006	.007	.003	.002	.003	.004	.001	.001

Figure 2. NINDS rt-PA Stroke Trial Early Improvement – Part 1.
Graph shows proportion of patients in each treatment group in Part 1 of NINDS rt-PA Stroke Trial who were either normal or had improved by the number of points on NIH Stroke Scale shown on the abscissa at 24 hours compared with baseline. Vertical bars represent 95% confidence intervals. P values from the Mantel-Haenszel test (stratifying for clinical center and time to treatment after stroke onset) are also shown. At 5 or more points improvement and above, the differences in proportions of successes favoring the rt-PA treated group are statistically significant, at least P < 0.05. (Reprinted with permission.[9])

patients (24.4 cm^3) showed only a borderline significance for an effect of t-PA (P = 0.06).[5] These results are largely due to the substantial variability in the volume of cerebral infarction as compared to the variability in the clinical scales in the NINDS trial. Thus, this large, well-done trial indicates that clinical scales are as powerful, and possibly more so, than imaging endpoints in acute ischemic stroke trials.

Techniques of diffusion and perfusion MR imaging and magnetic resonance angiography, as well as newer development in CT imaging such as Xenon CT and CT angiography, may have more use in the selection of patients for clinical trials than as surrogate endpoints. For example, patients who have a diffusion-weighted change consistent with an acute stroke in the internal capsule may not be the best candidate for a neuroprotective drug designed to effect cortical neurons. Computed tomography angiography or MR angiography also may be helpful in stratifying or selecting patients for different thrombolytic protocols.

The use of brain imaging as a selection tool or as a surrogate must also take into account the limited time to deliver effective therapies. Recent results from intravenous thrombolytic trials indicate that the highest likelihood of an effective therapy is in the first 3 hours or less after stroke onset.[8,10-13] Imaging, even echo-planar imaging, takes time to perform and can lead to substantial delays in the delivery of therapy.

At present, I think that clinical scales provide greater power to detect a drug's activity and are also much quicker and cheaper to perform than complicated MR imaging protocols. If MR imaging is to be considered a surrogate endpoint, proponents should pilot their imaging measurements at a few select sites. They should demonstrate the amount of variability in performance of the study as well as in the measurement of the volume of ischemic brain. They should assume that the variability of both will increase as more centers are added. An intent-to-treat analysis accounting for missing imaging data should be performed for imaging data as it currently is done for clinical endpoints. If these goals are accomplished, brain imaging surrogates may yet prove to be a useful and sensitive measure of the effectiveness of a given therapy.

Proponents of clinical measures of patient outcome also need to be more creative. We are currently evaluating all of the different clinical endpoints in the NINDS Stroke Trial to see what would be the most sensitive measure of t-PA's effect. We are even examining combinations of the clinical measures and imaging endpoints. To improve the design of phase I and phase II clinical trials, both clinical as well as imaging measurements need to be carefully chosen to provide the greatest likelihood of detecting the activity of potential therapies.

In the meantime, pharmaceutical companies, as well as other funding agencies, must recognize the substantial limitations of brain imaging as surrogate endpoints in clinical stroke trials. At present, studies using MR imaging endpoints will not require fewer patients to demonstrate a treatment effect than studies using clinical scales. The selling of MR imaging as a cheaper alternative to screen for effective stroke therapies is at best overstated and likely incorrect, at least at present.

References

1. Brott T, Adams HJ, Olinger C, et al. Measurements of acute cerebral infarction: A clinical examination scale. *Stroke* 1989;20:864-870.
2. Brott T, Marler J, Olinger C, et al. Measurements of acute cerebral infarction: Lesion size by computed tomography. *Stroke* 1989;20:871-875.
3. Broderick J, Brott T, Duldner J, et al. Volume of intracerebral hemorrhage: A powerful and easy-to-use predictor of 30-day mortality. *Stroke* 1993;24:987-993.
4. Brott T, Broderick J, Kothari R, et al. Early hemorrhage growth in patients with intracerebral hemorrhage. *Stroke* 1997;28:1-5.
5. NINDS rt-PA Stroke Study Group. Effect of rt-PA on ischemic stroke lesion size by computed tomography: Preliminary results from the NINDS rt-PA Stroke Trial. *Stroke* 1998;29:287.
6. Broderick J, Narayan S, Gaskill M, et al. Volumetric measurement of multifocal brain lesions. Implications for treatment trials of vascular dementia and multiple sclerosis. *J Neuroimag* 1996;6:36-42.
7. Broderick J, Gaskill M, Dhawan A, et al. Temporal changes in brain volume and cognition in a randomized treatment trial or vascular dementia. *J Neuroimaging* 2001;11(1):6-12.
8. NINDS rt-PA Stroke Study Group. Tissue plasminogen activator for acute ischemic stroke. *N Engl J Med* 1995;333:1581-1587.
9. Haley EJ, Lewandowski C, Tilley B, NINDS rt-PA Stroke Study Group. Myths regarding the NINDS rt-PA Stroke Trial: Setting the record straight. *Ann Emerg Med* 1997;30:676-682.
10. Hacke W, Kaste M, Fieschi C, et al. Intravenous thrombolysis with recombinant tissue plasminogen activator for acute hemispheric stroke. *JAMA* 1995;274:1017-1025.
11. Hacke W. ECASS II Results. Personal Communication – Werner Hacke. 1998.
12. Marler J, Tilley B, Lu M, et al. Earlier treatment associated with better outcome: The NINDS t-PA Stroke Study. *Neurology* 2000;55(11):1649-1655.
13. Donnan G. Streptokinase for acute ischemic stroke with relationship to time to administration. *JAMA* 1996;276:961-966.

Index

445